AF556698

FITNESS AND HEALTH EDUCATION

FITNESS
AND
HEALTH EDUCATION

Edited by
Dr. Sharad Chand
Badri Vishal Post-graduate College of
Physical Education, U.P.
Compiled by
Rachna Jain
Ekta Gothi

SPORTS PUBLICATIONS
7/26, Ground Floor, Ansari Road,
Darya Ganj, New Delhi-110 002
Ph.: (O) 55749511, 55257538
(M) 9868028838 (R) 27562163

Published by:

SPORTS PUBLICATION
H.O.: 7/26, Ground Floor, Ansari Road,
Darya Ganj, New Delhi-110 002.
B.O. C-13, Rose Apartment, Sector-14 Extn.,
Rohini, Delhi-110 085.
Ph. : (O) 55749511, 55257538 (R) 27562163, (M) 9868028838
E-mail: *ektathani@hotmail.com*
Website : www.sportspublication.trade-india.com

ISBN 81-89102-47-8

9 788189 102470

I.S.

PRINTED IN INDIA 2005

Laser Typeset by:
JAIN MEDIA GRAPHICS, Delhi-110035. Ph.: 27190244

Printed by:
CHAWLA OFFSET PRINTERS, Delhi-110052

Price: Rs. 750/-

CONTENTS

PREFACE

Fitness and Health Education is the latest effort by the author in the field of Fitness and Health Education being imparted in our schools, colleges and national curriculum.

Physical training is part of a well-rounded education. For this reason a comprehensive book like the present one, which outlines clearly the principles underlying physical fitness, physical education and health education, suggests means for achieving desirable objectives, will no doubt be sincerely welcomed by the school teachers.

To the traditional medical perspective on health and illness, there has been added in recent years, a psychosocial accompaniment—the frameworks of health psychology and behavioural medicine. The three approaches are considerably more in tune that they are dissonant—despite the sometimes strident voices within each calling for the subjugation of the others. For while medicine examines its subjects organically, and health psychology takes an intra-disciplinary tack and while behavioural medicine claims to wed behavioural science to medical science, the differences are often more apparent than real. In teaching health psychology and behavioural medicine courses to graduate and undergraduate students over the past 10 years, the author has drawn a multidimensional conceptual roadmap that highlights the what, why, and how of the terrain and shows quite clearly that the three distinct models converge in both their targets and their purposes.

The goal of this book is to present to the educated world, in India as well as abroad, the basic facts in fitness, health and physical education, a comprehensive picture of how physical education and its different branches are functioning at present.

The efforts is focused towards imparting fitness, health & physical education to the students of various classes viz., B.P.Ed., M.P.Ed. etc. The principles associated with the teaching-learning models offered apply to both viz., clinical as well as community delivery settings and their variations.

The motive of this book is to provide technical information in a sensitive manner, emphasizing the roles of parents, teachers, and other professionals in responding to the motor and physical fitness needs of infants, children and young adults with disabilities. In the development of any text, critical decisions must be made regarding the amount of information to be provided.

I owe my sincere thanks to all people who helped me in many ways in the preparation of this book and the publisher who have printed the book in a very nice manner.

All suggestions from users on omission or shortcomings will be most welcomed.

— Rachna Jain

1

FITNESS & PHYSICAL EDUCATION ACTIVITY PATTERNS—IMPLICATIONS

Physical Activity and the Prevention of Coronary Heart Disease

Jerry Morris and his colleagues were the first to attract serious attention to the hypothesis that physical inactivity may be related to CHD. Morris studied CHD in 31,000 London Transport workers, comparing the drivers with the more active conductors on double-decker buses. The conductors had a 50% lower rate of heart attacks than the drivers, and drivers suffered twice as many fatal heart attacks than as conductors. The findings of the study were, however, subsequently criticised on the basis of self-selection of occupation. Further, Morris's own analysis confirmed that the conductors were more lightly built than the drivers, a difference that was present from the time of taking up employment with London Transport.

Nevertheless, Morris's pioneering work stimulated the initiation of numerous epidemiological investigations into the effects of occupational activity on CHD. Inverse patterns of physical activity and CHD risk were found between letter carriers and mail clerks, farmers and sedentary towns folk, workers on different jobs in kibbutzim in Israel, railroad sorting yard workers and clerks, and San Francisco long shoremen loading cargo into ship holds or tallying it into warehouses. Contrasting or inconsistent results, however, were found in comparisons of Los Angeles civil servants, Chicago industrial workers and Finnish lumber-jacks. These

' occupational activity studies' have been extensively reviewed and have been criticized on several accounts.

The major criticisms include the self- selection of subjects, the inadequacy of CHD classification and the inability of broad job categorization to adequately distinguish between levels of physical activity. Paffenbarger's 22-year study of 3,686 California longshoremen is probably the best controlled and least open to the stated criticisms of the occupational studies. Job categories were carefully defined according to union agreements that required all employees to be highly active cargo handlers for at least their first 5 years of employment. Most men did heavy work much longer, 13 years on average, and shifted to less physically demanding jobs for reasons not of health but of higher pay and prestige. Paffenbarger argued that these work practices suggest that any differences in CHD rate for longshoremen in high -or low-activity groups could not be accounted for by self-selection alone or by job transfers that might have accompanied premonitory symptoms of impending heart problems. Physical activity patterns were verified by on-the-job energy output measurements, although cardiorespiratory fitness was not checked. Shifts in job assignments were noted annually, occupational activity was recorded in kilocalories per week, and mortality rates were derived from official death certificates and man-years of observation.

Multivariate analyses, incorporating cigarette consumption and systolic blood pressure as independent variables, suggested that the risk of a heart attack was about twice as great in longshoreman whose work demanded a low energy expenditure as in those with a high energy expenditure classification. By the 1960s it had become apparent that if physical activity was to contribute to the prevention of CHD, it would have to be predominantly through leisure time activity because mechanization and automation had reduced physical activity in the workplace. The research teams headed by Morris and Paffenbarger were again at the forefront of developments. Morris and his colleagues undertook an extensive 8.5 year prospective study of leisure activities in a group of about 17000 men in the executive grade of the British civil service. They found that those who reported vigorous leisure time physical activity and a CHD less than half of those who reported a lack of such activity.

Paffenbarger's group completed an equally extensive study, following almost 17000 Harvard University graduates, that related both certified causes of death and incidence of physician-diagnosed CHD to smoking habits and continued participation in various forms of physical activity. Analysis of the data demonstrated that current and continuing adequate physical activity, rather than only a history of youthful vigour and athleticism, was inversely associated with risk of CHD in all age brackets studied. The result of Paffenbarger's and Morris's research on the relationship between leisure time activity and CHD have been supported by numerous other studies. Recent critical reviews of the literature have concluded that physically active individuals arc at a lower risk for CHD than less active persons, but reservations concerning experimental design have been expressed. It is unfortunate that there have been few studies involving women as subjects. The results with women have been generally inconclusive, possibly because fewer women develop the disease before old age and the numbers are too small for significant results to emerge.

A recent authoritative meta-analysis focused on all papers published in the English language that provide sufficient data to calculate relative risk or odds ratios for CHD at different levels of physical activity. It seems that activity needs to be current to be beneficial and that habitual physical activity using large muscle groups for sustained periods of time is the only form of activity consistently and substantially associated with a lower incidence of CHD. An intensity of 7.5 kcal/min is of a lower intensity that normally prescribed in an aerobic exercise programme and approximately to only about 70% of maximal heart rate.

Paffenbarger, in his studies of Harvard alumni, placed less emphasis on how vigorous the activity was, and he was more concerned with total energy output but, as Morris et al.

pointed out, Paffenbarger reported more positive effects in men who undertook vigorous activity. An active way of life appears to prevent or delay CHD, but despite a vast research effort, there is no clear understanding of the mechanisms involved. It is generally agreed that appropriate physical activity has positive effects on coronary risk factors.

Other plausible mechanisms include improved cardiorespiratory efficiency, increased fibrinolytic activity, reduce platelet aggregation, reduced coronary thrombosis, increased resistance to ventricular fibrillation, increased myocardial vascularity and increased coronary artery size. The available evidence is, however, equivocal and several of these beneficial adaptations have yet to be convincingly demonstrated in human subjects. Nevertheless, although the debate over the precise underlying mechanisms may continue, the circumstantial evidence amassed by epidemiological studies and the known cardiovascular benefits of physical activity justify the present emphasis on CHD prevention through the medium of physical activity.

British Children's Habitual Physical Activity

Recognizing that the origins of many degenerative diseases are embedded in patterns of behaviour developed during childhood, the United States Department of Health and Human Services decreed that one of the health objectives for the nation is that by 1990, the proportion of the children and adolescents aged 10 to 17 participating regularly in appropriate physical activities, particularly cardiorespiratory fitness programs which can be carried into adulthood, should be greater than 90 percent. 'Appropriate physical activity' refers to the minimum frequency, duration and intensity with which an individual must participate in physical activity to maintain an effectively functioning cardiorespiratory system. Regular, vigorous and prolonged physical activity is generally accepted as essential for an effectively functioning cardiorespiratory system.

The definition adopted by the United States National Children and Youth Fitness Study referred to exercise involving large muscle groups in dynamic movement for periods of 20 minutes for longer, three or more times weekly, at an intensity requiring 60 percent or more of an individual's cardiorespiratory capacity. This definition appears to satisfy most expert recommendations and, with children, refers to activities that elicit heart rates equal to or in excess of 140 beats/min. This is in close agreement with research findings that relate activity to CHD prevention in adults. How may British children experience three 20-minute periods per week in which they sustain their heart rates above 139 beats/min? The available literature is relatively scarce and beset with problems of interpretation caused by the inherent difficulty of determining the quality and quantity of children's physical activity. Reliable data are limited and need to be interpreted in relation to the methodology employed. For example, self-assessment, through retrospective questionnaires or daily diaries, of the intensity and duration of periods of activity by children is especially problematic because children are less time-conscious than adults and tend to engage in physical activity at sporadic times and intensities. Ideally, the relative intensity and duration of activities should be simultaneously measured, and if a true picture of habitual activity is required, at least three days of monitoring are necessary. The technique used must be socially acceptable, it should not burden the child with cumbersome equipment, and it should minimally influence the child's normal physical activity pattern.

Before the Coronary Prevention in Children Project, no survey of British children's habitual physical activity that satisfied these criteria had been carried out. We utilize a self-contained, computerized telemetry system, the Sport Tester 3000, to continuously record the minute-by-minute heart rate of over 300 children. The Sport Tester 3000 consists of a lightweight transmitter, fixed to the chest with electrodes, and a receiver and microcomputer, worn as a watch on the wrist. It has been found to be a reliable and valid means of recording heart rates with children; a recent survey of the most popular commercially available heart rate monitors concluded that the Sport Tester 3000 was first choice because in addition to having excellent validity and stability it permits almost total freedom of motion. The Sport Tester is capable of storing minute-by-minute heart rates for up to 16 hours. If it is interfaced with a microcomputer, the development of a simple programme allows sustained periods with heart rates above 139 beats/min to be readily identified and recorded. During the initial phase of the Coronary Prevention in Children Project, we randomly selected a group of children from the total sample to participate in a sub-study concerned with monitoring heart rates on a daily basis.

A transmitter and electrodes were fitted to each child's chest, and a receiver was strapped around the wrist. The monitoring period lasted from about 9 a.m. until 9 p.m. The receivers were retrieved the following morning, and the data were analysed. The children were refitted with Sport Testers, and the process was repeated over three weekdays. Three-day traces were obtained on 63 girls and 34 boys. On the average the boys spent only 6.7% of their time during the monitored period with heart rates in this range. The interpretation of continuous heart rate data, however, is complex because heart rate not only reflects the metabolism of the child but also the transient emotional state, the prevailing climatic conditions and the specific muscle groups that perform the activity. The primary considerations should therefore be the number and length of sustained periods of appropriate physical activity rather than the total time in specified heart rate bands. Over 85% of the girls and 70% of the boys did not even sustain a single 20-minute period with their heart rates above 70% of maximum. Only two boys and none of the girls achieved three 20-minute periods with their heart rates above 139 BPM. Fifty per cent of the girls failed to achieve a 10-minute period of appropriate physical activity, and 2 of the boys and 11 of the girls did not even manage to sustain a single 5-minute period with their heart rates above 139 BPM. The boys spent significantly more 5-minute and 10-minute periods with heart rates above 139 BPM than the girls. To put these figures into perspective, it is worth noting that brisk walking on the treadmill elicited steady state hearts rates in excess of 139 BPM with the same group of children. Another sub-study involved primary school children, from the same distinct catchment area, who were monitored in exactly the same manner.

Three-day traces were obtained from 24 girls and 18 boys. Only about 30% of this group of young children managed to sustain a single 20-minute period with their heart rates above 139 BPM, and only one girls achieved three 20-minute period at this intensity. Twenty-five per cent of the girls and 17% of the boys failed to sustain a single 10-minute period of appropriate physical activity in 3 day, but only one boy failed to achieve a 5-minute period at this level. There were no significant differences between the boys and the girls in daily heart rate responses or in sustained 5 or 10-minute periods with heart rates above 70% of maximum. When the primary school children were compared with their secondary school counterparts, it was revealed that there were no significant differences between the relevant heart rate responses of the two groups of boys. However, the secondary school girls displayed significantly fewer 5-minute and 10-minute periods with heart rates above 139 BPM and significantly less total time in this range than the primary school girls. Monitoring the heart rates of the same children on a Saturday demonstrated that all groups were even less active during the weekend than during the week. Our data, the first to the generated from British children, indicate that children have surprisingly low levels of physical activity and that many children seldom experience the intensity and duration of physical activity associated with a lower incidence of CHD in adults. The activity level of teenage girls appears to be a particular problem. When the results are related to the marked decrease in activity with age that recent self-report surveys of adults appear to have identified in the United Kingdom, the magnitude of the problem becomes readily apparent.

The Implications for Children's Physical Education

The Community

Public awareness of the importance of increasing

children's physical activity patterns needs to be raised; we have found that local radio stations to be very willing to co-operate in doing this. Attractive and accessible sports facilities need to be made available at reasonable cost and at times when children can use them, such as during weekends and school holidays. Yet, at a time when local authorities and local education authorities should be extending multiple use of their facilities, evidence is accumulating to support the view that the problem of maintenance of facilities and resources for physical education is becoming serious.

Lack of opportunity to participate has not been identified as a major factor in the Coronary Prevention in Children Project, but many of the children we have studied have emphasized the value of a family approach to encouraging activity. They have particularly highlighted the importance of parental and sibling example. Attitudes towards physical activity are established at an early age; parents therefore have a prime responsibility to encourage their children to engage in active play, both spontaneous and formal, but the community must provide adequate safe, clean play areas for this to take place.

The Family

The value of parents as significant socializing agents influencing sport and activity involvement has been confirmed in several other studies. Family encouragement and the involvement of parents in vigorous activity have been found to be instrumental in the involvement of children, and parental attitudes towards activity have been shown to demonstrate a significant effect upon children's intentions to exercise. Perhaps the origins of the remarkably low physical activity patterns of teenage girls lie in the parental attitudes because parental behaviour appears to be more influential for increase in exercise frequency among girls than boys.

Parents elicit gross-motor behaviour at a young age more from their sons than their daughters. Because exercise and sport have been sex-stereotyped as masculine in our culture, boys have more parental reinforcement for exercise than girls. Boy's games are generally of longer duration, and the ceiling of skill is often higher. The type of game normally adopted by boys can be played in more simple versions at younger ages, becoming more challenging with age as higher levels of skill and strategy are incorporated.

In contrast, the types of games often adopted by girls seem to be less challenging with increasing age because the ceiling of skill was achieved at an earlier age. Parents should be encouraged to provide positive role models for their children's activity behaviour, and parental modelling may be especially important for girls.

The School

The primary school provides an ideal environment in which to further promote active lifestyles in partnership with the home. Children's natural curiosity can be used to help them understand how their bodies function, and the importance of physical activity can be emphasized and related to other aspects of education. The introduction of the National Curriculum invites primary school teachers to explore possibilities for developing aspects of the core subjects. This opportunity, in the present context, has been clearly recognized and illustrated in Science in the National Curriculum. Young children can be guided through a physical education curriculum that includes gymnastics, games skills, dance, swimming, athletics and outdoor education, with plenty of opportunities to explore the full range of available activities.

With a balanced, enjoyable programme, children can develop a repertoire of motor skills, achieve success at their own levels, and feel confident enough in their own abilities to want to pursue more active lifestyles. Leisure time activity can be encouraged by making equipment available at playtimes. Holiday activities and the availability of local clubs and facilities can be brought to children's attention, in an attempt to promote positive attitudes to physical activity. The recent Sports Council publication School Sport Forum advocates a daily session of vigorous activity in each primary school as part of the physical education programme or as a supplement to it, but this recommendation needs to be viewed with caution because children's resistance to participation in compulsory, structured programmes of vigorous physical activity is well documented. It is much more important to make children's early activity experiences enjoyable in order to foster future participation. In the secondary school it would be wrong to divorce physical activity from other aspects of a healthy lifestyle, so special provision needs to be made for a cross-curricular approach to activity education. Science, home economics, physical education, health education, school meals and school nursing staff should all be involved in a multi-disciplinary, integrated approach.

The emergence of the National Curriculum has provided a useful framework for projects of this nature. Physical education staff must grasp the opportunity to contribute to the many relevant areas discussed in the Science in the National Curriculum. Relevant parts of the programmes of study should be interpreted with the emphasis on the promotion of active lifestyles that will persist into adult life. Physical education by its very nature is the ideal medium for promoting physical activity, and physical education teachers have reacted positively to the recent emergence of health-related fitness in the curriculum. A survey by the Physical Education Association illustrated the increased importance teachers now give to health-related fitness as a major objective of the physical education programme. The same survey, however, reported that traditional team games continue to dominate the programme and pointed out that Her Majesty's Inspectorate Reports have both emphasized the imbalance that such a limited physical education experience may create and noted that there is a tendency for an overindulgence in games where supervision rather than dynamic teaching is in evidence.

An HMI recently commented that "we spend hundreds of hours teaching the skills of the major team games when in fact the vast majority of youngsters will not actively pursue these activities once they leave school". In fact, many children are discouraged from participating much earlier than this, perhaps through lack of competitive success simply due to their biological clocks running at different rates from those of their classmates. John Balding asked 18000 children, through the well-established Health-Related Behaviour Questionnaire, whether they had participated in various activities at least once per week outside school curriculum time. As expected, soccer was identified as the most popular sport with boys, but participation fell from 58.6% of first-year boys to 41.8% of fifth-year boys. The other major game for boys, rugby, had a participation rate that fell from 15.3% to only 6.3% over the same time period.

On the other hand, 44.8% of first-year boys played snooker at least once per week, and by the fifth year it had replaced soccer as the most popular sport. With girls, netball participation was reported to fall from a mere 19.4% of first-year girls to only 6.3% of fifth-year girls. Hockey participation fell from an even more dismal 10.1% to 5.7% over the same age range, yet the PEA survey revealed that heads of the girls's physical education department attached more importance, in terms of time allocated, to team games that any other area of the curriculum throughout the 5 years of secondary schooling. These figures lend strong support to the belief that competitive team games are of relatively little interest to the majority of adolescent girls. It therefore seems that although physical education teachers perceive the importance of promoting active lifestyles, their curricula may not be geared towards achieving this objective.

Fitness Testing

Within time allocated to health-related fitness, it appears that large chunks are devoted to fitness testing. Yet, the quantitative assessment of children's physical fitness is one of the most complex problems in exercise science. Furthermore, health-related fitness tests that are suitable for use in the school environment and that provide valid and objective measures of fitness are not available. All performance tests are primarily dependent upon the subject's motivation to do well, and several of most popular tests are not even based on sound physiological foundations. Many of the data generated by these tests are therefore more likely to cause confusion than analyse physical fitness or clarify relevant health-related concepts. The sensitivity of the components of health-related fitness to exercise is largely dependent upon maturation and genetic endowment; because each child grows and develops at his or her own rate, it is extremely difficult to separate the contributions of growth, maturation and exercise to any observed changes in performance. Cardiorespiratory fitness at a particular point in time can be assessed in an accredited laboratory.

It is widely recognized that the maximal rate at which oxygen can be consumed during exercise with large muscle groups is the best single indicator of cardiorespiratory fitness. We determined the VO_2 max of over 200 children, aged 11 to 15 years, by running them to exhaustion on a treadmill and simultaneously monitoring their cardiorespiratory responses to the exercise. Our results demonstrated that the boys were as a fit as the first boys ever to have their cardiorespiratory fitness scientifically assessed in a laboratory over 50 years ago. More detailed comparisons of our data with results from elsewhere have shown that British children are as fit as children from similar environments and that there is no scientific evidence to support the premise that the cardiorespiratory fitness of children has deteriorated over time. When we compared children's cardiorespiratory fitness with their habitual physical activity, however, we found no relationship between the two—and it is current physical activity, not cardiorespiratory fitness, which most epidemiological studies have related to coronary prevention. Fitness tests simply determine the obvious, at best only distinguishing the mature child from the immature child. The use of norm tables confounds the issue of relative fitness because tables constructed on the basis of chronological age cannot logically be used to classify individual children at different levels of skeletal and biological maturity.

Moreover, having different norms for boys and girls

results in different expectations. Norms are based on performances rather than capabilities; if teachers accept lower norms for girls as reflecting acceptable performance, girls will tend to meet these lower expectations. Any attempt to introduce fitness testing as a means of assessing levels of attainment in physical education should therefore be strongly resisted.

Motivating Students

It must be demonstrated clearly to children that activity can be enjoyable and that competition or athletic excellence is not necessary for the promotion of health. Children need to be exposed to a wide variety of individual, partner and team activities, and the emphasis should be placed upon developing a sound foundation of motor skills that can contribute to successful and enjoyable activity experiences in both the present and the future. Motivations vary; for example, despite recent progress in female emancipation, looking better remains a prime motivator for girls participation in relevant activity. The activity and leisure preferences of children and adults of different races and of different physical and intellectual capabilities are varied. These preferences need to be taken into consideration when designing a relevant curriculum. Although the provision of a high activity content should be an important component of most physical education lessons, the prime objective underpinning the inclusion of health-related activity in the physical education curriculum should be for children to achieve activity independence.

Teachers must help and encourage children to internalize the motivation to be active so that when the extrinsic motivation of the teacher is removed, the child will continue with an active lifestyle. To achieve activity independence, children should understand the principles underlying health activity and be taught how to become informed decision makers who can plan and implement individual activity programmes that can be periodically reappraised and modified as they get older. If teachers are to develop successful courses, they need to understand current concepts in exercise and health science and be cognizant of the growing body of knowledge associated with exercise adherence. This has far-reaching implications for both initial and continuing teacher education programmes.

Higher Education

Universities and other institutes of higher education must provide initial teacher-training students with a thorough grounding in both the practical and the theoretical aspects of exercise and health science. The potential cross-curricular contribution of physical education to the whole 5-to-16 curriculum must be emphasized, and suitable programmes of study must be integrated into current initial training courses. These courses should be underpinned and enriched with dynamic research programmes. In comparison to what we know about adults, we know very little about paediatric exercise and health science. Groups of scholars need to collaborate to address the exciting research problems on an interdisciplinary basis.

Optimum methods of delivery of courses, founded on research results, urgently need to be investigated. Universities, colleges, local education authorities, and schools need to work together to design appropriate postgraduate courses and to encourage school-based action research in exercise and health science as part of the continuing professional development of experienced teachers. The current level and pattern of children's physical activity is a cause for grave concern. Physical educators at all levels of education must collaborate with each other and with the community and the home to meet this challenge. The future health of the children depends upon it.

2

IMPARTING FITNESS, HEALTH & PHYSICAL EDUCATION— ART AND SCIENCE TOGETHER

Technology is everywhere. Microchips have changed the way we study data, communicate, travel, become entertained, balance our bank account, or select a running shoe. Everything has mathematical accessibility. It would seem that computers will eventually propel all things along a deterministic path, rule-bound like the planets, predictable like eclipses and tides. Science might reckon the future with absolute laws that will control its destiny. But what will always remain are the lessons of giving directions to this burgeoning cybernation, and of keeping technology in some sort of moral order.

Science does not automatically supply good sense and reason. Technology cannot, by itself, provide ethics. There still exists and always will an important place for visionary people to give critical perspective to the technical world. Science will not run without human aid and will not advance without social scrutiny. Nor will science replace the profound meanings of life that are found in the world of living experience. So now more than ever before, teachers, not machines, will arrange for the experiences that will provide people with enlightenment in ways that technology cannot. Teachers will, perhaps better than anyone else, give people completeness of life, and physical education teachers will offer equilibrium to an otherwise data-processed existence.

Components of the Job

Physical education is a process that enriches the senses of people through learning experience that forge the body, the mind, and the psyche. When properly administered, the provisions are lifelong aptitudes that sustain a sense of balance to the consciousness and a regard for one's own welfare. The consequences are life-living. But theory and practice are sometimes divided.

The actual job of the physical education teacher includes an entangled array of divergent affairs that often have no relationship to the act of teaching. For example, if one were to observe a teacher for a few days, the teacher might be seen performing most or all of the following tasks:

1. Explaining a skill
2. Demonstrating a skill
3. Patrolling a hall
4. Handing out tickets
5. Taking attendance
6. Counselling or guiding
7. Collecting money
8. Disciplining
9. Evaluating performance
10. Filling out reports
11. Talking with parents
12. Repairing equipment
13. Attending meetings
14. Arranging transportation
15. Making up tests
16. Planning lessons
17. Mediating an argument

18. Correcting tests
19. Distributing equipment
20. Collecting equipment
21. Unjamming a locker
22. Spotting for a performer
23. Explaining rules
24. Asking questions
25. Talking with teachers
26. Monitoring a study hall
27. Writing permission slips
28. Referring a scrimmage
29. Determining grades
30. Talking with students

A complete list might include a considerable number of other activities. Each of them might be necessary to perform the job of teaching, yet only a few are the actual acts of teaching. Consequently, the activities of teachers might be grouped into the following categories:

1. Instructional Acts

i. Explaining a skill

ii. Demonstrating a skill

iii. Evaluating a performance

iv. Explaining rules

v. Asking questions.

2. Managerial Acts

i. Taking attendance

ii. Disciplining

iii. Repairing equipment

iv. Arranging transportation

v. Making up tests

vi. Planning lessons

vii. Mediating an argument

viii. Correct tests

ix. Distributing equipment

x. Collecting equipment

xi. Unjamming a locker

xii. Spotting for a performer

xiii. Refereeing a scrimmage

3. Institutional Acts

i. Patrolling a hall

ii. Handing out tickets

iii. Counselling or guiding

iv. Collecting money

v. Filling out reports

vi. Talking with parents

vii. Attending meetings

viii. Talking with teachers

ix. Monitoring a study hall

x. Writing permission slips

xi. Determining grades

xii. Talking with students

There is obviously more to the job of the teacher than the actual act of teaching. In fact, observations of teachers in all fields show that the average work day consists of a greater proportion of time given to managerial affairs than to events that can formally be defined as instructional. It is not surprising, therefore, to find that some research indicates managerial effectiveness more than instructional competence to be determinative of how long someone remains in the teaching profession.

A Managerial Manifesto

Class management is now regarded as not only central to the task of teaching but critically supportive of its effectiveness. Physical education management covers a wide range of activities that re not instructional acts but may affect the amount of time given to instruction. Because of the nature of the setting, physical education teachers spend a greater percentage of time on management affairs than teachers in other subject areas. It varies considerably, but in general at the elementary level about 25 per cent of total class time is management, and in high school the proportion is about 22 per cent. Furthermore, research has used a wide variety of observational procedures and recording forms to reveal that the actual time students are actively engaged in learning experiences is often dismally small, perhaps averaging less than 10 per cent in elementary classes and only 5 per cent in high school.

There is considerable variation depending on the activity, but what is quite apparent is that overall the learning time in physical education is appealingly low compared to average learning time in classrooms. It is a hazardous judgment, however, for most of the observations have noted only the time that a student is actively engaged in learning. That is rather like counting only the time the ball is alive in football game. Learning includes not only overt acts of rehearsing a skill but also cognitions. Acquiring a golf swing, for example, incorporate plenty of mental thought about the mechanics of the action. Such covert, cerebral engagements may average more than 12 per cent of high school classes and over 20 per cent of elementary classes. Probably the most obstrusive of managerial act is the need to respond to disruptive students.

Evidence suggests that discipline problems are a major

source of frustration among teachers, the one factor that detracts more than any other from instruction effectiveness, a major reasoning why teachers leave the profession, a great concern among parents of students and the general public, and that the whole matter of discipline is getting worse. For students preparing to teach physical education, discipline is consistently ranked as the primary apprehension and continues to be a repressive factor once on the job. Since every event is unique, it is a difficult aptitude to rehearse.

No comprehensive theory of discipline management now exists. Ability to handle problems appears to accrue only from being in the workplace and discovering what does not achieve the desired results. However, one factor stands clear: Those teachers who have the lowest incidence of disruptive encounters are those who are effective behavioural managers. They have put their house in order. By judicious class management, they have reduced the probability of problems. They have suppressed discipline affairs with strategies of firm and fair codes of conduct that are consistently observed and have focused on optimal learning environments. In sum, the most organized and well-prepared teachers have the least difficulties.

Profile of an Effective Teacher

Are the best physical education teachers, then, the best behavioural managers? It is a prime ingredient, but not the only one. The search for the formula to effective teaching has been like the Holy Grail, often with the same illusive results. One earlier comprehensive volume concluded that teaching successes in the first place. Another text on master teachers pronounced that great teachers are often lucky enough to have had great students. Most of the earlier studies of good teaching focused on personality factors and generally assumed that effective teaching and personal magnetism were related.

Certain persona characteristics still appear to be supportive of effective teaching performance, mostly centring on the teacher being a skilled communicator and a compassionate person. But the absence of specific criteria by which subjectively derived, not necessarily agreed upon, and frequency vague in meaning. So the research has filtered to using student achievement as a major tangible rating tool. Results have thereby shown that some teachers make more of a difference than others, and we now have some idea of the teaching behaviours that lead to effectiveness in instruction. In summary form, they appear to be the following:

1. High expectations. Students tend to achieve according to the teacher's expectations of them, especially in the earlier grades. Accordingly, a teacher's expressed ideas about objectives can be a strong motivation for students, provided those expectations are reasonable and perceived by the students to be attainable. Furthermore, teachers must demonstrate confidence in their own ability to promote the learning and in the student's abilities to accomplish the stated objectives. Unfortunately, there is indication that physical education teachers sometimes form expectations of their students based on such subsidiary factors as physical attractiveness, gender and perceived effort. These perceptions then tend to bias teachers toward their students and differentiate the teacher-student interaction. Better looking students get more attention. Boys get more attention than girls. Skilled students get more positive feedback than the unskilled.

Thus, the implications are that physical education teachers need to be conscious of providing fair and equitable treatment of all students, with reasonable expectations for each individual.

2. Effective organization and management. A stockpile of earlier research had shown that effective teachers have a great sense of what was called orderliness. It meant having responsible, goal-oriented behaviour. Effective teaching was seen to be performed with intention and resolution, manifested through clear and definite objectives, with well-formulated plans for achieving those

objectives. It more liberally implies good organization and management. As already indicated, behavioural management is a great suppression of discipline problems while at the same time it is effective in stimulating student achievement.

Important factors within class management include the ability to minimize inactive time, presenting appropriate learning activities, a proper sequential ordering of activities, monitoring of student responses, and smooth transitions from one phase of a class to the next.

3. A supportive learning environment. Praise that is spontaneous and genuine, and given in relation to specific accomplishments, is a reinforcement for further achievement. A willingness to help students through their learning by giving them necessary time and undivided attention will produce accelerated progress. A positive learning atmosphere is, in fact, one of the elements of physical education that is highly valued by both teachers and students. A sense of humour also seems to be a good benefit. Conversely, a negative climate produces negative results. Criticism can repress learning to a greater degree than praise will promote it. Negative behaviour is the exact antithesis of effective teaching.

4. Active teaching. The best teachers are actively involved in the class via productive teaching. They are task oriented, focusing everyone's attention on the instructional content and objectives of the lesson, actively demonstrating, cuing performance, and providing ample feedback. They are rather like the referee who is in complete control of a game yet is accomplishing that dominion without attracting undue attention.

5. Logical pacing of the learning. Active teaching also tends to be related to instructional pacing that produces faster learning progressions than passive teaching. Organized teachers accomplish this with small steps that have a high probability for success and an overall plan of realistic stages toward the target objectives. Students are

taken through the steps, each one a gradation of the previous step, at a pace that can be adapted to each individual's capability.

6. Maximal active learning time. Active teaching produces active learning time. Generally speaking, the more time students have on task, the greater their achievements will be. Unhappily, observations of physical education classes have shown that students typically spend from 22 per cent to 32 per cent of their class time doing nothing. More organized teachers have managed to minimize this down time to provide for a greater percentage of involvement in learning. It relates, once again, to effective planning and class management. One research study concluded that active learning time is the single most important criterion of an effective teacher.

7. Providing for mastery learning. In the final analysis, active teaching coupled with proper pacing and optimal time on risk will produce a mastery of all phases of a skill. Monitoring of progress in skill acquisition is vital and is accomplished by objective measures that show to both teacher and student how things are going. Careful and realistic evaluations, given at periodic intervals, should allow enough time for each step of a skill to be sufficiently learned to support the next stage. The product will be more confident students who acquire more lasting aptitudes.

A Matter of Method

And what about the method of teaching? More preparatory attention is typically given to teaching methodology than to any other aspect of the job. There is good news. The instructional techniques now available are the most effective in the history of education. They have been researched and time tested. Best of all, they are supremely logical and direct. Interestingly, in spite of the variety of teaching strategies available, virtually every format has its origins in one of two systems.

One is a collection of philosophies generally referred to as humanism, and the other is a science based technique called behaviourism. Together these two systems have influenced educational thought more than any other previous approach. Their most positive feature is not only that they have made teaching more effective but that they have made learning more enjoyable and rewarding for the learners. The basic difference between these two approaches lies in their assignment of the responsibility for learning.

Humanists say students are quite capable of, and therefore responsible for, their own learning. In contrast, behaviourists state that teachers are more competent in stimulating learning and are consequently answerable for the process. Humanism places confidence in self-discovered learnings. Humanistic teaching is never a matter of telling things to students; instead, it is made up of movements when a teacher and a student reach some insight into the nature of the learning. It establishes a permissive atmosphere in which students can make discoveries. The teacher encourage students to explore, giving cues when necessary and leading them to conclusions, but never imposing the answers.

In physical education, this self-discovery method found a remarkable acceptance through a process called movement education, which relies on meteoric experimentation and problem solving as its means. A student is never told exactly how to perform a motor skill but is encouraged to experiment with the possibilities to find the most efficient techniques. The behaviourist model of teaching, on the other hand, is representative of a branch of psychology that attributes learning to the response to a stimulus. Given a set of circumstances, the reaction of people to those circumstances is predictable. Thus, all that is necessary is to organize the environment to provide the conditions known to produce the desired behaviours.

Consequently, a behaviourist teachers according to a set of educational strategies whereby learnings are precisely presented in increasing levels of difficulty. Students are, literally, told how to perform motor skills rather than left to discover appropriate techniques for themselves. The value in the two systems does not lie in the absolute use of only one method, but rather in the consolidation of the best elements of both. There are times when a teacher must allow for student experimentation and other times when the setting must be exactly organized. It varies in kind with the nature of the objectives of any given lesson. And appealingly, the judicious employment of appropriate methodology makes it more possible to be an effective teacher today than ever before.

Why Teach?

The major reason why people are attracted to physical education teaching is the opportunity it presents to be interactive with other people in a helping relationship. But there are an infinite number of other reasons why someone may want to teach. Following are a list of statements given by students in various preparation programs:

— Teaching seems to be a fairly safe, low-risk occupation.

— There are many attractive side benefits.

— I really like the idea of having control over a class.

— Being an influence on the lives of students is appealing.

— I cannot think of anything else to do with my major.

— The instruction I had in high school was so incredibly bad that I want to try to correct that situation.

— I really do not know what I want to do, so I'll teach until I find something else.

— I truly belief I can make a contribution to human betterment, especially through the positive outcomes that physical education offers students.

— I want to say physically fit all my life, and in this profession I can do it.

— I like activity.

— I like the idea of being able to be outdoors much of the time.

— My parents were teachers, and they would really be pleased if I became one too.

— I love kids.

— It is a chance for me to say young all my life.

— Teachers are my favourite people. I had good teachers all through high school, and it made me feel like I want to stay among them for a career.

— I want to coach, and I may have to teach along with it.

— It is something I've got to do until I can become an administrator.

— I like the respect that comes with the profession.

— I love sports, and I want to be around them as long as I can. At what other job can I be paid to be actively involved in sports?

— The vacations are great.

— It is a people occupation, where you can be with people all day—talking and relating—not like other jobs where your only contact is with machines or computers all day.

— It will allow me to express myself and share knowledge with others.

— I like the challenge.

— It is a profession rather than just an occupation.

— You can still enjoy growth and improvement in your own thinking and feeling.

— It is a chance to be creative and enjoy discovery.

— I really do not know why I want to teach; I just know that I do.

The reasons why someone can be attracted to the

teaching profession can range from conscientious desires to influence, society to such blithe logic as June, July and August. In any case, there is no more need to justify one's choice of teaching than any other preference.

The Matter of Money

It is no secret: Teaching is not the way to achieve financial independence. Low salaries are one of the major reasons why fewer persons are choosing to teach and may be the most important reason why one-half of those entering the teaching profession have left after seven years, two-thirds to three-fourths of them within the first three years of teaching. It is probably also the reason why nearly 30 per cent of teachers moonlight with a second job. Since the Second World War, the real purchasing power of teachers has declined compared to the national average. In one ten-year period, from 1974 to 1984, the average teacher's salary rose 30 per cent less than the average salary of other professional peoples. All things considered, teachers continue to lose about one per cent a year in their purchasing power. Furthermore, teaching is not an occupation that rewards service and experience with salary increments.

Raises are less for years of service rendered than the usual salary advances in other professions. In many cases, it takes a teacher a full career to double his or her salary. Worst of all, physical education teacher's salaries are below the mid-levels of the salary scale for teachers in general. An attempt at rewarding performance in teaching can be found in the establishment of merit play as an incentive system. In this regard, the better teachers would quality for the highest pay raises. Recommendations have included such supplements as bonus pay for teaching in disadvantaged areas and extra pay for all unused sick-leave days.

But as yet the merit play plans have received little support from the states. However, the teacher's salaries are normally quoted on the basis of a nine-month work year.

If the average salary is projected to a twelve-month equivalent, teaching salaries rank quite favourably with other professionals and rate considerably higher than the average industrial worker. Thus, the teacher who elects to teach during summer sessions earns a far more equitable salary. And in fact, the average teacher's salary is above the national average for all wage earners, even when computed on only a nine-month basis. Furthermore, certain job benefits are often available to teachers that may not be common in other occupations, such as paid health insurance, tax shelter plans, pensions, or tuition-free college educations for faculty children or spouses of college professors. In the final analysis, teaching does not offer the potential for untold wealth, nor for a quick accumulation of a sizable savings account. But the financial picture is more obliging than first believed. There is no fortune in teaching; nor is there financial famine. It just happens to be a median-level occupation in terms of monetary rewards.

The State of the Market

Throughout the 1960s and early 1970s, teacher turnover rates produced critical teacher shortages. The burgeoning school-aged population combined with an increased attrition from the profession and fewer new entrants, produced conditions in which the job market was wide open. But in the late 1970s and early 1980s, when school populations dropped, the demand for teachers diminished. During this time, the supply of public school teachers exceeded the demand by 88 per cent.

In physical education at one point as many as four qualified teachers may have been competing for every available job. A general discouragement ensues as teaching became viewed as a difficult market to enter. But now indications are that teacher shortages may again be resurfacing. Potentially, during the 1990s, there will be increasing shortages in science, mathematics, special education, computer science, English, and bilingual education. The situation for physical education appears less predictable, as projections do not always separate the field from education as a whole. It could therefore be speculated that vacancies might follow the trend of education in general, which would be favourable.

However, one report suggests that the supply and demand of physical education teachers will show no increase in demand. The picture is somewhat clouded by the way figures of supplying and demand are interpreted. Some announcements, reflect the number of teachers who, at present, should be employed according to a specified standard of educational viability, which is usually set by the National Education Association. Since this standard indicates the optimal teacher-student ratio that would in theory provide for the best educational outcomes, such a reference base will invariably show a shortage of teachers. On the other hand, the statistics that show an oversupply of teachers are often based on the number of qualified teachers who are available in a given year but do not indicate the number who actually seek employment in teaching. In this regard, it is possible that fewer than three of every four students seeking certification in teaching are actually planning to become teachers. So there is some room for interpretation of the supply/demand projections.

Assuming that not everyone in physical education certification programs is actually planning to teach, further assuming that the total number in the certification programs is decreasing, and adding the projection for a small but definite increase in the public school student population through the 1990s, one might arrive at a tentative conclusion that jobs in physical education should become easier to find. But the future is always disclaimed as a probable, which is the only thing it can be.

So, many teachers start their first job with little idea of what it is really like to manage their own classes. Some find the experience of frustrating. Initial difficulties in management may explain the high dropout rate among beginning teachers. But teachers who remain in the profession for seven years are likely to stay for many more, and consequently dropout rates are very low among experienced teachers. Management skills are an essential ingredient for success in the teaching profession. Although a number of personality factors seem related to effective teaching, the ability to be an efficient manager of class activities appears as a constant.

Unfortunately, the development of management abilities is a process that generally takes four to six years and this coincides with the fact that half of those who enter teaching level the profession within the first seven years, perhaps before this ability matures. Conclusively, then, it seems that the better prepared one is with management capabilities, the more likely the transition into teaching will be a successful one. Salaries continue to be a major issue in teaching and may in fact be the single most pressing reason for withdrawal from the profession. Yet curiously, money is not the most important factor for entry into teaching, and for those who remain in the profession beyond the initial transition period, money becomes even less of a concern as the rewards, and satisfactions of the job itself become the more encompassing aspects of teaching.

3

HEALTH-RELATED PHYSICAL ACTIVITY IN THE NATIONAL CURRICULUM

This may' seem to be a rather dramatic quotation with which to open a paper on the physical activity and health of children in Western society, particularly as Grant was referring specifically to children from the third world. Nevertheless, the changing trends of human mortality and morbidity in the 20th century necessitate a close look at the way adults involve themselves in physical activities and whether there are lessons to be learned, at least from a health perspective, for children's education and lifestyles. It is now well documented that the major public health problems of our society are degenerative, or lifestyle, problems rather than infectious diseases. If this is the case, it has important implications for the process of educating children about lifestyle and health habits. Recent evidence, to be reviewed later in this chapter, shows that physical activity can be an important part of this process. Given the evidence on physical activity and health from epidemiology, medicine and public health, has the wider community sought to bring about a greater emphasis on preventing medicine./ If so, has the physical education profession changed to accommodate this?

National and International Statements

The importance of placing greater emphasis on preventive health measures and policies can be highlighted with reference to several major statements. For example, the World Health Organization has set out the fundamental requirements for people to be healthy, to define the improvements in health that can be achieved for the peoples of European Region of WHO, and to propose action to secure these improvements. The U.S. Department of Health and Human Services set 223 health objectives for the nation, 11 of which were specifically related to physical fitness and exercise. Of these, 3 were specific to children. Impetus has also given to health-related physical activity in children by several organizations.

The American College of Sports Medicine has produced an opinion statement on physical fitness and children, and a joint position statement from the Sport Council and Health Education Authority also lists recommendations for action, including the need for more research into effective strategies for promoting exercise habits in children. In summary, there is a plenty of support and guidance for the promotion of HRPA in children. However, despite this apparent support, British literature on the topic has been diffuse and largely theoretical. This chapter therefore, attempts to draw together contemporary research findings in paediatric exercise science to produce a review of children, health and physical activity with specific reference to the British physical educator.

What is in a Name? Clarification of Terms

Physical education has adopted many terms for its work in physical fitness and health. Health-related fitness has been the most prominent because this is the term most often used in the United States. However, it could be argued that health-related exercise or health-related physical activity are better terms.

Physiological Outcomes of Health-Related Physical Activity

The physiological outcomes of HRPA are dependent upon

the mode, intensity, duration and frequency of physical activity. In this section we consider the health-related aspects of fitness and discuss the mode of physical activity, and the exercise prescription, required for the optimum development of each of the components of health-related fitness. We have discussed elsewhere the principles of training, the value of warming up and cooling down, and the importance of taking appropriate safety precautions.

Cardiopulmonary Fitness

Cardiopulmonary fitness may be defined as the ability of the circulatory and pulmonary systems to supply fuel and eliminate waste products during physical activity. Much more is known about children's cardiopulmonary fitness than about other health-related aspects of their fitness, but very few data are available from samples of British children. Any physical activity that is rhythmic and aerobic in nature, uses large muscle groups and can be sustained continuously for a reasonable length of time can improve cardiopulmonary fitness.

Typical activities include running, swimming, cycling, skipping, skating, some types of dancing and cross-country skiing. On the other hand, in the context of developing cardiopulmonary fitness, physical activities that involve the predominant use of small muscle groups or isometric contractions should be avoided because of the enhanced blood pressure response. Although a consensus exists concerning the mode of exercise in which children should engage to improve cardiopulmonary fitness, the minimum and optimum levels for intensity, frequency and duration of exercise have not been unequivocally identified. Recommendations for frequency of exercise range from 3 days per week. Recommendations for the duration of each exercise session range from 20 to 30 minutes. It is, however, important to consider children's attention spans, when determining the length of exercise sessions, and other commitments, when prescribing the number of exercise sessions.

We therefore feel that three 20-minute periods per week is probably the optimum for children. Some researchers have reported higher training thresholds for children than for adults. This is supported by Yates and Grana and in line with the application of Karvonen's formula to children. It appears that an exercise intensity that maintains the heart rate at about 80% of maximum produces the best results.

With children, jogging at about 8 km/h will raise the heart rate to about 160 BPM. When this type of programming is followed, children can expect changes in cardiorespiratory fitness very similar to those documented for adults. Maximal oxygen uptake, the highest rate of oxygen consumed by the body in a given period of time during exercise involving a significant portion of the muscle mass is widely recognized as the best single index of cardiopulmonary fitness. For reasons discussed elsewhere, the correct term to use with children is peak oxygen uptake, the highest oxygen consumption elicited during an exercise test to exhaustion. But for ease of exposition, the two terms will be used interchangeably in this chapter. Until the recent report by Armstrong, Balding, Gentle, Williams and Kirby data on the peak VO_2 of British children were sparse, derived mainly from cycle ergometry and based on small sizes.

Armstrong and his colleagues determined the peak VO_2 of 420 children, aged 11 to 16 years, and their resulted refuted the well publicized views that British children's cardiopulmonary fitness is deteriorating or inferior to children from other countries. Armstrong pointed out that the first laboratory-based scientific studies of children's cardiopulmonary fitness were carried out by Robinson and Morse, Schultz, and Cassels in the United States, and their results almost exactly reflect the current levels of cardiopulmonary fitness of British children. The relative stability of the cardiopulmonary fitness of North American children over several decades has also been noted. The cardiopulmonary fitness levels of British children were shown to be compared with the available United Kingdom data on other age groups, it was concluded that, in terms of peak VO_2, children are probably the fittest section of society.

Muscular Fitness

Muscular fitness has two components, muscular strength of and muscular endurance. Adult's muscular fitness and its improvement are well documented, but children, particularly prepubertal children, have been the subject of few studies. Nevertheless, our understanding of children's muscular fitness and the physiological outcomes of appropriate training programmes is gradually increasing, and several excellent reviews of the literature are available to the interested reader. Muscular fitness training involves repeatedly overcoming increasing resistances, and appropriate programmes can be structured around each type of muscular contraction. However, because of the disadvantages of isometric exercises, eccentric exercises and isokinetic exercises, we will concentrate upon isotonic exercises that use apparatus normally available in a school.

To develop an isotonic muscular fitness programme, the principles of training must be thoroughly understood, and in addition it is necessary to be fully cognizant of the concept of a repetition maximum. A RM is the maximal load that a muscle group can lift over a given number of repetitions before fatiguing. Although individual overload recommendations in the literature differ slightly, it is generally agreed that training with heavy weights should be avoided and the principle of progression strictly adhered to with young children. Specific optimal development of muscular strength would involve the use of heavier resistances than those necessary for optimal development of muscular endurance, but we believe that with children a reasonable compromise that would develop both muscular strength and muscular endurance is preferable to two distinct training programmes. For optimal physiological development we recommend that children perform about 8 to 12 repetitions to contraction failure. In practice this requires the 8 RM to be initial 8-RM resistance, a small increase in resistance can be made to bring the maximal repetitions back down to 8. For a balanced development, each session of exercises should consists of one exercise for each major muscle group.

It is advisable to start each session with large muscle groups and work down to smaller muscle groups. Upper legs and hips, chest and back and posterior aspects of legs, lower legs, shoulders and posterior aspects of upper arms, abdomen and then anterior aspects of upper arms would be a suitable rotation of exercise. We recommend one, gradually progressing to three, sets of each exercise per session, with not more than three training sessions per week, with at least 1 day's rest between sessions. Early studies of pre-pubescent children failed to show a significant increase in muscular strength following training programmes, and these results, combined with young children's low levels of androgens and immature nervous systems, caused many researchers to question whether pre-pubescent children were trainable. However, more recent research has indicated that pre-pubescent children are quite capable of increasing voluntary strength in response to resistance training, even though they experience more difficulty in increasing skeletal muscle mass. It is problematic to compare relative increases in training-induced muscular fitness between pre-pubescent and pubescent children and adults, as it is difficult to resolve the issue of using absolute or percentage gains in muscular fitness as the criterion measure.

Nevertheless, children and adolescents who follow our recommended programme can expect significant gains in muscular fitness, although substantial increases in muscle mass may be experienced only by adolescent boys. In the United Kingdom over 88,000 adults are unable to work each day because of back pain. Twenty-six million working days are lost through backache every year at a cost to the nation of £ 1000 million in medical care, sickness benefit and lost production. Improved muscular fitness will help to prevent or alleviate back pain and other postural problems. In addition, gains in muscular endurance, brought about through an enhanced microcirculation and positive effects on energy-generating enzyme systems, will promote resistance to fatigue during everyday tasks. There is also evidence to support the view that weight training may reduce the blood pressure of hypertensive adolescents, but this remains to be substantiated.

Flexibility

Flexibility may be defined as the range of motion about a joint. Less is known about children's flexibility than about any other component of HRF. Flexibility is joint specific and there is no single indicator of body flexibility. It is a popular belief that young children are very flexible and then gradually lose this flexibility as they grow olders. The scientific evidence for this premise is extremely limited, and flexibility seems to vary with the test administered.

Leighton reported a steady downward trend with age in the range of motion of a majority of the joint movements he measured with his flexometer. On the other hand, Renson, Beuen and Van Gerven studying 12- to 19-yeard-old boys, found a progressive increase in flexibility with age, as indicated by the sit-and-reach test, but this was not confirmed with either a trunk twist or an ankle flexibility test. Huprich and Sigerseth reported no significant differences among girls, aged 9 to 15 years, on six flexibility test items. Although the research evidence on changes in flexibility with growth is equivocal, it does appear that it is beneficial to initiate exercises for increased joint flexibility before puberty, as long as they are carried out with a concern to avoid damage to the joints and vertebral column. Flexibility may be increased by either ballistic or static stretching exercises.

Balistic stretching uses momentum to produce the stretch. The momentum is generated by a bouncing, bobbing or jerking movement, and because this produces a sudden and sometimes excessive stretch on the muscle, there is a potential for injury. Static stretching involves slowly stretching a muscle longer than its normal length and holding the stretch for a period of time. There is much less chance of teaching the soft tissue and less likelihood of causing muscle soreness. We therefore recommend static stretching for the development of flexibility and for including in warm-up routines.

The muscle should be slowly stretched beyond its normal length and the stretch hold for a minimum of 6 to 10 seconds. Each major muscle group should be stretched in this manner per set of flexibility exercises, and each session should consist of three sets of exercises. The exercise sessions should be repeated daily or not less often than every other day. More advanced techniques of improving flexibility, the problems of overflexibility and counter indicated exercises are considered in detail by Alter. Although unequivocal research evidence is not available, it appears that optimal flexibility is associated with the prevention of back pain and postural defects. It helps to prevent muscle, joint and connective tissue injuries, and it may reduce dysmenorrhoea. In addition, reasonable flexibility is required for the performance of many recreational and sporting activities.

Body Composition

Changes in body composition are a function of energy intake energy expenditure. Energy intake should be based upon sound nutritional principles, and several expert committees; Committee on Medical Aspects of Food Policy have recently made recommendations concerning diet. The principal recommendations are, in summary, to reduce fat, sucrose, salt and alcohol intake, increase fibre-rich carbohydrate intake and maintain protein intake. Energy intake must be defined in relation to maintenance of optimal body weight and level of physical activity. It must be recognized that adolescents who choose to severely limit their energy intakes might no obtain all the nutrients they require, and they should be particularly encouraged to adhere to the expert recommendations above.

On the other hand, many adolescents have large

appetites and high energy intakes, particularly from foods and snacks with a high energy content. Because adolescents seem to prefer to eat more of their food as snacks rather than as meals, they need to have access to snacks that are low in sugar, fat and salt. The accumulation of body fat is normally a result of long-term energy imbalance and should be addressed through a small reduction in energy intake and an increase in energy expenditure. Energy expenditure can be subdivided into basal metabolism, thermic effect of food, adaptive thermogenesis and physical activity. The greatest potential for increasing an individual's energy expenditure lies with his or her level of physical activity.

This increase in energy expenditure comes about not just from the direct effect of physical activity on metabolic rate but also from the persistent elevation of metabolism following physical activity. In a research study, Ward and Bar-Or estimated that a 30-kilogram child with an energy expenditure of 7,500 kJ/day can increase her or his daily energy expenditure by 20% to 25% through 40 to 50 minutes of jogging or swimming. Such an increase in daily energy expenditure, without an increase in energy intake, would result in a 1-kilogram fat loss within 23 days. Although the definitive study of the effect of physical activity and exercise intervention on energy intake has yet to be carried out, the weight of available evidence suggests that only very small changes in energy intake accompany exercise training. The mode and volume of physical activity described in the cardiopulmonary fitness section can also be recommended in this context.

When we are concerned with body composition, and in particular body fat content, not exceeding the recommended maximum level of intensity of physical activity is important. Exercising at intensities that elicit heart rates higher than 80% of maximum may be counterproductive. Such high-intensity exercise is significantly supported by anaerobic metabolism with a buildup of lactic acid in the muscles. The high anaerobic content will probably restrict the duration of the exercise and, in addition, because fat cannot be metabolized anaerobically, there will be an increased reliance on glycogen stores as the major source of energy.

To increase lean body mass in line with a reduction in body fat, it is advisable to supplement any aerobic exercise programme with a muscular fitness programme such as that described in the muscle fitness section. The assessment of children's body composition is problematic, and although there is some evidence to suggest that North American children are getting fatter, data on British children are sparse. Armstrong and colleagues assessed 357 boys and 350 girls, aged 11 to 16 years, and according to the criteria of the RCP, 13% of the boys and 10% of the girls could be classified as overweight. The magnitude of the problem of children's overfatness can be put into perspective when one realizes that obesity acquired in childhood is highly predictive of obesity in adult life. It appears that the later into adolescence the individual remains obese, the greater the persistence of obesity into adulthood. Abraham and Nordsieck concluded that the risk of an obese adolescent becoming an obese adult is 63% to 72%.

Psychological Outcomes of Health-Related Physical Activity

The identification of the psychological outcomes of involvement in sport, exercise and physical activity has proved to be a difficult problems for researchers over many years. Although ancient civilizations recognized the potential of the therapeutic benefits of exercise from a psychological point of view, and emotional development was discussed in the early sport psychology literature, it has not been until quite recently that researchers have been able to pursue a consistent line of research. Unfortunately, from a paediatric perspective, little is known about the effects of physical activity on children, whereas considerably more research has been conducted on adults in both clinical and non-clinical settings.

Psychiatric and Psychological Epidemiology

Vikan reported on the psychiatric epidemiology of 1500 children in Norway aged 10 years. The prevalence rate for psychological problems was 5%. More transitory mood swings were probably not included in this figure. However, this suggests that children are not immune from psychological problems, although the source of such problems will likely be different from that for adults, in many cases, and change across the life cycle through childhood and adolescence. In addition to negative emotions, positive psychological aspects, such as self-esteem, character development and cognitive functioning, have also been addressed in the context of physical activity. From an epidemiological perspective, the data provided by Stephens are important in identifying the possible links between exercise and mental health.

Stephens analysed data from four large population surveys from North America. These included over 56,000 people, and data were available on measures of physical activity and mental health. Thirty-two analyses were conducted, and in 25 of these the results showed a positive association between physical activity levels and mental health. These results were obtained using different measures of both activity and mental health, with the latter being defined as positive mood, general well-being and relatively infrequent symptoms of anxiety and depression. Unfortunately, the results by age only referred to those under and over 40 years, thus it is not possible to detect any trends for children. Overall, the effects were more positive for older subjects and for women. Such data do not allow clear statements to be made about the direction of the relationships. Are person with positive mental health more likely to be active, or does activity cause good mental health? Other evidence from biochemical, physiological and psychological sources supports the latter position.

However, it is likely that some people with particularly poor mental health such as those suffering depression, will have low activity and fitness levels. In short, mental health can be both an antecedent and a consequence variable in exercise and physical activity. Consensus. statements on exercise and mental health include the following:

1. Exercise is associated with reduced state anxiety.

2. Exercise has been associated with a decreased level of mild to moderate depression.

3. Long-term exercise is usually associated with reduction in traits such as neuroticism and anxiety.

4. Exercise may be an adjunct to the professional treatment of severe depression.

5. Exercise results in the reduction of various stress indices.

6. Exercise has beneficial emotional effects across all ages and both sexes.

Although evidence can be produced to support most of these statements, the research is not always without problems or conflict. For example, there is very little evidence to support statement 6 in terms of all ages. Indeed, Morgan and Goldston later acknowledge that the effects of exercise on the mental health of children need investigation. In short, we have very little evidence on children, although there is no indication, as far as we know, that the benefits reported for adults will elude children for youths.

Negative Affect

Much of the research on the mental health outcomes of exercise and physical activity has focused on negative emotion/affect and, in particular, anxiety and depression. Although adult data do suggest that positive changes in these factors can occur with activity, few data are available on children. Similarly, the reduced physiological response to psychosocial stressors thought to occur in subjects with higher levels of physical fitness. North, McCullagh, and Tran conducted a meta-analysis of the literature on exercise and depression. A meta-analysis is a quantitative summary of research findings across a number of studies and produces an effect size or index of magnitude, for a particular intervention. In this case, the ES shows the strength of the effect of exercise on the change in depression scores across studies. The ES is expressed in standard deviation units, and therefore an ES of 0.5 shows that the subjects receiving the treatment scored, on the average, one half of a standard deviation above subjects in a control condition. North et al. located five studies with subjects under 18 years old, although three of these were unpublished dissertations. These studies yielded 17 effect sizes, the strength of which can be compare for those of college students and middle-aged subjects. The underlying reasons or mechanisms for the effects of exercise on mental health are unclear, although a number of possibilities exist.

Biochemical mechanisms provide an intriguing possibility for explaining the effects of acute exercise. For example, some have suggested that exercise produces elevations in plasma endorphin levels and that this has been implicated in mood elevation. Similarly, physiological explanations can be offered, such as reductions in muscle tension after exercise, thus producing the postexercise relaxation effect. Finally, psychological factors have been suggested, such as increased self-esteem, mastery and competence from participation in an activity deemed worthwhile or where some success is perceived. In summary, it is quite likely that negative affect can be changed through physical activity and exercise, but the research on children is virtually nonexistent, and the mechanisms of such effects are still not clearly understood.

Positive Affect and Cognitive Functioning

How many school PE programmes in the past have been justified based on character and moral development? This argument supports the notion that participation in particular activities can produce positive changes in the individual's personality and moral behaviour. Regrettably, this assumption is largely untested and naive as far as character is concerned. In short, there is little evidence, that has scientific rigour, to support such assumptions or to delineate which children benefit under which circumstances. There is little doubt that positive changes can be brought about by professional, skilful leadership in most activities, but equally, character can be damaged through inappropriate strategies. Weiss and Bredemeier however, state that 'when structured purposefully and guided by sound educational principles, sport can build character and develop a sound mind in a sound body'. They go on to say that 'we strongly believe that physical education and sport settings provide children, adolescents and adults with ideal opportunities for realising optimal moral growth. The few studies that have been designed to effect changes in moral reasoning and behaviours through sport-related experiences have been optimistic'.

Further discussion of the role of sport and physical activity in moral development can be found in Weiss and Bredemeier. Another important issue in the study of psychological outcomes from physical activity and exercise is the development of self-esteem in children. The effect that physical activity might have on self-esteem has interested teachers and researchers for some time. Although evidence supports a link, it is far from clear under what circumstances SE is affected or what the underlying mechanisms might be that produce such changes.

Nevertheless, a meta-analysis of studies on physical activity and SE in children did find evidence for a positive influence on activity on SE. The greatest effect were found for children with disabilities and for children in aerobic fitness activities, although all of the types of activities studied demonstrated a positive relationship with SE. Recent developments in the study of SE suggest that SE is a hierarchical and multidimensional construct. In other words, SE consists of a number of subdomains, such as perceptions of competence in sport, as well as such domains as physical self-worth, in addition to global self-esteem.

Physical self-worth is also one of the many domains of SE, hence it has a multidimensional structure. The influence of HRPA on self-esteem, therefore, might be seen in this light. HRPA may affect some subdomains of the hierarchy and, over time, physical self-worth and global self-esteem. However, the complexities of such an approach are not yet understood fully. An issue currently arousing the interest of physical educators, and one associated with the physiological outcomes of physical activity, is that of enjoyment. It is recognized that activities that are enjoyable are more likely to be intrinsically motivating and therefore approached through free choice. However, from a research perspective, the concept of enjoyment has remained elusive. Perhaps the most comprehensive analysis of enjoyment has been made by Csikszentmihalyi who studied activities that were participated in for purely intrinsic reasons. He suggested that enjoyment, or a state of flow, was optimized when the demands of the activity were matched by the individual's abilities.

A mismatch produced either anxiety or boredom. Scanlan and Lewthwaite studied the factor of enjoyment in 9- to 16-year-old male sport participants. They suggested that enjoyment from physical activity was best described in terms of intrinsic/extrinsic and achievement/non-achievement dimensions.

The four quardrants identified by Scanlan and Lewthwait as follows:

I. Achievement-Intrinsic: 'predictors related to personal perceptions of competence and control, such as the attainment of mastery goals and perceived ability'.

II. Achievement-Extrinsic: 'predictors related to personal perceptions of competence and control that are derived from other people'.

III. Non-achievement-Instrinct: 'predictors related to (a) physical activity and movement such as sensations, tension release and (b) competition such as excitement.

IV. Non-achievement-Extrinsic: 'predictors related to nonperformance aspects of sport such as affiliating with peers'

Finally, physical educators have shown an interest in the potential effects of physical activity on cognitive functioning. Indeed, arguments for increasing the amount of time devoted to physical education, as through daily PE programmes, usually suggest that cognitive functioning will improve as a result of increased involvement in physical activity. The evidence is not convincing for older school students, however, as many potentially extraneous variables are rarely controlled for, such as teacher expectancy effects.

However, research in perceptual-motor development has suggested that early development of neuromuscular control and psychomotor function could assist academic learning in young children. One of the mechanisms for this could be the increase in cerebral blood flow that has been documented after physical activity, and, in particular, the increase in blood flow in the prefrontal somatosensory and primary motor cortices of the brain. So far, the discussion has centred on the possible outcomes of physical activity and exercise. However, an important issue here is that of children's actual physical activity patterns.

Children's Physical Activity Patterns

The evidence linking an active lifestyle with a reduced risk of some diseases is well documented for both adults and children. Regular weight-bearing physical activity is known to be essential for the normal growth and development of the skeleton. Most studies of physical activity as a preventative modality have, however, been carried out in relation to coronary heart disease. There is no clear understanding of the mechanisms involved, but it is generally agreed that physical activity has positive effects on other coronary risk factors, and other plausible theories include physical-activity-induced changes in blood coagulability, platelet function, fibrinolytic activity, myocardial vascularity and coronary artery size. Very few propective studies have been carried out, the available evidence is equivocal, and several of these beneficial adaptations have yet to be convincingly demonstrated in human subjects.

The well-documented improvement in cardiorespiratory efficiency, at rest and during sub-maximal exercise, brought about by appropriate physical activity may also offer some protection against CHD. Nevertheless, the circumstantial evidence amassed by epidemiological studies associating an active lifestyle with a low incidence of CHD is incontrovertible. A recent analysis of all published papers in the English language that provide sufficient data to calculate a relation risk ration for CHD at different levels of physical activity concluded that "the inverse association between physical activity and incidence of CHD is consistently observed, especially in the better designed studies; this association is appropriately sequenced, biologically graded, plausible, and coherent with existing knowledge. Therefore, the observations reported in the literature support the inference that physical activity is inversely and causally related to the incidence of CHD." The form of physical activity that is consistently and substantially associated with a lower incidence of CHD involves large muscle groups for sustained periods of time. The hypothesis that participation in HRPA in childhood increases the likelihood of such participation as an adult is compelling.

Although research data are sparse and results equivocal, evidence to support the view that children's physical activity patterns persist into adulthood is accumulating. Engstrom appears to have carried out the only published prospective longitudinal study of physical activity through to adulthood. He interviewed 2464 randomly selected 15-year-olds about their sport activities during leisure time and followed the same group through mailed questionnaires 5, 10 and 15 years later. He obtained a full set of data on 2072 subjects, and his results indicated that early experiences of physical activity are important for psychological readiness to participate in keep-fit activities in later life. These findings reinforce the importance of adopting an active lifestyle during childhood. Simons-Morton et al. reviewed the published 'physical activity recommendations for children' and concluded that appropriate physical activity involves large muscle groups in dynamic movement for periods of 20 minutes or longer.

They emphasized that this type of physical activity should occur at least three times per week and that it should be of sufficient intensity to elicit heart rates equal to or in excess of 140 BPM. We have shown that for children, brisk walking on the treadmill at 6 km/h equates with steady-state heart rates of about 140 BPM. It appears, therefore, that there is a close agreement between the volume of physical activity recommended as health-related for children and the volume that is coronary preventive for adults. The assessment of adult's physical activity is one of the most difficult tasks in epidemiological research, and the estimation of the daily physical activity patterns of children is even more problematic. The technique used must be socially acceptable, it should not burden the child with cumbersome equipment, and it should minimally influence the child's normal physical activity pattern.

Ideally, the relative intensity and duration of activities should be monitored, and if a true picture of habitual activity is required, some account of day-to-day variation must be taken. Bar-Or suggested that with children a minimum follow-up of 3 days, including 1 weekend day, should be employed. A range of methods for assessing the level of adult's physical activity has been developed, and several of these methods have been used with children without due consideration being taken of the differences between children and adults. The vast majority of studies have used self-report techniques, and it is well documented that these techniques are particularly problematic with children as subjects.

Few studies of children's physical activity patterns have satisfied the criteria outlined above, and it is only very recently that objective evidence of British children's level of HRPA has become available. Armstrong et al. carried out the first study to unobstrusively monitor heart rates of British children for extended periods of time. They estimated the volume of physical activity of 266 children, aged 11 to 16 years, using a self-contained, computerized telemetry system. The Sport Tester system is capable of storing and replaying minute-by-minute heart rates for up to 16 hours; when it is interfaced with a microcomputer, sustained periods with heart rates above 139 BPM can be readily identified and recorded. This methodology does not give a direct measure of physical activity, but more importantly in this context, it measures the stress placed on the cardiopulmonary system. Armstrong et al. monitored each child from about during a normal school-day. The receivers were retrieved, replaced and refitted the next morning, and the process was repeated over 3 days. In addition, 212 of the children were monitored from 0900 to 2100 on a Saturday. Seventy-seven per cent of the boys and 88% of the girls failed to elicit a single 20-minute period with their heart rate equal to or above 70% of maximum over the 3-week-day monitoring period.

Only four boys and girls averaged a daily 20-minute period of HRPA. 36% of the boys and 52% of the girls did not even experience a single 10-minute period of HRPA during the 3 weekdays of monitoring. During Saturday monitoring, 88% of the boys and 97% of the girls failed to exhibit a 20-minute period of HRPA, and 71% of the boys and 94% of the girls did not even experience a 10-minute period of physical activity equivalent to brisk walking. These data demonstrated for the first time that British children exhibit very low levels of habitual HRPA.

When the data were analysed by sex, it was shown that boys were significantly more physically active than girls. Furthermore, the girl's level of HRPA significant decreased with age. These results provoked the research group to recruit a group of 42 primary school children, aged 10 years, from the same catchment area as some of the secondary school children already surveyed. The physical activity patterns of the younger children were monitored using the same techniques, and a comparison of HRPA levels revealed that although there was no difference in the level of physical activity of primary and secondary school boys, the primary school girls were significantly more physically active than their secondary school counterparts. The research team concluded that children have generally low levels of physical activity but that teenage girls appear to be particularly inactive. More detailed analysis of the primary school data revealed that there was no difference between the physical activity patterns of 10-year-old boys and 10-year-old girls. Armstrong and Bray confirmed this finding in a further study of 67 boys and 65 girls, but their results illustrated the relatively low levels of physical activity of even 10-year-old children. Sixty-one per cent of the boys and 66% of the girls failed to experience a single 20-minute period of HRPA during 3 days of heart rate monitoring. 19% of the boys and 25% of the girls failed to elicit even a 10-minute period with their heart rate about 139 BPM. During Saturday monitoring the children appeared to be even more sedentary, with 75% of the boys and 65% of the girls failing to experience a 10-minute period of HRPA. The results of these studies clearly demonstrate the British children currently exhibit sedentary physical activity patterns and that many children seldom experience the intensity and duration to physical activity associated with health-related outcomes.

This suggests that a real deal more emphasis needs to be placed on the underlying reasons for such patterns of behaviour. Strategies and interventions designed to promote increased participation in HRPA will now be discussed.

Promoting Health-Related Physical Activity

Motivating Participation

The issue of motivation is a complex one. Sallis and Hovell in a review of the determinants of exercise, suggest that a natural history model is useful. This model is probably more applicable to adults, because children will be more sporadic and informal in their activity patterns. Nevertheless, the Sallis and Hovell model provides a useful base from which to consider the psychological correlates of HRPA in children. This section will focus on the processes of maintenance and dropout; little is known about the adoption of exercise in children.

Motives for Participation and Reasons for Dropout

Several papers have reported data on why children participate in or drop out of sport. The motives most commonly identified by children are to have fun, to learn or improve skills, to be with their friends, to have excitement, to win, to be successful, and for health and fitness. The Canada Fitness Survey showed that young aged 10 to 18 years rated a mix of physical and psychological health factors as very importance reasons for being active. Reasons cited for giving up sport include a lack of playing time, a lack of improvement, not having fun, or an overemphasis on winning, parental pressure and dislike of the coach. A study by White and Coakley on school leaves in South East England, revealed a number of influences on why older teenagers did not take part in community sport programmes. Such decisions were influenced by negative perceptions of competence, constraints such as lack of money, lack of support from significant others, and past negative experiences in school PE.

Negative memories of PE included boredom, perceived lack of choice, feelings of incompetence, and negative peer evaluation. Girls reported feelings of discomfort and embarrassment, dissatisfaction with the physical environment in school PE, as well as the rule relating to kit and showers. The reasons cited by children for participating in sport and exercise do not, of course, necessarily reflect the initial influences or determinants of their involvement. For example, a child may start playing badminton at the local sport centre simply because he or her friends are there. However, once the child is involved, the reasons for continuing playing may change to, say, skill development. Teachers are encouraged to ask children why they do or do not participate in certain activities and use such information to their advantage in motivating and planning participation. Where a matching of activities with motives occurs, participation is more likely to be sustained. Similarly, despite the emphasis on competitive activities, not all children are motivated by competition.

Telema and Silvennoinen found that motivation toward competition and performance declined across the teen years, whereas recreation and relaxation motives became more important.

Intrinsic Motivation

Intrinsic motivation is motivation related to participation for its own sake rather than for external rewards such as badges or money. Intrinsic motivation has been conceptualized in a number of different ways, but Deci and Ryan say that it is concerned with self-determination and competence and with feelings of enjoyment and interest. The belief that IM is important for participation in HRPA in children is probably correct, although the relationship between IM, other influences, and behaviour is far from simple.

For example, the use of external rewards or other external events have been shown, under some circumstances to reduce IM. Whitehead and Corbin investigated the effects on IM of giving norm-referenced feedback to children after a fitness test. Children were told they were in either the top or the bottom 20% for students of their age. In reality, the scores were bogus. The results showed that IM declined for those told they were in the lower group, and IM increased for those in the upper group. Analyses showed that this was due to perceptions of competence held by the children. Intrinsic motivation, and the accompanying feelings of self-determination, interest, and enjoyment, are not likely to accrue to large numbers of children when externally referenced criteria are used for judgments. This was supported by Vallerand and colleagues for children in competitive situations.

From a health-related perspective, an important aim is to have as many people participating as possible. A re-orientation of the way some activities are presented may therefore be required.

Perceptions of Success and Goal Orientations

A number of researchers in both the United States and Britain have highlighted the importance of recognizing that children may differ from each other in terms of the goals that they may have in achievement situations. Two of the most commonly found goals are those labelled mastery-oriented goals and ego-oriented goals. The former refers to children who measure their success in terms of the extent to which they improve or master the activity, and this is independent of the success of other people.

Ego-oriented goals are help by children who judge their success by winning and losing. Social comparison then becomes the important factor. Some researchers have suggested that these goals will focus children on either effort or ability judgments. Ego goals will create a situation whereby the child considers others and her or his ability to do better, and therefore ability is the main attribution used to explain success or failure. Under failure conditions this can be debilitating. For mastery goals, because the motivation is to improve or master a task, personal effort becomes more salient. This is a controllable attribution that allows the child a possibility of success after a failure situation. This would suggest that a mastery orientation to HRPA will predict higher participation levels. These notions have support in the education literature but require support in health and physical activity contexts.

Exercise Motivation: Support

Motivation is a complex topic, and space does not allow justice to be done to some of the issues raised. Nevertheless, educators need to be the aware of various approaches to motivation and sport and exercise in children. These include recognizing children's motives for participation, the possible reasons predicting dropout, the nature of intrinsic motivation, children's various goals orientations and the possible consequences of these for participation.

Intervention Strategies

Attempts at increasing children's involvement in HRPA can be made at both the individual and the institutional level. Both of these will be addressed briefly here.

Institutions

Parcelt et al. suggest that schools should use social learning theory and organizational change if the impact of a health programme is to be felt. Interventions based on social learning theory would include modelling, behaviour reinforcement and cognitive change. In addition, organizational changes in the school may be required. Parcel et al. suggest for major stages in this: institutional commitment, structured alterations in school policies and practices, changes in the role and actions of staff, and the implementation of learning activities for students. One intervention frequently cited as a possible remedy for low activity levels in children is the introduction of daily periods of physical activity or physical education, particularly in primary schools.

However, it is not clear whether this would simply be a daily training session or constitute a more educational use of time by teaching physical education. More time is not necessarily the answer, and studies evaluating the physical fitness outcomes of daily PE programmes have been relatively unsuccessful in demonstrating major changes, probably due to the current lack of valid and reliable field tests and the problems of assessing children's fitness in the field. Similarly, daily PE/PA studies have attempted to demonstrate that academic performance is at least unaffected, and probably improved, as a result of the extra physical activity. Regrettably, the methodological problems inherent in these studies precludes firm conclusions being drawn. In short, we believe that daily vigorous PA is not the answer.

What is required is a quality teaching programme emphasizing the processes and benefits of HRPA across the life span and how such activity can be accommodated in an individual's lifestyle One of the problems of approaches such as daily PE/PA is obtaining a balance between short- and long-term objectives: If such an institutional intervention is applied because children have low activity levels, it is the role of the school to promote physical activity, exercise and fitness in the short term or to encourage and develop long-term behaviour-change strategies that will be used by the students once they have left school? Current pleas for extra time in PE are often based on the assumption that PE teachers require this time to get children fit. Such an approach could lead to negative experiences for many pupils. The goals must be reoriented towards the achievement of longer-term aims and objectives, such as behaviour change. This is not to say that children should not experience exercise appropriate for fitness development, but teachers will realize that time does not permit genuine long-term fitness development in curriculum time. Physical education teachers may wish to consider the use of homework assignments to make up for the erosion of PE time in thc schools in the last 2 decades.

Individuals

There are a number of strategies for individual-behaviour change that can be implemented in schools to help children learn about long-term involvement in HRPA. Space here permits brief discussion only. Teaching children self-regulatory skills holds an important key to future participation in HRPA. One of the main elements of this is the ability to understand and set personal goals. The goal-setting process can be complex, but the following guidelines should be taught to children:

1. Set short-, medium, and long-term goals. See goal setting as a stairway, with long-term goals at the top of the stairs.

2. Set goals that relate to the process of exercise rather

than just the product. In other words, focus on goals that encourage participation over and above fitness or performance outcomes. This is particularly important for those less fit or willing. Indeed, some have advocated that for the initial stage in an exercise programme, fitness improvement should be discouraged so that time is allowed for gradual and comfortable changes in behaviour to be made. We concur with such an approach for children.

3. Set goals that are specific, realistic and reasonably challenging. Goals must act as a stimulus—not too hard and not too easy.

4. Goals must be accepted by the participant, and he or she must be committed to achieving them. This can be enhanced by having the participant set the goals or at least be involved in the goal-setting process. Goals set externally, by the teacher for example, often have less impact.

5. Monitor the goals by writing them down, and obtain feedback on progress.

In addition to goal setting, children should be taught how to programme exercise into their lives. This should include programme-planning exercises where children are introduced to the following ideas and topics:

— Why people exercise

— Why people may quite exercise, and the barriers that can inhibit participation

— How to construct an exercise timetable

— Which activities may be appropriate from the point of view of individual motives and interests, convenience and likely adherence, and health/fitness requirements

— How to set appropriate goals

Other self-regulatory skills might include positive self-talk, where negative thoughts about physical activity are modified to be more positive; planning and understanding the process of temporary dropout so that exercise can restart again; and self-reinforcement. Further discussion on these and other techniques can be found in Knapp.

Health-Related Fitness Training and Monitoring in Schools

The availability of cheap equipment and elementary computer software packages, seem to have restimulated interest in performance tests of health-related fitness. A number of PE departments are administering their own fitness test batteries and developing norm tables or percentile charts against which to compare their students. Some departments are including scores in student profiles, and others are using them as a means of evaluating the effectiveness of their teaching programmes. The Council of Europe Committee of Ministers has recommended that member states adopt the Eurofit tests of physical fitness for the purpose of measuring and assessing the physical fitness of school-age children in the range 6 to 18 years old. The Inner London Education Sport recommended that all pupils from 10 to 18 years old should be tested for fitness at regular intervals and parents informed of their children's fitness rating assessed against accepted norms. A nationwide survey of Northern Ireland children's physical fitness has recently been published, yet there has been little informed debate about the validity of the using HRF tests with children. This section will evaluate the role of HRF testing and monitoring procedures within the school PE curriculum. The quantitative assessment of children's HRF is one of the most complex problems in exercise science, and HRF tests suitable for use in school environment that provide valid and objective measures of HRF are currently not available

All fitness test scores are influenced by a number of factors. Fox and Biddle have discussed these at length. In short, only part of the score obtained from performance tests is related to HRF. The dependence of test scores upon the subject's motivation to do well, for example, was vividly illustrated by Schwab's 1953 study. Schwab required subjects to hang from a horizontal bar in a manner similar to the test recommended to assess local muscular endurance in the Handbood for the Assessment of Physical Fitness. He found that with instructions to hold on as long as possible, the average length of time before letting go was less than 1 minute. With a $5 reward promised for beating their previous records, subjects managed to hang on for an average of nearly 2 minutes. So their local muscular endurance was doubled with a financial inducement. Several advocates of HRF testing emphasize the use of norm tables, but norm tables confound rather than clarify the issue of relative fitness.

Norms are based on performance rather than capabilities, and for example, if teachers accept lower norms for girls as reflecting acceptable performance, then girls will tend to meet these lower expectations. The constant comparison of children on the basis of test scores is likely to negatively affect those who score low. Furthermore, how can tables constructed on the basis of chronological age provide worthwhile information about children at different levels of skeletal and biological maturation? With 13-year-old boys, a teacher may be testing a group in which 10% are prepubertal, 10% are in pubertal stage, 5 full mature and the remainder are somewhere in between. The effects of growth and maturation on performance and children's responses to exercise training are well documented. Each of the components of HRF could be used to illustrate the futility of HRF testing from a physiological viewpoint, but as cardiopulmonary fitness is arguably the most important component, we will for the purpose of this chapter, concentrate upon the testing of children's cardiopulmonary fitness. No one parameter can fully describe cardiopulmonary fitness, but it is widely recognized that the best single physiological indicator is the maximal rate at which oxygen can be consumed.

The results of any test claiming to measure children's cardiopulmonary fitness must be correlated strongly with peak VO_2 if the test is to be judged valid. The determination of peak VO_2 requires sophisticated apparatus and expertise usually only available in a well-equipped exercise physiology laboratory. However, several performance tests designed to predict cardiopulmonary fitness using cheap and simple apparatus have been developed and are currently in use in schools. The most commonly used procedure is to predict peak VO_2 from a single sub-maximal heart rate measurement and the corresponding oxygen consumption or power output on a step bench or cycle ergometer, using the Astrand nomogram, which is often supplied as a computer program.

The nomogram was, however, derived from data on an adult population, and several incorrect assumptions are made when it is applied to children. The cardiopulmonary responses of children to sub-maximal exercise do not parallel those of adults, and children's maximal heart rates are often much higher than those of adults, with a much greater range. Realizing the obvious problems involved, the Åstrands have never seriously tested their nomogram with individuals below the age of 20 years, but others persist in doing so. Wilmore and Sigerscth found the prediction of VO_2 max to be questionable with girls aged 7 to 13 years. Hermansen and Oseid concluded that an indirect method of estimating VO_2 max should be used only when accurate individual values are not required. Washburn and Montoye commented that the prediction of an individual's VO_2 max from sub-maximal data was subject to large errors. Woynarowska tested 80 boys and 43 girls and reported that the Åstrand nomogram underestimated the measured VO_2 max in boys by an average of 26% and in girls by an average of 23%.

Buono and colleagues reported similar results and suggested that 'use of the Åstrand nomogram to predict VO_2 max in children and adolescents is not warranted at this time'. Koch, Karlegard, and Fransson obtained extensive cardiovascular and lung function data annually on a group of 10 boys from the age of 12 to 17 years. They investigated the accuracy of predicting VO_2 max from data obtained at sub-maximal exercise, including the Åstrands methodology, and concluded that in the age group of 12 to 17 years, true VO_2 max cannot be properly evaluated from sub-maximal measurements but has to be directly determined. Binkhorst, Saris, Noordeloos, Van't Hoff, and de Hann summed up their studies with the recommendation that 'it is therefore strongly advised not to use prediction formulas for an accurate individual VO_2 max determination'. In our laboratory the standard error of prediction using either the Åstrand nomogram or the similar Margaria, Aghemo, and Rovelli procedure with young boys has proved to be 10% to 12%. A substantial volume of data concerned with children's PWC170 has also been accumulated, and most published fitness surveys from the United Kingdom and Ireland have relied on this measure.

The PWC170 first promoted by Wahlund, is a measure of physical work capacity at a heart rate of 170 BPM during cycle ergometry. There are, however, many problems with the use of the PWC170 test, and it is of limited value as a measure of cardiopulmonary fitness in children. The fundamental assumption of a constant mechanical efficiency during cycling is not valid. In adults the mechanical efficiency of cycling is assumed to be 22% to 23%, but with children it has been shown to vary from 14.5% to 34.4%, cited in Shephard. This variation is due to the facts that most children are not accustomed to pedalling at a slow and constant speed against a heavy resistance and that the posture required on a cycle ergometer differs from that adopted on most modern bicycles.

Mechanical efficiency improves with practice, and familiarization with the test has been demonstrated to increase scores by as much as 10%. Furthermore, in our experience the coefficient of variation of children's maximal heart rate during cycle ergometry is about 5%, which makes the PWC170 data very difficult to interpret in terms of children's peak VO_2. Some investigators have used maximal performance tests, such as the 12-minute run, to predict VO_2 max, but this type of test is not a reflection of the environment, the child's pace judgment and the potency of the motivational conditions under which the test takes place than of VO_2 max. Kemper and Verschuur studied the relationship between VO_2 max and the 12-minute run on a longitudinal basis and discovered that in boys, 12-minute run performance increased with age, whereas VO_2 max in relation to body weight remained constant, and in girls the decrease in VO_2 max in relation to body weight was not accompanied by a fall in 12-minute-run performance. They concluded that the 12-minute run and VO_2 max in relation to body weight were measuring different fitness factors. Following his review of the literature, Cunningham concluded that performance tests such as running for 12 minutes were relatively weak predictions of VO_2 max. Leger recently introduced a performance test, the 20-metre progressive shuttle run, that has been enthusiastically adopted by the National Coaching Foundation and the Health Education Authority/PEA Health and Physical Education Project.

The validity of the test with children is not well documented, but initial results with small groups of boys and girls were initially encouraging. However, we examined he relationship of directly determined peak VO_2 to peak VO_2 predicted from progressive shuttle-run performance in 77 boys, aged 11 to 14 years, and found that the common variance between the two scores was only 29%. This is not better than can be achieved from other simple field tests, and it was concluded that the use of the 20-meter progressive shuttle run as a valid substitute for a direct determination of an individual's VO_2 max cannot be supported. Cumming stated that in normal children the prediction of VO_2 max is little better than can be obtained from height, weight and skinfold measurements. He felt that performance tests distinguish the obvious and can tell the athlete from the non-athlete but are of limited value in the evaluation of physiological functions in the average population.

Shephard commented that performance tests are a complicated way of identifying tall or fat pupils. Recent research results are therefore unequivocal and confirm that with children there is no valid substitute for a direct determination of peak VO_2. In earlier sections of this chapter we described the analysis by Armstrong et al. of children's physical activity patterns through continuous heart rate monitoring. They also examined the same children's cardiopulmonary fitness determined during the either treadmill or cycle ergometry. When these researchers compared peak VO_2 with heart rate indicators of habitual physical activity, they failed to detect any significant relationship between the two.

This, they argued, was not an unexpected finding when one considers the presence of an as yet unquantified genetic component of peak VO_2 and the influence of the body size/maturation interaction on the development of peak VO_2. However, it does put the use of fitness testing, whether the tests are valid or not, into perspective. If one is interested in physical activity as a means of preventing degenerative diseases, numerous epidemiological studies have demonstrated that it is current physical activity, more than cardiopulmonary fitness, that should be emphasized.

The simple fact is that few children experience the recommended volume of physical activity, and even fewer children exhibit the levels of physical activity associated with the improvement of peak VO_2.

Pedagogical Issues

The discussion so far has centred on the problems inherent in measuring children's fitness. Our conclusion is that valid and reliable measures in the field are not available and that tests currently in use are too reliant on factors unrelated to current exercise habits. This renders fitness tests obsolete in the curriculum unless other objectives can be stated and justified. One objective proposed by Fox and Biddle and Whitehead, Pemberton and Corbin is the educational development of the child. In other words, if performance tests can be justified from an educational perspective, then the problems associated with measurement become less of an issue. It is our belief that if the performance of some kind of HRF test takes place in PE sessions, such as running the 20-metre progressive shuttle, and can be justified on the grounds that it helps children to learn about exercise and health and assists in the promotion of HRPA, then that HRF test is an acceptable use of time.

It is likely, however, that the value of such HRF test will lie not in any scoring or classifying procedure but in the feedback provided by the teacher. PE often emphasizes performance, but a different philosophy is required to properly use HRF tests, where the emphasis should be on learning, self-improvement and motivation. Regrettably, certain types of feedback are as likely to demotivate as to motivate. Teachers and students must be aware of the severe limitations of HRF test in the complex analysis and assessment of children's fitness. Teachers must ask themselves why they are testing children's fitness, and if the answer is to classify children, then perhaps they would be better employed seriously addressing the problem of children's sedentary physical activity patterns.

Towards the National Curriculum

In earlier sections of this chapter we argued the case for HRPA and described the psychological and physiological outcomes associated with an active lifestyle. On the surface it appears that physical educators have taken on board the issues we have raised, and the 1980s saw a re-emergence of emphasis upon the health-related fitness within the physical education programme. A survey by the Physical Education Association illustrated that heads of department rated the promotion of physical development the 2nd most important objective of physical education. A previous survey had ranked physical development 7th in order of importance.

The PEA commented that this major shift represents accurately the recent and positive encouragement being given to the movement for health-related fitness in the physical education programme. The following year the Inner

London Education Authority School Sport Working Party concluded, 'Enthusing and informing the young about physical activity to be the top priority for teachers of physical education' By the end of the decade Her Majesty's Inspectorate had endorsed the view that to "develop an understanding of the importance of exercise in maintaining a healthy life' is a fundamental aim of physical education. Although heads of PE departments may perceive the importance of promoting HRF/PA, their curricula may not be geared to this objective.

Recent attempts to promote active lifestyles through the PE programme or supplements to it have generally been unsuccessful. In this chapter, we have documented unequivocal evidence, from studies in the PEA Research Centre, that despite 10 years of a supposed emphasis on the promotion of active lifestyles, both primary and secondary British schoolchildren exhibit very low levels of habitual HRPA. We have therefore reaffirmed our view that physical educators must promote active lifestyles more explicitly and that HRPA must be a central issue in physical education, HRPA should underpin the physical education programme, and we endure the view of the British Association of Sports Sciences. These experiences need to be supported by a theoretical framework, and pupils should develop understanding of HRPA's beneficial effects and the ways these benefits can be achieved and sustained through adult life.

4

VITALITY OF FITNESS, PHYSICAL AND HEALTH EDUCATION

We are living in an era during which people in the United States have changed fundamentally their perception of human life and of how it can be lived. It is now clear that lifespan involvement in sport, fitness and physical education is possible and desirable. Persons can become involved in purposeful physical activity very early in life and can continue to pursue these interests throughout their lives. That possibility has not yet been realized for many people. What an extraordinary era this is for persons interested in sport, fitness and physical education. There certainly has been no period in the history of the United States to match it.

Sport is central to much of our cultural life. The neighbourhood turns out to watch a youth soccer game. The community is brought together as it follows the fortunes or misfortunes of the high-school basketball team. Students, alumni, and fans rally around sports teams from universities. Professional teams draw more spectators than ever, and in a good season capture the imagination of an entire region. Watching events such as the World Series, Super Bowl, or National College Athletic Association basketball finals has become a national ritual of immense proportion. But do not get the idea that we are simply a nation of spectators. As spectating has increased, so good has participation. More adults than even before are participating in sports such as soft-ball, golf, bowling, running, cycling and swimming. If you are a fitness buff, then you already are aware of the current trend of getting into shape. Fitness centres and sport clubs with fitness facilities have sprung up everywhere. Whereas the slim look was the fashion of a generation ago, the athletic look is clearly the fashion today.

The current fitness movement, however, is by no means simply a manifestation of the latest fashion. Rather, it is part of a larger lifestyle trend that has a strong health basis. Looking good, feeling good, and increasing your chances of living longer are all part of this movement. Slowly, but surely, we are changing our eating habits and our exercise habits. These changes are all aspects of the wellness movement, which recommends adopting a lifestyle that helps you to feel well and to stay well that emphasizes prevention of illness rather than remediation of disease. Wellness is not just for the benefit of the individual, nor is lack of wellness merely an individual problem. The active, healthy lifestyle is also a public-health issue because the enormous costs of health insurance and health care have made it so.

The U.S. Public Health Service has dealt specifically with this issue in its landmark publication Healthy People 2000, which has the specific goal of motivating more citizens to become and stay more physically active. Physical education in schools is obviously one important setting for achieving the goals of a healthy lifestyle. Recognizing this, the U.S. Congress passed House Concurrent Resolution 97 in 1987, calling for quality, daily physical education in schools. The fact is, however, few students participate in daily physical education, and there is considerable question about the quality of what is done in physical-education classes. In the area of fitness, particularly, school physical education has come under severe criticism within its own ranks for its failures to provide programs that provide children and youth with the knowledge and activity experiences that lead to adoption of a healthy lifestyle. It is clear that physical education is undergoing serious examination and needs to develop stronger programs that achieve higher status in the school curriculum.

Watershed Periods

This is not the first time in American history when a sense of optimism and expansion has permeated sport, fitness and physical education. There have been several historical periods when great leaps forward have been made. Four such periods merit mention here. First, the early to mid nineteenth century saw the removal of many religious sanctions against sport and play. Historians refer to this period as the era of muscular Christianity. Because religion and religious thought were so central to American life at that time, it must have been very exciting for sport, fitness and physical education professionals not only to have religious sanctions removed but also to have their subject matter begin to be strongly approved by the religious community. The second watershed period was in the late nineteenth century, when organized sport emerged in America.

The first intercollegiate baseball and football games were played. Professional sport developed and began to spread quickly. Tennis and badminton were first introduced in the United States. Basketball, volleyball, and softball were invented in America and became popular not only here but throughout the rest of the world as well. The third period we shall describe occurred in the early twentieth century and was marked by the development of the sport, fitness and physical education professions. Many national sport associations were formed. The Amateur Athletic Union was founded. The group that would eventually become the American Alliance for Health Physical Education, Recreation and Dance formed and expanded rapidly.

The NCAA was organized. Colleges and universities developed programs to prepare professionals in sport, fitness and physical education. All of this organizational development was accompanied by professional meetings and by the emergence of a professional literature. The fourth important period was more recent, in the 1960s and early 1970s when the academic study of sport, fitness and physical education emerged. College and university programs were changed substantially in this period. Research and scholarship in all areas was recognized and began to grow. Whereas preparation for teaching and coaching had dominated previous eras, this period was marked by the addition of a broad array of career options—adult fitness, worksite health promotion, cardiac rehabilitation, academic sport disciplines, and sport management, to mention just a few. In each of these four eras, there was the sense of excitement and optimism that accompanies rapid change.

Yet the changes in each of these periods were limited compared to those that are currently happening in sport, fitness and physical education.

Lifespan Involvement—A Revolution not Limited By Age or Gender

Historians will someday describe and interpret the current era as a watershed period best characterized by the emergence of the possibility of lifespan involvement in sport, fitness and physical education. We have not achieved lifespan involvement yet, but the possibilities for us to do so are clearly there. When you consider the topics of sport, fitness and physical education, what groups come to mind? Traditionally, our thoughts might turn to children at play, youth involved in sport, young adults perhaps continuing for a time in recreational sports, with involvement slowly diminishing as people grow older. Very young children would not typically be included in such a scenario.

We might be less likely to imagine the involvement of girls than we would that of boys. And, although we might think of men continuing their recreational involvement as they age, many of use would be less likely to think of older women being involved in strenuous activities. The stereotypic view is that people in their senior years play a bit of shuffleboard and perhaps take a leisurely stroll in the afternoon. The point is that, historically, sport, fitness and physical education have been limited primarily to older children and youth, with adult participation decreasingly rigorous with age. Furthermore, the participation of girls and women has always been viewed as different from that of boys and men, especially by the persons in positions of power and leadership, who typically have been men. Those are the stereotypes with which many of us entered this incredible era in which we now live and those are the stereotypes that we have not begun to dismantle. We are replacing our old ideas with a vision of lifespan involvement in sport, fitness and physical education—not only for adolescents and young adults but also for very young children, for older people, not only for adolescents and young adults but also for very young children, for older people, not only for boys and men but also for girls and women. It is those changes in perception, and the changes in opportunity that accompany them, that lie at the heart of the revolution we are now experiencing—and it is those changes that make this era unlike any before it. The possibility of lifespan involvement potentially touches every person. This revolution is not limited by age or gender. Does this vision mean that every person has to be a committed athlete from childhood through to old age? No, clearly not. What it does mean, however, is that people who want to follow such a course now have the opportunity to do so. And it means that we will increasingly see some fitness and/or sport involvement as a fundamental part of living well, regardless of age or gender. The purpose of this chapter is to provide glimpses of the kinds of opportunities available in sport, fitness and physical education that together constitute the possibility of lifespan involvement. Each vignette presents a particular point in their life and in particular places. None of the scenarios have been contrived; each is based on real programs or persons. Together, they paint a picture of lifespan sport, fitness and physical education.

The Early Years

Physical movement is the basic language of the early childhood years, from birth to age 6 or 7. Moving about and physically exploring their immediate surroundings are the main ways young children learn about their world. Providing opportunities for physical movement and, later, for motor play has long been recognized as fundamentally important in fostering a child's physical, social and mental development. Traditionally, the movement experiences of young children have been only informally arranged and monitored, often with no specific purpose other than to keep the child involved in some activity. Furthermore, these early movement experiences have been almost exclusively the responsibility of parents, most of whom have little knowledge of and no training in motor development or early childhood physical education.

Preschool Motor Programs

Now, that model seems to be changing. Typical of the change is fit by five, a franchised preschool for children ages 2 to 5 years. In this skill and fitness program, children learn motor skills, improve their coordination, and take part in activities designed to increase their confidence at motor tasks. Because activity is the medium through which all things are learned, children are frequently and active and, as a result, fitness is improved. Children attend classes twice weekly. Sport opportunities are being made available to children at an earlier age than in the past. It is no longer unusual to see 5-year-olds enrolled in a children's soccer or gymnastics program. Many infant swimming programs are available. Children's playgrounds are increasingly being designed with apparatus to accommodate activities that are developmentally appropriate for young children and that encourage children to explore and use their entire movement repertoire. Most evidence indicates that children who have enriched motor experiences as infants tend to be more fit and more likely to participate in sport throughout their lives. Sport psychologists even speculate that the drive to excel in sport may originate in infancy, when early motor efforts are recognized and responded to lovingly by parents or child-care workers. There seems little doubt now that fitness habits originate in childhood and that the longer learned bad habits are allowed to persist, the more difficult they are to change. There is much debate about the nature of early-childhood motor activity programs. Should they be mostly exploratory, with adults providing only encouragement, support and reinforcement? Or should they aim to develop specific skills? At the moment, there is not enough evidence to decide the issue.

Experts all agree, however, about the importance of providing rich, stimulating motor experiences for very young children: "Enhancing and expanding the movement vocabulary of a young child is just as important as improving word and reading vocabularies. Since movement is the child's first language, a variety of experiences will help make that language as precise and expressive as possible.

Children's Sport

Sport opportunities for children have grown enormously in the recent past. Both the number of children participating and the kinds of early sport opportunities available to these children have increased. Some sports, such as swimming and gymnastics, have age-group programs that are highly specialized, with children sometimes beginning to train year round in their early elementary-school years. Typical of this boom in children's sport are the many children's soccer programs that have sprung up across the land.

The quality and appropriateness of these programs differ dramatically from place to place. Typical of the better programs is one in a mid-sized metropolitan area, in which 2000 boys and girls learn and compete. This soccer association was started by parents and is maintained by them. Together, they purchased a 76-acre tract of land on which they gradually have built a huge soccer complex to accommodate their age-group program. The program begins as an instruction only program for boys and girls aged 5 years. From ages 6 to 12, the children are given continued instruction and are involved in intramural competition.

Teams are separated by age and sex when sufficient children are available and children from the same neighbourhood typically are grouped together to make the transportation easier for their parents.

A 10-week season costs $30 for the first child, $20 for the second and $10 for the third. No family pays more than $60 for any season. All children are guaranteed to play at least one-half of each game, and teams are kept fairly small so that most children get a great deal of playing time. The demand for participation is so strong that leagues are typically formed by age and gender; for example, there is a league for 10-year-old boys and league for 7-year-old girls. This soccer program is an all-volunteer association.

Parents, of course, provide the main bulk of the volunteers, serving as referees and coaches. Individuals or businesses can sponsor teams for $85; all players wear shirts that bear the team name.

Elementary Physical Education

Not all elementary-school children attend physical education programs; and nearly one-half of those who do are taught by their classroom teacher rather than by a physical education specialist. In many schools, elementary physical education is hardly more than a recess recreation period; in some schools, recess actually is counted as physical education. There are nonetheless school physical education programs that are extraordinary. In one school of 670 children in the South, there are two teachers who are physical education specialists, as well as one physical education teacher's aide. Each child, from kindergarten to sixth grade, attends physical education classes daily. Part of the program is fitness-oriented. Teachers have adopted the "Fitnessgram" to communicate regular fitness-test results to parents on a regular basis. In addition, any one who walks down the schools halls will see posters listing children's names and adjacent different coloured stars. Closer inspection reveals that each poster shows the level of performance each child has attained in a specific fitness activity. Children also learn what are most often called adventure skills.

In the gymnasium, there is a climbing wall, which is brightly coloured to represent a mountain scene. At the top of the climbing course, there is a place for each child who makes it to write his or her name. Children also participate in cooperative games and group initiatives, learning the value of working together and depending on one another to reach specific goals. Sports are part of the curriculum too. On one side of the gym is a volleyball schedule for the fourth- through sixth-grade intramural program, which takes place during the recess after lunch. Next to it is the schedule of games for the floor-hockey unit in which the fifth- and sixth-graders currently play. A visitor to a first-grade class finds the children playing in a unit in which they explore different ways to strike objects. They strike balloons, yarn balls, very soft rubber balls, and balls that bounce more like tennis balls. They strike with different kinds of implements, some of which look like stubby tennis rackets, others like paddles. As the teacher directs their exploration, the visitor can begin to see that the children will eventually explore forehand stroking, backhand stroking, overhead stroking and even something that begins to approach a tennis serve.

The children are all active and they seem to enjoy what they are doing—for its own sake, not as an activity they eventually will utilize in sports. We can see this second benefit, however.

Youth-The Transition Years

It is not difficult to think of many different ways in which adolescent boys and girls are involved in sport, fitness and physical education. Many of us find that our memories of our own youth are dominated by those kinds of experiences. In fact, those experiences may have been so influential that we decided to explore a professional career in these fields.

The High-School Interschool Sports Program

Virtually every high school in the nation has some kind of sports program for its students. The programs differ based on the financial resources of the school district and on the stage regulations under which they typically operate. They are all, however, more similar than different. The program described here exists in suburban high school with an enrolment of 2200 students.

The school competes in thirteen varsity sports, both in a local league of suburban schools and in state competition. In major sports such as basketball, there are ninth-grade teams, reserve teams, and varsity teams, all for both boys and girls. In other sports, there are only reserve and varsity teams. In the spring, over 400 students compete on teams. The school has recently built a year-round weight-training facility. Next year, for the first time, the district will employ a full-time athletic trainer at the high school. Nearly every sport has a parent's or Booster club, which supplies extra funds for the program and acts as a communication link between coaches and parents. The school district has difficulty finding enough people to act as coaches, especially from the ranks of certified teachers in the district. Recently, that allows them to hire noncertified persons to coach if they cannot find certified teachers to fill the many vacancies.

Out-of-School Sports

Not all high-school students participate in the inter-school sports programs. And some of those who do not participate have an active sport involvement outside the school. Two examples are Andrea and William. Andrea owns her own horse and has trained and competed for years in equestrian sports. She boards her horse at a nearby stable and goes there nearly every day after school to train and care for her horse. She hopes some day to compete in equestrian Three Day Event competitions. Thus, she trains both in dressage and in jumping. Last summer and autumn, she competed in 15 separate events, most of them against boys and girls her own age, but sometimes in more open competition against adults. It is true that her sport involvement is quite expensive. Yet her training and competition are every bit as intense as are those of her school-mates who play on the school basketball or volley-ball teams. Many of her classmates do not even know that she is such an accomplished athlete. William has taken karate lessons for six years. He has slowly advanced in local karate competitions and is beginning to make a name for himself. He trains at a small karate studio that occupies a store-front in one of the area shopping malls. He has grown very strong and can make very quick movements. His room at home is filled with trophies that he has won in local competitions.

Like Andrea's, however, his athletic accomplishments are not known by many of his classmates. He, too, has never played on a school team.

The Young Adult

Young adult means women and men who have finished high school and have gone on to further education or have entered the work force. They are in a time of separation from youth and of establishment of patterns of work and play that will last a lifetime. There are so many that young adults participate in sports, fitness and physical education that they can only be sampled here.

The University Recreational Program

For the many thousands of undergraduate and graduate students of Ohio State University, an important part of campus life is spent in intramural and recreational facilities. More than 100 activities are offered each year, running the gamut from individual-oriented activities, such as weight lifting, to traditional team sports, such as soccer. League play in a variety of sport activities generates enormous enthusiasm, as do the more special events, such as the H-O-R-S-E tournament in which more than 300 men and women compete each year.

Billiards, bowling, rowing and ice hockey offer opportunity to learn and compete in activities not often available in high school. The two swimming pools seem to be busy every hour that the building is open. It is not uncommon to see more than 600 women and men taking part in the several scheduled aerobics sessions each day. The recreation and intramural-sports department also organizes sport clubs and sponsors special events for them. Last year, more than 40 such clubs were registered, with a total membership of over 6000 students. The Ski Club went on a winter trip. The Scuba Club arranged a large sprint outing. And the Biking Club has tours in the local area at least once per month. In the 1991-1992 academic year, nearly 56000 students, faculty and staff played over 13000 contests in 104 intramural activities on more than 4400 teams.

The level of "drop-in" activity in intramural facilities, such as the indoor running track, weight room, swimming pools, and the like, can only be estimated but the numbers are substantial. The estimate for participation in the conditioning rooms alone was over 489,000 for the school year. There are ten full-time professional staff members in the university recreation program, and more than 200 student assistants.

Each student in the university pays a $45 fee each term to support the program. Students, faculty and staff pay no direct user fees for any activity. The recreation facilities on this campus are the most widely used facilities of any in the university. Opportunities to learn, train, and compete are available to faculty, students and staff.

Community Recreation

Most towns and cities have recreation departments that organize learning and participation opportunities for citizens within their geographic boundaries. Although children and older adults often take part in these programs, it is the young adult who is the main consumer of community recreation services. Recreation opportunities are provided in different ways.

Classes are organized for people to learn new skills. Drop-in recreation is often provided—times when facilities are open and available for persons who want to get a fitness workout, to play a game of tennis, to swim laps, or to take part in a quickly organized, noon-hour volleyball game. Community-recreation departments try to provide a wide variety of activities, much in the same way as does a university program. Rather than describe the scope of such a program, as was done for the university program, in this section we shall describe in more detail the organization for one sport—softball. Softball is the most popular participation sport in America.

In one city recreation department in the summer of 1993, 223 softball leagues competed on 123 city-owned softball diamonds, involving 1750 teams with more than 34000 participants. There were men's slow-pitch leagues, women's slow-pitch leagues, church leagues, men's and women's fast-pitch leagues, and co-ed slow-pitch leagues. On any given spring or summer evening in this city, thousands of men and women compete in softball. The calibre of play from league to league varies tremendously, depending on the purpose for which people participate.

Some of the leagues are social, and everybody is out to have a good time. Other leagues are competitive, with fancy uniforms, skilled players, and an atmosphere more like a college or professional game. The city employs and trains umpires. The city maintenance department spends a great deal of time keeping the facilities in top shape. As in the university, the entire operation is administered by a professionally trained recreation staff.

Fitness Involvement

All across the land, fitness facilities of various kinds have sprung up in recent years. Some are franchised; they run television advertising campaigns and display familiar logos on their facilities. Others are more local, often occupying storefronts in shopping areas. Some offer a range of fitness activities, often including workouts using the latest in exercise equipment. Others focus more on group of activities, such as the many variations of aerobics. Still others focus more on strength development, with weight lifting as the primary activity. The young adults who constitute the main clientele for these establishments are concerned with how they look and what their levels of fitness are. This increased concern with fitness is an important phenomenon in current American life. As is true of sports participation, some people's fitness involvement is as much social as it is physical. Other people, however, undertake serious workouts. Like sport involvement, the various fitness facilities allow a range of participation modes and motivations.

Informal Participation

Although young adult's participation in organized sport and fitness is impressive, it pales compared to their levels of participation in informal activities. Accurate statistics on informal participation are difficult to obtain. The evidence that informal participation levels are high, however, is visible all around us. Increasingly, young adults are incorporating some aspect of sport and fitness in their lifestyle. They seek out opportunities to learn or improve their skill in activities, thus, they pursue a continuing physical education.

The Older Adult

One of the myths that pervaded physical education and sport as late as the 1940s was the athlete's heart. The myth was that vigorous exercise was inappropriate for young persons because of the potential damage to the heart. We now know, of course, that lack of exercise is more likely to be detrimental. Similar myths kept older adults from participating in many kinds of sport and fitness activities. What have traditionally been considered appropriate for older adults are nonvigorous sports such as golf or bowling. If older adults cycled or jogged, they tended to do so in leisurely fashion. The prejudices accompanying these traditional myths have been breaking down rapidly.

The Masters Athlete

In the late summer of 1989, more than 4900 athletes from 58 nations gathered in Eugene. Oregon, for the eighth World Veterans Track and Field Championships. Masters sport competition begins at age 40 years and proceeds in 5-year age divisions through age 95. The women and men competing at the World Championships represent the best of the hundreds of thousands of people who participate in Masters track and field worldwide. Although the competition is friendly, it is also extremely serious. Athletes in their fifties, sixties and seventies train diligently to perform at top levels. Many former Olympians from many nations have extended their athletic careers through the Masters movement. The performances of Masters athletes are extraordinary. Sprinters in the group aged 60 to 65 run below 12.5 for the 100 meters.

Male long jumpers in the ground aged 50 to 55 regularly jump farther than 20 feet. Women in the group aged 45 to 50 run below 26.5 for 200 meters. Women in the group aged 55 to 66 run below 19:00 for 5,000 meters. The Masters track and field movement is perhaps the largest of similar movements in many different sports. It is no longer uncommon to find vigorous competition among groups of older adults in swimming, volleyball, and basketball. What has changed most dramatically is our conception of what is possible for the older adult. Vigorous training and serious competition are not for youth and young adults only.

Fitness Forever

People now live longer than ever before. We are more knowledgeable about the contributions that fitness makes to the quality of life and, perhaps, even to the length of life. Although many fitness centres are populated primarily by young adults, it is no longer uncommon to see senior citizens taking part. Some seniors prefer low-impact exercise in the form of aerobics, walking, cycling, or jogging. Others work out in much the same ways as do young adults, using Nautilus machines, running of serious cycling. Senior-citizen centres now often offer fitness facilities to their clients. The men and women who now constitute our senior generation grew up in a culture that did not promote fitness in the same ways as our current era does.

Women particularly tended to be socialized away from vigorous activity and were exposed to the prejudice that it was not feminine to exercise or to compete vigorously. The detrimental effects of tobacco smoking and of eating a poor diet were less well known. Thus, the current senior generation is actually learning to be more active. The generations that follow them who grew up in the current climate of knowledge about and support for sport and fitness as lifetime endeavours are likely to alter further our perceptions of what is possible for the senior citizen.

The New Settings for Sport, Fitness and Physical Education

Traditionally, sport, fitness and physical education have been restricted primarily to children, youth and young adults. Facilities, therefore, have most often been those associated with schools, communities, and family-oriented organizations, such as the Young Men's Christian Association. These agencies still provide such facilities and are expanding their programs. There is, however, a host of facilities more widely available to more people than ever before. Many of these sport and fitness facilities are in the private sector, with users paying direct fees for the opportunity to use them.

Multipurpose Athletic Clubs

Historically, the term athletic club has referred to a social club for wealthy men in a big city, but these facilities have changed. The modern multipurpose athletic club is one of the most important examples of the shift toward life-span sport, fitness and physical education. The new athletic club attracts singles, married couples, and families. The facilities include indoor and outdoor swimming pools, racquetball courts, several exercise rooms, a sportswear shop, a snack bar, and locker rooms that include a steam room, sauna and jacuzzi. At any time during the day, the facilities bustle with activity. At peak hours—from 5 to 8 in the evening for example—virtually every piece of equipment and every inch of space is utilized. The multipurpose athlete club provides more than just facilities.

Racquetball leagues are formed. Aerobic classes take place several times daily. Swim and jogging clubs meet regularly. Special competitions are organized, as are classes to help people learn and improve skills. In the exercise areas, individuals can track their progress on computer-based records and can receive guidance from a staff member on what exercises to do and how to use the exercise machines appropriately. A supervised nursery cares for young children while mothers and fathers work out. The typical price range from a family membership for 1 year is $400 to $850.

Classes and racquet-ball-court time are changed on a peruse basis. The private, multipurpose athletic club is a modern version of what for years has been offered in family YMCAs. The YMCA has also updated its operations and now offers a similar range of instructional participatory opportunities.

Sport Clubs

Private-sector sport clubs are now regular features of any metropolitan area. Tennis may account for the largest number, but there are many different types of clubs, ranging from foci on skating to trap-shooting to racquetball. Typical is the Olympic Tennis Club, where 2,500 tennis players of all ages play each week, primarily outdoors in the summer and indoors in the winter. Sport clubs offer three primary services: instruction, organized competitions and social play.

At the Olympic Tennis Club, 350 adults take lessons each week. Lessons might range from a 30-minute private lesson for $24 per lesson to a 1½-hour group lesson costing $13.50 per lesson. Beginner lessons are typically given in groups of six, last for 1 hour, and cost $8 per lesson. Competitions are organized in several ways, but primarily on the basis of skill level, that is, beginners, intermediates and advanced. Leagues are formed so that players can participate regularly for an extended period of time. Social play and practice requires only that members sign up for court time. The cost of court time depends on the hour of the day and day of the week, with popular times more costly than off times.

Many members have regular court-time reservations and often play with the same person each week, thus emphasizing the social element often associated with adult involvement in sport. Sport clubs often have attractive lounges, weight-training facilities, and child-care services available, as well as some kind of food service. The falsities are typically bright, clean and attractive. The service at sport clubs is typically quick, courteous and friendly. Amenities such as these keep customers returning.

Specialized Sport/Fitness Centres

While multipurpose centres have grown in importance, so too have the specialized sport and fitness centres. These centres are differentiated from the public type of facility, such as a golf course or bowling alley, where participation is defined mostly by a pay-per-use arrangement. More recently, sport/fitness centres have developed that are defined by a monthly or yearly membership, and participation is restricted to members. Typical of these are swimming clubs, racquetball clubs, indoor tennis clubs, weightlifting and body-building clubs, aerobics centres, and gymnastic centres. Activities are often organized by these specialized centres.

Lessons and classes are available, as are regular competitions, such as tennis leagues or water-polo tournaments. The membership feature of these centres tends to produce a social network in which friendships develop and are sustained around the common activity interests of the members.

Sport-Medicine Centres

People who participate in sport and fitness activities

often need health-care treatment and rehabilitation—sometimes to remediate problems and sometimes to prevent problems from developing. Unheard of 20 years ago, specialized sport-medicine facilities and programs are now common in metropolitan areas. A sport-medicine program serves varied clientele. It might provide care for high-school athletic programs, serve adults who have sport-related injuries, implement sport/fitness education programs, or treat children both in remedial and preventive modes. The staff of sport-medicine organizations might include orthopedic surgeons, family-practice physicians, paediatricians, nutritionists, physical therapists, X-ray technicians, athletic trainers, and even sport psychologists. Initially, sport-medicine programs were attached to hospitals or were operated out of a regular group medical practice as an additional service to clients. As their popularity has grown, however, they have tended to become separate facilities, specialized to serve clients of all ages.

Home Gymnasiums

As sport, fitness and physical education grown in lifespan importance, adults find ways to accommodate these interests within the home or, by extension, in public facilities available within their immediate area. Ellis has noted that the do-it-yourself approach that has traditionally characterized some leisure activities, such as gardening, is spreading quickly to sport, fitness and physical education. Just as we are seeing increased use of private-sector sport and fitness facilities, people also are developing informal sport and fitness opportunities within their homes and immediate neighbourhoods.

Many new houses include small areas for exercise equipment. Many more basements and family rooms have been converted to accommodate exercise bicycles, rowing machines and weightlifting setups. While many people are paying to gain access to sport, fitness and physical education opportunities in private facilities, others are developing the capability to produce these opportunities themselves, often at home.

Worksite Programs

Increasingly, employers are converting older facilities into space for recreation and fitness programs. Newly constructed buildings often include specially designed fitness and recreation centres. Corporations have found that a healthy and physically active work force is a more productive and less expensive work force. The costs of employee health care can be reduced substantially by an effective fitness program. Employees who have the opportunity to use company fitness and recreation facilities at times convenient to their workday tend to be not only more productive but also more loyal to the company. Tenneco Inc. is one of the larges companies in America. If you are fortunate enough to be an employee at their corporate headquarters, you could take part in Tenneco's Health and Fitness Program, housed in a 25000 square foot portion of the Tenneco Employee Centre. The Centre houses fitness equipment, exercise bicycles, racquetball court, and a large space for four-lane walking-jogging track encircling the building. A computer based information system stores records for each individual in the program and provides employees and management with information. A staff of eight fitness professionals supervise the program and, along with a nursing staff, a cardiologist and nutritional consultants, provide educational and prescriptive information for employee fitness programs.

Although improved fitness is the primary goal of the program—and is important from the corporation's point of view—racquetball, volleyball, and softball leagues are also organized, and participation is high. The Centre is open from 6 A.M. to 7 P.M. each workday. Employees can make regular activity part of their workday; in so doing, they can make fitness a part of their lifestyle. Tenneco employees express greatest interest in weight control and stress relief. Nearly 70 per cent of the more than 2,500 employees are involved in weight lifting, 51 per cent in jogging and 48 per cent in regular exercise classes, all representing participation rates that are much higher than is typical for corporate fitness programs. There is now considerable agreement among authorities in the fitness field that fit employees are happier and more productive, are absent from work less often, and cost less in health-related medical expenses.

Sport/Games Festivals

One phenomenon that illustrates the theme of lifespan involvement is the recent development of state sport festivals, including participation from youth through senior citizens in a variety of sports. The first such event, New York's Empire State Games, attracted 5,000 participants in 1978. By the summer of 1992, the movement had swept across the nation with 40 state sport festivals attracting more than 500,000 athletes of all ages. In Montana, a state with only 800,000 residents, more than 10,000 competed in the finals of the Big Sky State Games. State sport festivals typically include a wide variety of sports in which a number of age divisions compete. In the Empire State Games, there is competition in 28 sports, with festive opening and closing ceremonies. Athletes of all ages and skill levels come together to participate and to celebrate their involvement.

The Emerging Characteristics of Lifespan Involvement

Lifespan involvement in sport, fitness and physical education is an emerging phenomenon, How it will continue to develop and mature is difficult to predict, but we can identify certain characteristics from its early, developmental stages:

1. The importance of an early start. It seems increasingly clear that habits of participation begin early in childhood. It is also clear that a foundation of motor skill development, established in early childhood, can be used throughout the lifespan. On the other hand, basic skills are increasingly difficult to learn with age. Also, many fitness problems may have a paediatric origin; that is, unfit children tend to grow up to become unfit adults.

We should expect that programs will soon develop that aim at producing super-baby and make many exaggerated claims. Some of these programs will, no doubt, do more harm than good. Nonetheless, the increasing recognition of the importance of infant and early-childhood physical education comes at precisely the time when day care and early-childhood education are becoming important social and political issues; there will be an opportunity to make important gains.

2. Breakdown of gender stereotypes. We may finally be approaching an era when girls and women will have opportunities for lifespan sport, fitness and physical education similar to those men enjoy. Being fit is not a gender-specific phenomenon. Being an athlete does not require being male. Physical education can no longer afford to stereotype activities or roles based on gender rather than skill or interest. We hope that future generations of girls will be socialized into sport, fitness and physical education in ways different from their mother's and grandmother's experiences.

3. Breakdown of age stereotypes. People now live longer than ever before. They also spend a significant portion of their lives in retirement, when time is more readily available for leisure activity. Clearly, the health problems related to aging represent a major national issue, if only because of the enormous costs of health-maintenance programs. The traditional stereotype of appropriate activity involvement for older person's was, "Do not do it too much and do not do it too vigorously".

Although scientists have known for some time that this stereotype is inappropriate, it has been the many role models provided by active senior citizens that have begun to break down the stereotype. When you see older people who are really fit and are involved in regular activity, you can no longer delude yourself into thinking that their activities are inappropriate. More important, when older people see their peers involved in activity and maintaining a high level of fitness, they too begin to see different opportunities for themselves.

4. Shift in emphasis from youth to adults. The median age of our population increases with each passing decade—America is getting greyer. The median age is now over 30 years, will reach 35 in the next decade, and will above 40 by the year 2020. Sport, fitness and physical education have traditionally been viewed primarily as programs for children and youth. It is quite clear now that they are undergoing an important transformation, becoming industries that primarily serve adults rather than just children and youths. This transformation will require new programs, new facilities, a newly trained group of professionals, and an entirely new outlook in terms of program goal and of the processes through which those goals can be achieved.

5. Shift to the private sector. Historically, opportunities for sport, fitness and physical education have been most widely available in the public sector; in schools, community recreation, and in public facilities such as parks. In the past several decades, we have witnessed the emergence of an enormous private-sector industry dealing with sport opportunities, fitness and physical education. The emergence of this new industry has brought bright new prospects for participation; it has also exemplified certain problems, such as the increasingly strong relationship between wealth and opportunity in sport, fitness and physical education. There is no doubt, however, that sport, fitness and physical education now represent major industries in America. And, like most other industries, these are market-oriented, catering to the interests and desires of the consumer and trying to influence those interests and desires through creative advertising.

6. Increasingly strong scientific base. Within the past 25 years, a science of sport, fitness and physical education has emerged. Our health and fitness practices are coming to be informed by reliable scientific evidence, rather than being influenced by accumulated experience and myth. Many consumers of sport, fitness and physical education services are highly educated. As they become more

knowledgeable, they will demand that practices represent the best of what is known. Their concerns range from appropriate and inappropriate exercise strategies to questions about what might be the best kind of program for a young child.

7. More information, more readily available. Spend some time at a bookstore or video store in your local shopping mall. Pursue the books and videos within the sport, fitness and physical education areas. The first thing that will impress you is the sheer number of them, particularly the how to books and videos—how to play better golf, how to learn to scuba dive, how to stay fit, how to build a weightlifting program, how to help you child become more skilled or fit in a sport.

Not all of these books and videos would stand up to the increased scientific knowledge now available. Some present strategies and practices that are quite simply false by any scientific standard. The information is there, however, form people who want to avail themselves of it, and the number of books, magazines and videos indicates that many people do want to.

8. The new professionals. Many of the occupational roles described in this text represent fairly recent developments in professional life. For some time now, there have been professional opportunities to become a physical education teacher, a health educator, or a community recreation specialist. Now, however, there are many more and different professional opportunities available—in sport management, adult fitness, cardiac rehabilitation, athletic training, early-childhood motor development, worksite health education, and sport/fitness marketing. Each of these new professions requires somewhat different preparation. Some now require certification. As lifespan sport, fitness and physical education become more of a reality in our culture, professional opportunities should continue to grow. A real issue emerging is the degree to which preparation should be specialized or generalized.

Limitations

As the possibility for lifespan involvement emerges, it will not do so evenly for all people. There is no doubt that socioeconomic status and race are limiting factors in the current sport and fitness scene. Persons from low socioeconomic groups have little information about the benefits of physical activity and even less opportunity to engage regularly in beneficial activity. Currently in the United States low socioeconomic groups are also more likely to be blacks or Hispanic. As the possibility, and desirability of lifespan involvement has emerged, it has done so primarily as a matter of individual responsibility. Most of our people are unfit or inactive, it is most often considered an individual problem. Although the notion of individual responsibility is important, it is just as important to recognize the structural or collective responsibility we all have to make lifespan involvement more likely and available regardless of race or socioeconomic status. To accomplish this structural goal, we have to make sure that more and better information and education is available and that facilities and programs are accessible and affordable for these portions of our population.

A Framework for Understanding the Possibilities for Professional Service

A major purpose of this text is to provide you a framework within which you can understand the prospects, problems and possibilities for professional service in sport, fitness and physical education. The choice of a professional role should be informed not only by the immediate framework for that professional role but also by the larger history from which the role has emerged and the alternative possibilities derived from that history. Within this text, sport, fitness and physical education sometimes are treated separately and sometimes are integrated. This presentation reflects the reality of professional life today. Clearly, professionals in sport are concerned with fitness and physical education Just as clearly physical educators teach sport and fitness. The separation of these areas is, therefore, somewhat artificial and arbitrary.

On the other hand, preparation for these professional roles is typically specialized in today's colleges and universities. If you major in adult fitness, you will receive a curriculum substantially different from that offered to students preparing to become physical education teachers, the curriculum leading to a degree in sport management is different again. Thus, the seeming ambiguity that results from treating these areas separately in some instances and together on other occasions simply reflects the ambiguity of professional life in these disciplines today. The consumer of sport, fitness and physical education activities will not recognize the differences that form the structure of this text.

The woman or man who goes to a local fitness club or recreation centre for an aerobics class or a volleyball match typically does not know or care about the distinctions between sport, fitness and physical education that form the structure of this text. For the average consumer, the field of health, recreation, sport, fitness and physical education are all the same. For the persons studying these fields, however, it is important to understand the differences that do exist and the history from which these differences have emerged.

So, in last it can be concluded that:

1. Recognition of the possibility and desirability of lifespan involvement in sport, fitness and physical education represents a fundamental change in our perception of human life.

2. Sport and fitness are in boom eras, whereas school physical education has perplexing problems but bright prospects.

3. There have been four watershed eras in American history for the sport, fitness and physical education professions—those of muscular Christianity, the emergence of organized sport, the emergence of professions, and the academic study of sport, fitness and physical

education.

4. The era of lifespan sport, fitness and physical education represents another wathershed period—one not limited by age or gender.

5. Physical activity in the early years represents a new and exciting field for the sport, fitness and physical education professions.

6. Sport, fitness and physical education for children occur in both the public and private sectors; each has its own problems and prospects.

7. Activity programs for youths are extensive, with opportunities within and outside schools.

8. The young adult finds many outlets for activity in community programs and in the growing private-sector activity and fitness industry.

9. Adults increasingly have activity programs available at their worksite, and the adult fitness and sport industry has become big business. The Masters sports movement has shown that older persons can stay active as competitive athletes throughout their lives.

10. The new setting for sport, fitness and physical education include multipurpose athletic clubs, sport clubs, specialized sport/fitness centres, sport-medicine centres, home gymnasiums, worksite programs and sport/games festivals.

11. The emerging characteristics of lifespan involvement include the recognition of the importance of an early start, the breakdown of gender and age stereotypes, the shift in emphasis from youth to adults, the shift from the public to the private sector, the increasingly strong scientific base, the increased availability of information, and the creation of new professional roles.

12. Although the consumers of sport, fitness and physical education typically does not recognize the specialized nature of each field, professional specialization is typical of career preparation.

5

UNDERSTANDING SKELETAL MUSCLE AND PROPERTIES

It has been argued that the single most important topic in the field of exercise physiology is the muscular system. While it is indeed true that muscles will fail to function normally if innervation is withheld or if the circulation is impaired, the fact remains that the total organism is put into motion and remains there because of the action of skeletal muscles. In a very real sense, then, it is essential that the structure and function of muscles be understood in some detail, so that an adequate explanation may be available concerning practical matters of exercise and training.

Structure of Muscle

The student of kinesiology will immediately recognize the human skeletal muscles are arranged in a variety of configurations, depending upon the function for which they are intended. It is common to think of muscle as being composed of fibres that seem to run directly from tendon to tendon, such as in the biceps broccoli, but in reality a large number of muscles in the human body are small, with their fibres arranged in a variety of ways. In one example, the longitudinal type, the fibres run approximately parallel to the long axis of the muscle, although they may not reach the entire distance covered by the muscle.

In the longissimus muscle, for instance, the fibres need not be very long, running from the spinous processes of vertebrae to the transverse process and lateral surfaces of the ribs, a distance of only a few inches. In the unipennate form, the fibres approach the tendon from only one side, as occurs with the tibialis posterior muscle, while the bipennate muscle has fibres converging on both sides of the tendon, as illustrated by the rectus femoris muscle. An example of the multipennate muscle is shown by the deltoid, where internal collagenous sheets divide the muscle into three parts, thus providing a mixture of the first two pinnate forms. The advantage gained by these variations is easily seen, as there is provided a means for initiating movement, particularly for joints that may be involved with large masses, such as the trunk where the surface area is large, or in other specialized areas of the body where range of motion may not be great.

One can compare the function of the trapezes with that of the biceps to realize the great differences in joint function that are served. The fact that the fibres in penniform muscles shorten less than longitudinal muscles probably only attests to the types of functions they are intended to serve. The contractile portion of the muscle gradually gives way to connective tissue, which is continuous with the tendons of origin and insertion, and forms a rigid adherence to bone so that it may bear the full tension of contraction. As the structure of the tendon interweaves with the muscle, the collagenous threads form a network that binds the muscle itself together with interfering either with contraction or the fibre arrangement.

Fibre Characteristics

In order to understand the complexities of total muscle contraction, it is first necessary to understand the detailed characteristics of the muscle fibre. Since the thrust of exercise physiology necessarily implies external work and usually movement, the discussion will be restricted to skeletal muscle. Skeletal muscles are composed of rather large numbers of fibres, amounting in large muscles to many thousands. In fact, individual fibre count of an older adult engaged in a lifetime of hard work revealed that the biceps contained over 316,000 fibres, arranged in more than 3,300 fascicles. This would leave nearly 100 fibres to each fasciculus for that muscle. The fibres themselves range in size from 10 to 100 microns in diameters, and are surrounded by the sarcolemma, the muscle cell membrane found just beneath the endomysium. It is not the individual fibre per se that is crucial to understanding of the contraction characteristics of muscle so much as it is the constituency of the fibre. An individual muscle can be further subdivided into the following parts: (a) The fibres (b) have the striated appearance that characterizes skeletal muscle, and a single fibre (c) is composed of a number of myofibrils. The myofibril (d) can be further resolved into a series of repeating light and dark patterns known as sarcomeres (e). The sarcomere reveals that it consists of protein microfilaments, the thin filaments of actin and the thick filaments of myosin (f).

A great deal is known about the various mechanical properties of muscle, as they have been favourite topics of physiologists for decades. Some of the characteristics to be described are so classic in nature that they have become suitable subjects for laboratory experiments in undergraduate physiology courses. These experiments are ordinarily conducted on isolated vertebrate muscle, such as that of the frog. Considerable progress has been made in learning about muscle tissue, but the crucial tests for human physiology will come when more complete information is available on muscle characteristics in vivo—that is, in the intact organism, not only with normal blood and nerve supply but with the muscle or group of muscles exerting tension through the usual muscle-tendon-joint complex.

Length-Tension Curves

The amount of tension that a muscle can obtain depends upon its initial length, the maximum tension generated is not at resting length but when the muscle is slightly stretched beyond equilibrium length. A muscle that is foreshortened is at some disadvantage, as the amount of active tension produced becomes reduced. Even lengthening has its own built-in limitations, for excessive stretching can result in a decrement of active force. Considering the position of the actin and myosin filaments, one can understand how extreme stretching can place actin just out of reach of the myosin cross-bridges. The lower curve describes the tension produced when a resting muscle fibre is lenghtened. Changing the joint angle effectively alters the muscle length, and for this particular test it reveals that 115 degree is the most effective angle for obtaining maximal tests of strength. Force drops off on either side of this value.

Force-Velocity Curve

The muscle has been examined for speed of shortening after being loaded. The relationship is curvilinear and has been found to be mathematically predictable. When there is no load on the muscle, maximum velocity occurs. It also reveals that under essentially isometric conditions, where the velocity is zero, the force becomes maximal. It is difficult to load intact human muscles in quite the same way as the frog sartorious muscle, although the force-time curves of hand-gripping muscles have been examined when the muscles have adopted a preliminary tension varying from zero to 30 kg. There is a curvilinear nature to the curves, also, the best force being obtained when the performer begins with very little or no preliminary tension. If he adopts some force to begin with, the velocity of contraction noticeably slows, and there is likely to be some reduction in the amount of maximum tension achieved.

Elasticity

For muscle to exert tension it must activate its contractile components. What may not be apparent is that the effective force generated is dampened by viscoelastic properties of the muscle and tendon. These elements must first be overcome during the uptake of force. The result of their activity is a reduction in the force measured externally, as compared with actual forces created by the contractile elements themselves. These elastic components are arranged both in series and in parallel and represent the portions of the muscle that do not contract. The series elastic component is so named because the elastic elements occur directly in line with the contractile components; it is thought that these elastic elements are located in the tendons into which the muscle fibres are inserted, and are probably present at the Z-line region of the sarcomere. The parallel elastic component does not lie in series with the contractile mechanism, but in parallel, located specifically in the sarcolemma.

The contraction of the muscle imparts a given force, but this can be increased, if, at the time of stimulation, the muscle is first given a quick stretch so as to pull out the elastic elements. The increase in measured tension, results from the elimination of the elastic elements. These elements smooth out changes in tension, lessening to some degree the sudden force invoked by the act of contraction.

Reaction Latency

A term often employed in physical education and athletics in reaction latency, or reaction time. The latent period is the time elapsing between the onset of the stimulus and the initiation of response by the contractile mechanism. It represents the duration of the nerve impulse. The reaction time, on the other hand, may include other factors that makes its duration somewhat longer than pure latency. The typical method of measuring reaction time is to present eh subject with a stimulus, either auditory or visual, which starts a timer As soon as the subject is able, he initiates some movement, which immediately stops the timer. The elapsed interval is reaction time. If the mass to be moved is large, the RT is longer than if the mass is small. Thus, finger RT is shorter than leg RT, because included in the measurement is time for the muscle contraction to move the mass of the limb involved.

Since more motor units must be activated to move the heavier leg than the lighter finger, there will be a slight delay while this is being accomplished. This has led to use of the concept of promoter and motor reaction time, in which we separate RT into two components, employing an electromyograph to detect the instant that depolarization of the muscle cell membrane occurs. The premotor time is the time that elapses from the onset of the signal to initiation of the muscle action potential, and motor time is the time remaining for the actual response to be initiated. It should also be pointed out that the onset of the signal is usually external, a sound or light stimulus, so some portion of the response time must be taken up with signal detection, to be followed by descending motor patterns to the appropriate body parts.

Having the performer make a choice usually lengthens RT appreciably while he sorts out extraneous stimuli and decides upon the correct ones. Reaction time may be subject to some learning over a series of trials, the amount of this learning being greater if the individual must make a choice between alternatives in his response. The actual act of moving the body or its limbs is not a part of reaction time, since, this is usually referred to as movement time. The time consulted by a ball carrier to the line of scrimmage is preceded by his reaction time; the time it takes for the action to be completed once it has been initiated is movement time. It may seem surprising, but a number of experiments indicate a low correlation between reaction time and movement time. In other words, an individual who has a fast reaction time does not necessarily have a fast movement time.

Summation of Contraction

Strength of contraction can be increased in two different ways. Since the motor unit is the basic contractile entity, consisting of the motor nerve and all of the muscle fibres that it innervates, then it follows, first of all, that the force generated can be increased by bringing more motor units into play. However, a second factor involves the rate at which individual motor units are contracting. If a muscle stimulus is followed by a second one before the first is over, the total tension produced is increased. Thus, increasing the rate of firing up to 60 per second successively increases the maximum tension, and is an example of wave summation. However, at a firing rate of approximately 60 per second, the successive contractions fuse together—a state of tetanus; further increases in rate lead only to slight increases in maximal tension. The individual motor units that become active contract rhythmically, but it turns out that they are out of phase with each other and so contract asynchronously. This serves a useful purpose by making the overall contraction appear to be smooth, even during weak contractions.

Staircase Phenomenon (TREPPE)

When a series of maximal stimuli are delivered to a muscle below a frequency that would cause tetanus, an increase in the tension during successive stimuli occurs, resulting eventually in a uniform tension. This is known as the staircase phenomenon, or treppe, from the German word for staircase. Undoubtedly, some sort of activation facilitation within the sarcomere allows the actin and myosin filaments to interdigitate more effectively.

Site of Muscular Fatigue

Repeated muscular exertion will soon lead to a fatigued state, greatly reducing the ability of the muscle to contract. There seem to be three potential sites where the focus of the fatigue process comes together: (i) the synapses of the central nervous system, (ii) the neuromuscular junction, or (iii) the muscle itself. It is difficult to imagine how the central nervous mechanisms could actually become fatigued during voluntary effort, although the following type of experiment would seem to indicate otherwise: voluntarily fatigue a muscle by a series of maximal contractions and then stimulate it directly by electrical means. It will be observed that the muscle seems to respond with renewed strength.

Merton, however, indicated that perhaps in humans some fibres are not under control of voluntary effort, and demonstrated that a muscle does not contract by electrical stimulation after it has fatigued by voluntary effort. Employing the adductor pollicis muscle of the hand, he compared voluntary strength with maximal tetani and found them equal. As strength declined during the exercise bout, electrical stimulation of the motor nerve did not restore the tension, thus suggesting that the site of fatigue was peripheral—that is, in the muscle itself. Further support was given this position by the finding that muscle action potentials evoked by nerve stimulation were not significantly reduced even in extreme fatigue, meaning that the wave of depolarization was successfully crossing the neuromuscular junction. Moreover, recovery from fatigue did not take place if circulation to the muscle was occluded.

Asmussen has stressed that local muscular fatigue involves the many chemical reactions, both aerobic and anaerobic, that are responsible for delivering energy to the contractile mechanisms of the myofibrils.

Form of the Uptake and Release of Force

There have been very few efforts to study the characteristics of muscle contraction in the human with normal innervation and all other mechanical factors which produce maximal effort intact. The question involves how fast a maximal contraction can be made and what is the shape of the contraction curve. The force reaches half its maximum in approximately 0.8 sec, and three-fourths its maximum in .15 sec. By .4 sec the contraction is essentially compete. This compares with the mechanical responses of mammalian skeletal muscle fibre to a single maximal stimulus of .04 sec for the gastrocnemius and .1 sec for the soleus. The release of tension, on the other hand, is much more rapid. Half the drop occurs in only .04 sec, and by approximately .15 sec resting tension has been achieved once again.

Thus, release can take place some four times faster than contraction. As might be expected, the ability to exert force is affected by such things as prior activity and temperature. It is not surprising to find that immersion in cold water will reduce tension and markedly slow the rate of contraction, since this is a common experience encountered in cold weather. Its effect is to cut the speed of contraction approximately in half. A passive warm-up effect is less pronounced; that is, immersing the muscles in hot water does not lead to a very large change in contraction speed or strength. The release phase is lengthened by cold, but not by heat.

Muscular Fatigue

Since the turn of the century, there has been great interest in problems of muscular fatigue, and several experimental approaches have been tried. A complete understanding, however, has not been achieved. Such things as type of exercise and rate of work are crucial concepts. For example, is the exercise performed to be isometric, with no change in joint angle, or isotonic, employing a full range of motion? If the latter, is the resistance to be lifted a fixed amount, or some percentage of the person's maximum strength? Will he perform contractions according to some prescribed rhythm? If so, how much? If isometric, what is the criterion of fatigue? The topic is of practical significance to the teacher or coach, who should know something about the manner in which strength declines as a result of repeated effort. After a bout of exercise, the resulting decrement must be paid back in the recovery period. This is payment of the strength debt, analogous to the oxygen debt that involves the oxidative processes of recovery from exercise.

The strength debt, or recovery, from fatiguing work has not received the same attention as the exercise phase itself, even though a number of practical problems in dealing with training and adjustment to optimal working conditions are involved. In a study by H.H. Clarke et al., subjects isotonically exercised the elbow flexor muscles until fatigue occurred when lifting a load equal to three-eighths of their strength. The recovery curve showed an initial rise during the first two minutes, followed by a slower gain for the next ten, so that recovery was still not complete for most subjects two hours after the cessation of exercise.

Lind found fast and slow components in the ability of subjects to perform additional static contractions following fatigue. The process of recovery from isometric and isotonic exercise is difficult to compare, since the two exercise forms can easily result in quite different levels of fatigue. However, this can be controlled, so that the pa-off of the strength debt can begin at about the same value.

Residual Muscular Soreness

One of the handicaps associated with the resumption of exercise after an extended layoff is the usual experience of soreness in the exercised muscles. It ordinarily appears anywhere from 8 to 24 hours after activity and can be rather debilitating. This residual muscular soreness should be differentiated from the local discomfort that may be experienced during exercise. Residual soreness may last for several days, depending upon the degree to exercise and the type of activity engaged in, and there is the assumption that no acute injury has occurred, since this would be reflected in immediate symptomatology. The causative factors are now known, although minute tears in the muscle and connective tissue have been implicated, as well as an increase in extra or intercellular fluid, and the existence of tonic muscle spasms. Apparently not just any form of exercise leads to the same degree of residual soreness. Talag found the acentric phase of exercise to produce the most pain.

Muscular Training

A great deal may be said about the many aspects of training for muscular strength and endurance, but there are limitations in a text of this scope. Therefore, we shall briefly consider the training techniques and then the physiological effects of training. The individual will select his exercises from a system involving either isotonic or isometric forms. Isotonic exercises involve raising and lowering a load, whereas isometric require a static contraction to be held against a resistance. A number of factors can still be considered. For example, the isotonic exercises, usually known as progressive resistance exercises, are generally given in sets, or groups of repetitions, based on some criterion ranging from 6 to 15 repetitions maximum. Since no really definitive standards have been established, a great deal of individual preference apparently exist, based on customs and convenience.

There is reason to believe, though, that an optimal combination may be to train at 6 RM for three sets, three times a week. Isometric exercise, popularized as an effective strength-improving procedure, has not proved as effective as at first supposed. The reader will find references to the early 1950's which seemed to indicate that strength gains as much as 5 per cent per week could be expected when isometric tractions of two-thirds maximum were held for 6 sec per day. Confirmation of these findings has not been forthcoming, and it seems much more realistic to expect up to a 2 per cent gain per week with these exercises, and the duration of contraction lasts at least 5 sec.

When two forms of exercise have been compared, it is difficult to draw clear conclusions, particularly since it has been so difficult to equate the amount of effort involved. It may be a safe presumption that the isometric exercises are particularly helpful for individuals who are beginning training and have a long way to go to become conditioned, and also for those who have a limitation in range of motion. However, even in the former case it may be desirable to engage in typical resistance exercise of an isotonic nature, since the results seem to be clearly successful in increasing muscular strength and hypertrophy. Still another form of exercise that has been inaugurated in recent years is what has come to be known as isokinetic exercise, or accommodating resistance exercise. It resembles the isotonic contraction, in that the joint moves through its range of motion, but the device that is used holds the speed of movement constant. Thus, the desired rate of limb motion may be preset, causing any effort to encounter an equal opposing force.

An increase in exertion fails to increase the acceleration, but merely raises the resistance throughout the movement. This means that there is a high force applied at all times during the exercise. Typical weight lifting is subject to great fluctuations during the range of motion as the mechanical advantage changes. This means that the effort is often difficult at certain angles, and is relatively easy at others. The isokinetic exercise tends to equalize this factor. We might raise the question of whether this form of exercise makes any difference in training. Thistle and colleagues compared isokinetic training with isotonic and isometric procedures, and after eight weeks found that the isokinetic group gained approximately 35 per cent in quadriceps, strength, as compared with increments of 27.5 per cent for the isotonic group and 9.2 per cent for the isometric group. A control group decreased 9.4 per cent over the same interval.

A similar experiment was performed by Moffroid and co-workers utilizing quadriceps and hamstring muscles. Significant increases in isometric strength of the quadriceps occurred at the end of the fourth weeks in subjects who trained with isokinetic, isometric and isotonic procedures, although the latter group failed to show a change when tested at a knee joint angle of 90 degrees. When the hamstring muscles were tested at this angle, only the isometric group gained significantly in isometric strength, although at 45 degrees both the isokinetic and isometric groups were significantly improved. When an isokinetic test was employed at the end of the training period, no improvement was noted for the quadriceps muscles, but the isokinetic group was significantly better than the other groups when the hamstrings were tested. Thus, it seems reasonable to conclude that isokinetic exercise provides a training stimulus that is comparable to or even better than isotonic exercise.

Strength vs. Endurance

It is often very confusing to the student to differentiate between strength and endurance, since they are often used interchangeably. Yet the differences should be pointed out. For example, a test of maximum effort against a dynamometer or tensiometer can be considered a test of strength, since it seeks to learn the outcome of a maximal voluntary innervation and subsequent contraction of the available motor units. It can be argued that employing a series of repetitions gradually introduces muscular endurance.

The maximum number of sit-ups or push-ups, for example, are tests of muscular endurance. No doubt each is important in its own way, but remember that different physiological events accompany the two forms. The endurance event must be supported by the circulation; the energy requirements will be very different than those for the single-effort test of strength. It is typical to develop strength by deemphasizing endurance—that is, by employing a weight training regimen involving a high resistance but few repetitions. Endurance may be more satisfactorily developed in the opposite way: keep the resistance low and increase the number of repetitions. While this may be a satisfactory generalization to begin with, it may be inadequate when we examine their relative influence in delaying fatigue.

Maximum Strength

It is interesting to contemplate the actual amount of tension that can be developed within a muscle during its contraction. Since the usual tests are administered by attaching straps to limbs and connecting them to some measuring device, they becomes estimates of external force, and not true measures at all. They are instead subject of the reduction associated with the mechanical application of resistance and force arms of a particular joint and muscle arrangement. A standardized system for strength testing of individual muscle groups is available however, and the reader may wish to consult these procedures before beginning an exercise program. Though the true measure of muscle force is difficult to calculate, several attempts have been made.

Such findings are generally expressed in kilograms per square centimetre, of cross section of muscle, and Ralston and his associates point out the wide variability that exists from one muscle to another. In the cat quadriceps it may average 1.23 kg/cm^2, and in the cat gastrocnemius some 6.36 kg/cm^2 Their own data on human imputes with surgically prepared muscles was 1.63 kg/cm^2 for pectoralis, 2.38 kg/cm^2 for biceps, and 1.31 kg/cm^2 for triceps. It may be useful to conclude that the maximum tension varies from 1.5 to 2.5 kg/cm^2 in vertebrate, nonhuman muscles, and perhaps slightly higher in the normal human. If one assumes a value of 3 kg/cm^2, and assuming that large muscles of the thigh may have 100 cm^2 of cross section, the resulting internal force that could be developed would be 300 kg, or 660 lb. This is a large force, as one can readily appreciate.

Hypertrophy

Muscular hypertrophy, an increase in the number or the size of individual fibres, is normally attributed to the long-term effects of heavy-resistance exercise. The prevailing view is that there is no formation of new muscle fibres, even though some rather bizarre changes can sometimes occur when muscles are placed under unusual stress. Goss explains that grows in response to external demands. This functional unit is the smallest irreducible structure that can still carry out the basic physiological activities, and for the muscle this would refer to the myofibrils, or more specifically, the sarcomeres.

One of the prime questions, then, would be whether the myofibrillar portion of muscle increases as a result of training. Helander, employing guinea pigs, found a 15 per cent increase in the nitrogen component of the myofilament as a result of training, when compared with control muscles in animals now exercised. Other investigators have also shown increases in the myofibrillar portion, which can be interpreted as enhancing the contractile ability of muscle fibers. Penman worked with college students in a progressive-resistance program aimed at developing the quadriceps muscle. Muscle biopsies revealed increased myosin filament concentration, a reduction in the distance between myosin filaments, and fewer actin filaments in orbit around a myosin filament. In other words, there would seem to be an increase in the packing density of the interdigitating filaments within a cell, plus a changing ratio of actin to myosin. It is quite well established that eventually a change in the cross section of muscle will occur if heavy-resistance exercises are carried out systematically.

These alterations are reflections of ultrastructural changes, which have been observed only with the use of biochemical or histochemical analysis. However, in practical terms, the use of limb circumference has proven to be helpful for reflecting changes in hypertrophy. Provided that a tape measure is employed carefully, with exactly the same tension on each occasion, changes in hypertrophy can usually be expected from isotonic exercise. Such changes do not always accompany isometric training.

Resistance to Fatigue

Recently the concept has been challenged that strength training and endurance training always lead to different results. When a fixed weight is used, one that can be handled readily, it is obvious that trained muscle can perform more work for each unit of time than can untrained muscles. However, when strain-gauge ergography is employed, where the individual exerts maximum tension rather than lifts a weight, the picture is somewhat different. It apparently does not matter whether the training involves low resistance and high repetition or the opposite. Both forms of training lead to increases in absolute muscular endurance, but also they result in approximately the same strength gains.

In other words, the fatigue curves after training closely resemble those to speculation that the main result of both strength and endurance training is an increase in strength. Endurance changes may be secondary outgrowth.

Recovery

Training also improves the strength recovery rate after exhaustive exercise. In an experiment utilizing an ergograph loaded with weight equal to three-eighths of each subject's elbow flexor strength, the recovery of trained muscles was much faster than that of untrained muscles. Moreover, the strength recovery of trained muscles was more rapid when the subjects were permitted to move about and generally increase their circulation than when they were required to lie quietly during the recovery period.

Effect of Training on Connective Tissue

The changes that result from muscular training can also be seen in the connective tissue. Of particular interest has been the strength of ligaments supporting various joints. Specifically, a primary target has been the knee joint, partly because it can be isolated for study rather easily, and partly because leg action is so important in exercise and athletics. It is not surprising to learn that the subjects have often been experimental animals, such as the rat.

In such a study involving male white rats, Zuckerman and Stull examined the effect of a nine-week training program of swimming and running on the amount of force required to separate the medial and lateral collateral ligaments of the knee joint. Forced physical activity was found to increase this separation force, showing that training affects the strength of the ligaments as well as the muscles. With the prevalence of knee injuries so high in athletics, it serves as a further reminder of the importance of adequate physical conditioning.

Ingelmark summarizes the general area by indicating that exercise increases the thickness of ligaments, tendons, and other connective tissue in muscles; in fact, the hypertrophy of the tendon may be as great as that of the muscle. The hyaline cartilage, which covers the articulating surfaces of bones in joints, shows similar changes. Bones increase the amounts of calcium phosphate and calcium carbonate in response to training.

Effect of Training on Muscle Skill

One of the important questions to be asked relates to what changes can be expected to occur in the skill of movement, or the motor performance. It is one thing to demonstrate changes in strength, but quite another to translate these alterations into some form of coordination. It is not unusual for athletes and others to engage in weight training in the off-season, with the expressed belief that such activity will enhance their motor performance. In general terms, it seems clear that such activity is preferable to participating in no conditioning at all, and in fact, there may be some truth to the concept that other things being equal, the performer with the greatest muscular strength will probably have an advantage in athletic events.

There are undoubtedly many situations in which strength is a very important ingredient, so that enhancing the strength component establishes a foundation for the element of skill. However, the question is whether or not increasing muscular strength will result in improvement in motor performance per se. Investigations reveal that prediction is really not possible, even though occasionally improvement in certain events has been found to occur. Isotonic exercise is more beneficial than isometric, but the best method is clearly to practice the task itself, especially when the skill element is pronounced. In one investigation where the two variables were isolated, the correlation between gain in arm strength and gain in arm speed was found to be quite low. Apparently, changes in strength cannot very well predict changes in speed of movement.

6

PHYSICAL FITNESS AS A MEANS OF SPORTS

In this Olympic year, when virtually everyone is talking about the virtues and vices of sport, it may be timely to ask: What is sport all about? Who originated the idea of throwing sticks and stones at the nothingness of empty space? What motivated him to devise rules for the performance of this absurd action? What emotions were generated by his attempts to perform this empty action in accordance with the rules he had devised for himself? And why were those emotions so complex? And why were they so often ambivalent? In all truth, no one knows how it all began. But certainly the custom of holding stick-throwing contests at funerals was well established by the time of Trojan Wars—which were fought some three thousand years ago; and fortunately Homer repeated the legendary story of one of these funeral contests in the Iliad—so we may start our speculations about man's involvement in sport-type competitions. As you probably remember, Patroclus was a nobleman, a warrior, and a hero, who fought and died on the bloody plains of ancient Troy.

In his brief lifetime, he did well and gloriously all that the gods and other men might expect such a man to do; and so, at his funeral, his companions thought it fitting to remind the gods of the excellence of Patroclus by calling attention to some of his most glorious deeds. Thus, his companions threw javelins, hurled stones, drove horse-drawn chariots at full speed, ran as fast as a man could run, and wrestled with each other in hand-to-hand combat. But they did not perform these glorious deeds in the same way that Patroclus had performed them in the heat of battle. On the battlefield Patroclus had seldom had an opportunity to demonstrate how far he could throw a spear. On the battlefield he had to throw on the run, and he had to throw at other men who were running toward him with their own spears at the ready; so he had to adjust his aim and force to the requirements of the moment, always keeping his own guard up to ward off the enemy spears and arrows.

As he threw, other warriors often jostled him, or his feet slipped in the muck, or his throw was hampered or hindered by any one of the countless circumstances and necessities of war. In the funeral competitions, the companions of Patroclus tried to rule out all of those hampering and hindering circumstances; and they tried to give each warrior a fair chance to demonstrate his own maximum spear-throwing ability. They did this by converting the deadly act of spear-throwing into the harmless act of throwing a stick at empty spaces, and they identified this non-consequential act as a wholly voluntary action which a man might choose to perform for his own reasons. Then they set aside a time and a place for the performance of this action, and announced a set of rules which would impose the same conditions on all competitions, and they appointed an official judge, giving him the power to impose those same conditions on all men who entered into the competition. Thus as each warrior stepped up to the starting line, he knew precisely what he was going to try to do; he knew he would have a fair chance to perform that action as well as he could perform it; and he knew how the outcomes of his efforts were to be evaluates and by whom. Freed of all the hampering circumstances of war, he was free to go all out, holding nothing back, he was free to focus all the energies of his mortal being on one supreme attempt to hurl his own javelin at the nothingness of empty space. He was free to throw his own stick as far as he could throw it; or he was free to run as fast as he could run, to hit as hard as he could hit, to leap, to jump as high, as far, as he could leap and jump.

In short, he was free to use his own human powers in open contest with the powers of other men; he was free to bring all the forces of his own being to bear on the performance of one self-chosen human action. The Greek warriors created this moment of freedom for themselves—and for all men—by devising the paradoxical rules of sport competition. These rules impose restrictions on human behaviour by defining one set of actions and by specifying how those actions may be performed; but within those restrictions they offer every competitor an opportunity to know the feeling of being wholly free to go all out—free to do his own utmost—free to use himself fully in the performance of one act of his own choosing. These paradoxical rules created this man-made moment of freedom by ruling out the conditions that cloud the realities of man's earthly existence.

They created this moment of freedom by ruling in the pattern of an idealized world in which every man might have an opportunity to make full use of himself—an ideal world in which every man might make full use of all the energies of his mortal being, unhampered and unhindered by the necessities of his life. And so we must note that the Greek warriors did not show the gods how well Patroclus had actually performed the glorious actions of his life in the heat of battle. Rather, they showed the gods—and other men—how well each warrior could perform the empty action of throwing a javelin at the nothingness of empty space under ideals conditions which offered him a fair chance to do his own utmost as a man among men. What values did the Greek warriors find in the performance of these idealized and non-consequential actions?

Here we may turn to the experiences of their modern counterparts, letting three college students speak for all devotees of sport competition.

Sport and Modes of Meaning

It might seem semantic playfulness to ask whether meaning gives structure to individual existence, or if it is structure that lends meaning to life. But if culture is seen as a prearranged, imposed and somewhat restrictive design for man's potential actualization, then the meaningfulness of his activities is inspirable from this structure. Whether culture is, in fact, acting to free man, in the sense that he does not have to replicate countless formulations and decisions, or to restrain him within its social order, it is the notion of pre-designed structure which is compelling. Experience itself cannot be said to be wholly culturally formed.

But insofar as man's confrontation with reality is symbolic, experience does have a dimension of cultural content. Since human experience is essentially an outgrowth of the capacity for abstraction, it is both formulated and interpreted within a pervasive system of symbols which is culturally structured. As man both creates and is created by culture, there is an ongoing process by which the individual internalizes culture and absorbs both its content and modes of thinking, feeling and acting. Although we may speak of such generalized human motivations as drives or needs, or even instincts, and somehow conceive of these as sources of meaning, it is only the culturally shaped modes of expressing, fulfilling or gratifying them that may be explored or understood.

Our concepts of human selfhood and its expression depend on the same capacities for abstraction that have given rise to culture. The individual experiences his own motivations, but he has come to seek their fulfilment and expression in ways that are learned as generally appropriate. And, ultimately, meaning must be viewed as modal; that is, related to the unconscious, perhaps, but absorbed dispositions formed by cultural experience. Generically and specifically we may refer to sports as subcultures, and in doing so imply the existence of another structured and abstracted reality. In fact, the symbolic reality of sport is generally recognized more easily than that of culture as a whole. The only point that may need to be reaffirmed is that abstraction does not imply bloodlessness, and the symbolic reality of sport, though organized in an action or effective domain, is structured for most in relation to affective factors. Sport is a personal-social phenomenon and to examine modes of meaning in the sport experience as either only personal or only social may be inadequate. In some sports, of course, there is no actual social interaction involved in performance, but there are socializing agents and models, social roles and statuses, and a pervasive social context. On one obvious level, social values and norms simply becomes a mode of meaning for the individual in sport.

There is little doubt that people pursue sport for the satisfaction of many social motives and achieve gratification of many related drives and needs through sport participation and success. Similarly, success in sport can be used as a certain kind of self-adequacy affirmation. Either because of personal achievement-need or because of its relationship to such things as popularity and prestige, sport simply is a potential proving-ground for the self. There are, however, many areas of human endeavour other than sport in which modes of meaning based on concepts of socialization and self-validation can function. Despite the fact that we can talk about a generalized kind of culturally imposed appropriateness of meaning-expression, experience is modified and created and more importantly, chosen by the individual. In order to understand modes of meaning particularly or singularly related to the sport experience, perhaps we need to examine the structure of it as freeing the individual rather than retraining him.

The fewer the variables or alternatives which are not prescribed, the greater the freedom the individual has within those alternatives. Where a great deal of the activity in a situation is prescribed, or governed by pre-existing rules, performance becomes focused on those aspects which are not so ordered. The individual may be said to have been freed by the restraints within which he must operate. In sport, the individual is free from having to deal with a host of situations and variables. These are covered by the rules and, furthermore, usually enforced and affirmed by over-responsibilities. In both our sport and our society, this kind of freedom is lately symbolized as being free to do your own thing. But the question must be raised about the difference in modes of meaning of choosing to do your own thing as a hippy, with as few restraints as is culturally possible, and as an athlete within a context of defined and enforced restraints.

Obviously, if the feeling of freedom is the source of meaning the mode of meaning is defined by the choice. The structure of sport exemplified in pre-designed and replicated experiences also provides the means for continual refining of responses. If the sport experience was, indeed, the same each time, we can only assume that eventually it would become boring rather than interesting; that is, it would not have continual meaning. This element of challenge, either because there are no upper limits established or because there are pervasive better ways to do things, becomes another potential source of meaning within the structure of sport.

Response to challenge and mastery are related concepts of meaningfulness to most people. Although both of these may be seen in their relation to self-validation, the repetitive and continual challenge of sport experience suggests that this is not the only mode of meaning involved. In sport, challenge is defined and perceivable. It is related to the areas of freedom, that is, whereas many variables are held constant, both freedom and challenge exist in relation to those variables which are not held constant. Certainly, some notion of mastery is a more likely source of meaning when the challenge is at the level of successful participation in general, rather than when it is more sophisticated and related to freedom.

In the sense that the freedom becomes the challenge, or at least its focal point, the mode of meaning is defined in the structure. One of the most important aspects of meaning in sport is involvement that relates to the complexity and kind of structural demands. Sport may even be defined as involvement; to choose to enter and re-enter the structured reality of sport is to be involved in it—to care about it. If the sport choices of individuals or societies are expressive if some kind of cultural life interpretations, then the mode of meaning is that which is demanded by involvement in the sport.

These demands are related to the structure of specific sport as well as to the general affective dimensions of all sports; that is, to the importance of winning and losing, scoring or not scoring, improving one's mark or performance, and the whole perceptual frame of self as a sportsman or competitor. The notion of involvement is not restricted to sport. Many activities are engrossing and compelling enough in their challenge, complexity and mystique so that they endure as areas of human significance. It is true that sport involvement is not only individual but is manifest in cultural and social ways, and perhaps there is another characteristic of sport that further clarifies its compelling modes of meaning. It is the effective realm that truly characterizes sport, and movement is real, not symbolic; the body is a source of sensation, and in human experience it is sensation which has the least cultural content.

The sensations produced in movement in sport are related to the feelings of power to affect the environment; to act. In the sense of its use of movement, sport is the effect of man's biological technology on the environment, and on that level, sport is inherently meaningful. The question of whether meaning yields structure or structure lends meaning is, finally, ad hoc. Why would man develop and impose structure, except that something was initially and inherently meaningful? Structure and meaning are, thus interactive and sport, based on man's inherent power to act, embodies his modes of meaning in its structure.

Physical Education and the Good Life

The previous speaker has done, appropriately and sensitively, what it would be presumptuous for me to undertake. It has always been proper for an educational group to ask itself what ends it should serve. Often, however, the query is made perfunctorily; habit having so established the answer that further investigation, while recognized as part of the ritual, is unnecessary. But the meaningless habit will no longer prove adequate. Education is under attack on every hand. Critics are emerging from every nook and cranny of the culture. Some of them, because they speak from a background of professional concern and insight, must be taken more seriously than others; yet none should be ignored, whether speaking from a background of insight or of ignorance, since all speak as members of a public which, properly, has a stake in the schools of the nation.

Their right to speak makes the educational situation somewhat messy and does the legitimate educational expert less honour that he deserves; it represents, nevertheless, the burden the educator has to bear in a free world. And this burden is now considerable, what is at issue is nothing less than the continuity of the free world itself. We are confronted today by a brute fact. A determined and, by our standards, a ruthless nation is on the march. Its intention is nothing less than world supremacy and it rightly sees that this country alone, of all of the countries that prize freedom, has the strength to stay its hand. Moreover, its leaders, unhampered by a need to please an electorate, are able to more toward their goals with a directness that would be the envy of the heads of government within the free world—did not the latter know that, were they able to act with comparable ease, they would no longer be representatives of freedom. Turmoil and anxiety have characterized the years since the end of World War II. The peace we thought we had secured at war's end yet eludes us.

We have had the comfort of knowing, however, that we were an advanced nation and it has been disconcerting to discover, as we recently have, that the Russian people, thought by many to lack either the knowledge or the incentives to catch up with our scientific and technological know-how, have made clear in fact what too many of us have heretofore treated only as theory—namely, that no nation has a monopoly on intelligence. Sputnik I and Sputnik II shagged our complacency and brought us down to each aruptly, if may phrase it so, there to watch these instruments, seen always as potential agencies of destruction, move in their orbits around us. Our own Explorer and Vanguard have given us a measure of reassurance but Russia's invasion of outer space, catching us not only grounded, but also bickering about how best to take off economically, made it evident that we are involved in a contest of brains. This is the latest cause for criticism of our public schools.

We are hastily comparing our curricula with those of the Russian schools. We are demanding that more scientists be trained. We are insisting that the frills and froth in education be eliminated. We are pleading that education become an intellectual endeavour and that the merely social and physical emphases be eliminated. We are told all this without sufficient recognition of the fact that the Russian pattern of education would be inappropriate in the free world. The excited critics seem not to know that more than curriculum content is at issue. We cannot assign students to the niche we want them to occupy. We cannot move them from the classroom to, say, a collective farm if they lag behind in their studies. We will not support fully all students of promise, whether their educational interests are in science or in the Russian language, and then place them in government service upon graduation. Nor are we prepared to pay the salaries teachers are said to get in Russia, and despite the occasional cry that we appoint a czar of this or of that, our leaders; there being no czars, in fact, and hence no single will.

We face, in short, no mere problem of schooling, a term much narrower than education, yet one which the critic constantly confuses with the latter. A way of coming at life—

a conception of the good life—is at sake. The terms of the good life, of course, have been set forth in many patterns, including, in our culture, a pattern that permits men to conceive the appropriate terms differently. It has been said that the Academy, was completely free to go another way if he chose, leave his master and follow his own path. There were no fixed dogmas in the Academy; everything was open to discussion, to attack and defence. No one claimed to be teaching the truth; all were seeking it. Here is the root idea of our culture, the freedom of individual man to follow the challenges to, and the leads of his thought. We have held as worthy the aspiration that man should rise above a servile state. We have found life good when men were free to follow their own paths, no longer compelled to tread paths others approved as proper and right.

We have seen no reasons to quarrel with Aristotle's conclusion that the essence of being a slave is to be without either the opportunity or need for thought. We need seek no further to discover why our forebears took education so seriously that they created a system of public education to serve all of the children of all of the people. There is no freedom to think when men so lack knowledge they are compelled to accept as true that which the informed claim to be true. There is no freedom to think when men have no habits of questioning, when they have been conditioned by their culture to accept custom uncritically. The right to think freely comes into being only as men, collectively, prize the goods that flow from this ability sufficiently to work to create and to maintain the conditions that make such learning possible on the part of all. The free man, to remain free, has to work continuously to share his achievement with others who, should they find the good life somehow reflected in their ability to suppress thought, may deny him what he has come to look upon as right.

The price of liberty is, indeed, eternal vigilance. Thus, our interest is at one and the same time in the individual, since it is his development which is paramount; and in society, since, apart from nourishing social conditions, the individual's growth as a reflective being will not be valued. A bottom, then, for free men, the individual and the social interests are identical and, if this were but better grapsed, we would quarrel less at the political level about which interest is being represented and would be less critical, as we examine education, about the social emphases it currently expresses. As men have lived with idea of freedom they have realized that its acceptance has consequences for more than what is often called man's inner life Men can, as the courageous lives of prisoners of war attest, create a world of thought which helps them survive when all that surrounds them is calculated to degrade them, if not to destroy them. But their selfhood will flower, as they well know, when, released from restraining conditions, they are free to move about as they wish; to work at that which tests the adequacy of their aspirations, to give expression to ideas and thus test them against the ideas of others, to associate with those in whose company they find fulfilment, to remain quiet and refrain from speaking when they wish to do so.

Further, as men have made the educative act a matter of study, they have learned that more is involved than the conditions of the classroom, if the end of the education is to incorporate more and more of youth in the shared life of freedom. Irwin Edman summed up this point when he said: "It is no accident that in the United States, from Thomas Jefferson down, public education has been considered a primary business of democracy if democracy is to survive. But such education does not mean, obviously, the mere provision of the central business of education. Neither information nor indoctrination, even of democratic ideas, is enough. The temper of intelligent criticism is the essential not only of a liberal culture but even of a free society. And that temper can be cultivated only in those sufficiently well clothed, well housed, and well fed to be able to think with composure and alertness and to sense a share in the general welfare". A further conditioning factor, one that has increasingly disturbed the public conscience since Edman wrote these words in 1941 is this: one must be sufficiently well integrated into the full life of citizenship "to be able to think with composure and to sense a share in the general welfare" And this means more than clothing, housing and food, as the United States Supreme Court has recently recognized.

Man is not educable, in the full sense of the good life as free me have conceived it, if he is arbitrarily cut off, by virtue of the conditions of his birth and of his growth, from free participation in the affairs of his culture. Nor, on the other hand, are those who insist upon restricting the development of others as free as their sense of power leads them to believe. We are caught up in an associated life; and this, without any planning on our part. If we are to make it a good life, we shall need to engage in a creative, shared effort. Any restriction placed upon any individual, or any opportunity to achieve freedom granted him, means, in fact, restriction or opportunity for all. Freedom, as I have been arguing, is an achievement—a social achievement—as well as an individual one. It is not a gift.

Yet the achievements of prior generations make the problems of freedom easier for later generations. Most of our citizens, for instance, gain the right to vote today simply by living long enough to meet the requirements of the states in which they live. Were they called upon to fight for the right, generation by generation, the right to vote would be a limited right, indeed. This is a fact that the women of this country should readily recall; it is a fact that some citizens of this country are painfully aware of today. The achievements of past generations to provide a cultural inheritance that extends the opportunities of later generations to participate more fully in the co-operative task of building a free world.

But, unfortunately, as the rise of the authoritarian state in its new form in this century has shown, any generation may create social conditions that will deny freedom to the unborn for generations to come. It is small wonder, whatever mistakes modern education may have made and however, harsh the voices of the critics, that our schools have been concerned to create educative conditions that exemplify the essential qualities of free and democratic men. Information alone, on matter what the quantity transmitted, will not promote the good life for free men. Again, to turn to Edman, we find him saying correctly that it is "only on the basis of institutions nourishing the ancient ideals of freedom, justice and equality the men will be liberated to come to their full stature, to live richly in themselves and in mutually stimulating and understanding peace with one another". And one of these institutions, of course, is education, as the school men of this country have rightly seen. A word of caution is in order here. We are not the sole inheritors of that vision of the good life which has been created as men over the ages have struggled to attain these conditions of decency and humaneness upon which the gaining of freedom depends.

Nor are we alone today as the struggle continues. The specific character of our inheritance has made it possible for us to maintain and extend the conditions of freedom for ourselves, but it has challenged others to a comparable achievement, men whose initial opportunity for development was not as favourable as ours. The challenge has been accepted and, from one quarter to another, there will be tension and struggle until the ends of freedom and independence are gained, or until a contrary approach to life prevails. We too often forget that what we have achieved, by a combination of fortunate circumstances and determination, has become for others a vision of a life good to live and that, therefore, the leadership expected of us is a leadership so devoted to freedom that it works ceaselessly to help all men experience it. Arnold Toynbee, attempting to forecast what the historian will say of this century 300 years hence, has said this age will be remembered chiefly for having been "the first age since the dawn of civilization in which people dared to think it practicable to make the benefits of civilization available for the whole human race".

In the development of this idea, Toynbee contends that this "vision of a good life for all is new one, and—whatever our success or our failure may be in the attempt to translate this vision into reality—this new social objective has probably come to stay. That the ideal of welfare for all is new is surely true; for, as far as I can see, it is no older than the seventeenth century West European settlements on the East Coast of North America that have grown into the United States. And it has surely come to stay with us as long, at any rate, as our new invention of applying mechanical power to technology, for this sudden vast enhancement of man's ability to make nonhuman nature produce what man requires from her has, for the first time in history, made the ideal of welfare for all a practical objective instead of a mere utopian dream".

Finally, he notes the moral obligations which this vision of the good life imposes upon those who have thus far been its beneficiaries, saying, "When once the odious inequality that has hitherto been a distinguishing mark of civilization has ceased to be taken for granted as something inevitable, it becomes inhuman to go on putting up with it—and still more inhuman to try to perpetuate this inequality deliberately". We identify this vision of the good life with democracy and, in so doing, run the danger, as is always true when a covering label is handy, of obscuring its essence, the continuing quest by all for a life that is good to live.

We are not dealing with a completed vision, with a way of life so complete that, viewing it as finished, we may set out to teach it as we may teach an unquestioned body of fact. It was for this reason that earlier I used the expression a way of coming at life in referring to our conception of the good life. We know that we are dealing with an open world, not a closed one. We know that we get our directions from an active and probing intelligence, not from a recipe book. We know that concern for others, respect for ideas and for the individuals who express them, and readiness to consult and compromise as the differences we cherish conflict, are principles that help us keep on the right track as we find our way amidst the ever-new problems which arise. We know, even as we at times forget it, that callous action which excludes either appropriate persons or relevant ideas is always a denial of the spirit of democracy, whether this occurs on a playing field or at a summit conference of world leaders.

We do, in short, have ways of testing ourselves as to how well we are living up to our commitments in the daily round of our lives. Some years ago, John Dewey asked whether we could find supporting reason for our preference for democracy or whether, as many thoughtful people insist, we hold this preference simply because we were born where the concept was rooted historically, in much the same way that some people prefer strong seasoning in their food, to the distress of those whose tastes were differently developed. This is a basic question, if we are dealing with no more than a matter of taste, of unreasoned preference, it is sheer lunacy to claim that what we find good will be good for others.

Dewey's answer moves us from the plane of tastc, provides supporting reasons, and in my view, sums up the principles that should guide us as we come at life for the purpose of securing more completely the conditions of freedom for all. "Can we find any reason", he asks, "that does not ultimately come down to the belief that the democratic social arrangements promote a better quality of human experience, one which is more widely accessible and enjoyed, than do nondemocratic and antidemocratic forms of social life? Does not the principle of regard for individual freedom and for decency and kindliness of human relations come back in the end to the conviction that these things are tributary to a higher quality of experience on the part of a greater number than are methods of repression and coercion or force? Is it not the reason for our preference that we believe that mutual consultation and convictions reached through persuasion, make possible a better quality of experience than can otherwise be provided on any side scale?" If I have laboured long over my point about the nature of the good life, I have as an excuse only my conviction that it was important to do.

We have heard, much of late about making education consistent with the nature of man, though those who press this point often write as if man in the study of man had learned nothing in the last two thousand years. Interest is centred on a strong mind, with the strength of the vehicle, the body, being left presumably to inheritance or, perhaps, to you. We hear much, also, of the need to provide an education that will be appropriate for all times and for all places, a position that considers the prevailing conceptions of the good life as these emerge with differing cultures to be irrelevant and which, to take a case in point, would give the United States and Russia identical educational patterns.

Your place in this scheme of things is surely restricted, since it is doubtful that you have been provided for within the immutable and unchanging principles said to be directive of this pattern of thought. And, at another level, much is said as I noted earlier, of clearing the schools of the debris left over from a once-held enthusiasm for progressive education in order that proper subject matter may again be emphasized. This case could be argued, if its adherents did not use the label progressive so loosely as to make it meaningless, and if they did not act as if subject matter had an inherent power to educate people on contact. Of course, subject matter is important but, in the classroom, it becomes important only as it enters the reflective experience of students and leads them to an understanding of their talents and to a grasp of its social significance.

As the case is argued, however, the uncritical acceptance of organized knowledge as the focus of educational effort should given pause to those who know how this conception at an earlier time led to so much boredom in the classroom. As for your field under this view, I am afraid you will be benched, unless you are permitted to enter the game from time to time to serve as traquilizers for overwrought students. But perhaps I need not turn to the present day critics of education to uncover the problem of your place in the scheme of things. A well-known professional book that deals with the high school curriculum, the second edition of which was issued in 1956, contains almost 600 pages and is divided into 32 chapters. The 31st chapter discusses the place of health education in the curriculum; the 32nd the place of physical education. I spoke to the high school teachers of the academic subjects in a large city school system while, at the same hour, meetings were being held for the elementary school teachers and for the teachers of special subjects, including health and physical education. Am I right in asking myself these questions: Are you part of the public school show, but not essential to the development of its basic educational program? Now, I a aware, of course, that you are concerned with more than muscles, that you do not ask students to put their mental life in their lockers during their hours with you. I know that such matters as health in general, or health specifically, sanitation, immunization, hygiene, special and corrective exercises, understanding of and respect for a self that is manifested through behaviour, an appreciation of what it means to be of one sex and to grow in relationship to the other, skill in individual exercises or in competitive games, and the like, are all matters that concern you are teachers.

I know also as Jesse Williams has stated, that your thinking is directed by such principles as these: "Physical education will be an education through the physical rather than an education of the physical"; "Recreation belongs in the good life"; and "The qualities included in the term sportsmanship are primary objectives of certain physical activities". And I am aware that what you do is tested against carefully formulated criteria, and that you are sensitive about certain hazards in your field, such as the ease of slipping into regimented drills and of permitting sports to be exploited commercially. But I recall, also, that Williams has said of games, sports and athletics that, "these are the heart of the program" and I am afraid the public generally and the critics specifically think of them as the total program. Moreover, the public and the critics tend to associate you with playing fields and physical activity, rather than with classrooms and mental activity. If the public has been misled, your academic colleagues must share with you some of the blame for this.

They have been only too happy to be looked upon as the guardians of intellectual halls, even as they have joined the public in increasing the hazard of exploiting those whose talents lead them to significant participation in games, sports, and athletics. They have found it good, on the one hand, to be identified with the essential intellectual centre of education, and, on the other, to be associated with schools that gain enthusiastic public support because of their excellence in athletic events. But this only means that we are dealing with an area of human activity in which it is hard to keep an eye on the ball. No activity of a school is warranted that does not have educative consequences for those to whom it is directed or, to state if differently, in which the intellectual component is not central. This is as true in a science classroom as it is on a playing field, when either involves meaningless, repetitive acts, though its absence in the former may not be equally meaningless, repetitive acts, though its absence in the former may not be equally obvious.

Classroom teacher may call the signals as readily as playing field teachers. They are, then, equally guilty of the exploitation of human material, of degrading the educative process. The fact is, of course—and this is the point of my argument throughout—that your field should either contribute to the good life we aspire to or have no place in the education of the free men. But this conclusion applies to all fields of knowledge. All that we teach should liberate the individual from binding custom and uncriticized habit and move him into the larger life of shared insight and understanding. Whatever is thus liberated is, in the essential meaning of the term, liberal. And here is to be found the ground on which you stand equally with other fields of knowledge. However, each field differs in specific concerns, all stand together in advancing the common quest for the good life. We should expect the critics to see the problem more clearly than the public. And in many respects they do, especially when they consider educational aberrations of the following sort: First, a failure to understand that the doctrine of interest should neither exalt the passing whim of the student nor eliminate hard work for the program. Second, the false assumption that to emphasize conformity, or adjustment to things as they are, instead of, as John Dewey pointed out, to be concerned with an adjustment of conditions so that plans of action may be tested and the conditions that initiated them reconstructed. Third, a misinterpretation of the place of doing in learning, so that any activity is viewed as educative, so that any activity is viewed as educative, when, in fact, it is only as the method of intelligence is operative that reaction is turned into response, into meaningful behaviour. Fourth, the inability to maintain perspective, illustrated, on the one hand, when athletic programs overshadow educational endeavours; or, on the other, when sentiment so dominates the proper emphasis upon individual development that the freedom given young people denies the teacher, as Dewey once remarked, the freedom to direct this development.

That these aberrations have occurred in a fact to reckon with, and it is proper that critical guns be turned upon them. Such guns were rolled into position, in fact, before the newly emerging critics started firing—as they should know. My repeated reference to John Dewey in the above paragraph was deliberate. He is currently being held responsible for most of the ills of public education. None seem to realize, however, that John Dewey, commenting on the difficulty of changing either individual or institutional habits in 1952, noted the way in which the latter tend to assimilate and distort new ideas into conformity with themselves and concluded emphatically. This drive or tendency in the educational institution is perhaps most glaringly evident in the way the ideas and principles of the educational philosophy I have had a share in developing are still for the most part taught, more than half a century after they began to find their way in various parts of the school.

In teachers colleges and elsewhere the ideas and principles have been converted into a fixed subject matter of ready-made rules, to be taught and memorized according to certain standardized procedures and, when occasion arises, to be applied to educational problems externally, the way mustard plasters, for example, are applied" (i) The aberrations may be facts of the situation. They bear no necessary relationship to the ideas and principles of Dewey's thought, however; nor does their presence invalidate these ideas and principles. By ignoring this, it is convenient for the critics to sweep Mr. Dewey from the scene, an act which inadvertently illustrates his point that the habits of individuals and institutions change slowly. The bearing of this upon your area is more direct than may at first seem apparent.

Modern, or progressive, or current, education is said to be anti-intellectual; and, by implication, Dewey's philosophy is held to be the responsible agent. Oddly, it would be hard to find anyone whose writings were more concerned to bring a liberating intelligence into the daily affairs of man and who wrote more pointedly to reveal the function of education in advancing this end. He did not think of intelligence, however, as a peculiar possession which a person owns, with each individual having a given quantity of birth, nor did he think of it as the highest faculty of a mind that was given to all alike. He knew that each of these views had its day in court, that each had been repudiated.

Intelligence, as a term, meant to him a shorthand designation for great and ever-growing methods of observation, experiment and reflective reasoning. He was concerned, therefore with the process of inquiring. Within it, he found qualities of behaviour that differentiated it as an act from acts of routine or of impulse. Hence, his interest was in the distinctive qualities of this way of behaving. He found it no longer necessary to refer to a separate entity that caused the behaviour, that served in Gilbert Ryle's admittedly abusive term, as "the Ghost in the Machine". He concluded, rather, that the "conceptions of behaviour in its integrity, as including a history and environment, is the alternative to the theory which eliminates the mental because it considers only the behaviour of the mechanism of action as well as the theory which thinks it ennobles the mental by placing it in an isolated realm"

He thus moved beyond the long held dualistic conception of separate realms of mind and matter without succumbing either to the mechanisms of recent behaviourism or to the futility of a preceding mentalism. Where present-day critics of education are concerned with the aberrations, the excesses, found in our schools, we should join hands to bring about their elimination. We have no dogmas to protect. If there has been an unreasonable emphasis upon mere activity, upon doing that which is without meaning, whether in a laboratory or shop, a classroom or gymnasium, upon a stage or a playground, this does not mean that education should swing to an extreme of mere contemplation. Where there is learning there will be doing but the doing will not itself be the learning though one may learn, as William H. Kilpatrick has put it, what one does.

Doing, in short, is not restricted to overt bodily activity; nor is learning restricted to the operation of an inner mind. If there has been an over emphasis upon social adjustment, leading either to the false view that the purpose of education is to conform to things as they are or that its end is exclusively to help the individual be a jolly, good fellow, this does not mean that we should suddenly loss interest either in the social deal that has given significance to the lives of free men or in the social significance of that which the student learns. It has seemed to some that there is not sufficient respect for knowledge in education as it is presently conducted, this does not mean that classrooms should become places where information and inert ideas should be paraded before young people endlessly

Information becomes knowledge for the student, when it does, as it bears upon what he is trying to do and helps him do it with an enlarged understanding and extended control. When this happens, students respect knowledge, without benefit of parchment. If schools have seemed to be so concerned with health that responsibility has been taken away from the family, the alternative is surely not to ignore health, since at this point in many instances may be found the critical factor that has led teachers to look upon a student as uneducable.

If education has been too practical, the contrast we seek is not an impractical education. The issue here is to teach whatever is taught so that meaning is progressively added to the life of the student. It is in this sense that theory may be more practical than activity. But this is true only when the theory illuminates activity in which the individual engages. Both the merely practical ad the merely theoretical, untouched by meaning, will seem abstruse to the student. The danger is that we shall permit our present anxieties to throw us off balance. The critics have found weak spots in our practices. But we had better watch their proposed remedies, especially when they emphasize intellectual activities as if they were cut off from the stream of physical life.

The temper of intelligent criticism as Edman has noted, is dependent upon many factors. It will not be cultivated simply by the study of a certain body of subjects, nor will it be cultivated when what we know about man and his learning is ignored because we are intrigued by a noble and historic, though wrong conception. The physical is in the educational picture to stay. It is one aspect of the total individual with whom we deal. Our problem is to differentiate inquiring, reflective, purposeful behaviour, that is illuminated by the consequences it forecasts and that is checked against what in fact occurs, from behaviour that is irrational, irresponsible, capricious, or blind. We cannot lift ourselves above behaviour into a realm of pure experience, since there is no experience worthy of the name where there is no meaning, and meaning, finally is grounded in the individual's ability to do what his ideas assure him that he can do. Intellectual development is central in an educational program that is designed to create men who may, in turn, create the conditions that enhance freedom for all.

But this is not to suggest, as I am afraid many critics do, that only an assumed intellect is the object of educational interest. Far from it. What is of interest are active individuals whose present level of interests, concerns, and knowledge make it possible to arouse them to engage in further activity within which what they presently know will be reconstructed as new information, ideas, insights are encountered. In these terms, physical education may make a major contribution to the achievement of the good life on the part of free men. Indeed, the basic potential of your area is distinctively a human potential. Many of our activities bring individuals together intimately, both competitively and co-operatively, and place them under the discipline of living up to established standards and rules.

Moreover, the failure of many, even at the teaching levels, to live up to the rules brings to the force something more than an interest in skills. Questions then arise from experienced problems, not from manufactured ones, questions that cannot be answered by a rote application of rules. Choices, and hence moral decisions, have to be made; since rules cannot substitute for intelligence. Rules do carry over into the present, however, what men in the past have found good, and thus serve as the means to help individuals become intelligent and sensitive in dealing with new problems. They make possible the games to which they apply and, also, make it possible to judge both the claim of validity of those who want to change the rules and the integrity of those who claim to live under their direction. The physical education teacher, without announcing it, may help young people continuously, if his eyes are lifted above the levels of skills and performances, shape up a conception of the good life.

Problems that confront the student with the need to make choices will arise, also, when rules of health are under discussion. In fact, whenever the function and appropriateness of a rule is considered, differing conceptions of life are then weighed one against the other. The intellectual and moral components of your field are potentially high. They will not be realized, however, without insight and understanding and effort on your part. They will not be realized at all, if the notion prevails that intelligence may arise only in classrooms that claim to be turned into the realm of mind, a realm that will be disturbed if the body is too much with us. You have a further opportunity, to the degree that games, sports and athletics are the heart of your program, that is given to few teachers.

You engage them in activities where their learning makes an immediate difference, a difference they can grasp and understand immediately. You do not have to keep assuring your students, as other teachers must, that some day they will be glad you made them study. The game is the thing and they can play at once. But even more is involved. The necessity of co-operation brings together into joined effort all of the diversities among our people. The individual is judged by what he does, by what he contributes to the common effort. He is not asked to show credentials of birth, of economic status, of religion, or of race. On this score, indeed, you have helped the average citizen, often without intending to do so, to gain an appreciation of others, whatever their background. You have provided, where your work has been properly conceived, an opportunity for the individual to be a person, a person gaining respect for himself as he understands what he can do and what he represents, as well as a person who contributes freely to the gains of others. Difference of backgrounds and diversity of talents are joined in the exciting effort to achieve together what none could achieve alone, and yet the sad fact is that men may compete or co-operate under the guidance of degrading ends. You cannot rest your case, therefore, on these abstractions. You must bring them to life as they serve an appropriate educational end. This end, it should be clear, is to help students rise to an appreciation of how their growth is ultimately related to their ability and willingness to create and maintain the conditions within which the spirit of freedom for all will be forever nurtured.

7

THE NOTION OF FITNESS, HEALTH AND PHYSICAL EDUCATION

Fitness, and Physical Education: An Academic Discipline

College physical education in developed countries like USA owes much of its genesis to the concept that exercise and sports are therapeutic and prophylactic. In fact many directors of physical education of the preceding generation were medical doctors. The school program probably received its greatest impetus as an effort to reduce draft rejects and improve the fitness of youth for military service in World War I. This objective was of course re-emphasized in World War II. It is understandable that our professional concern has tended to centre on what physical education can do for people rather than the development of a field of knowledge. Since most of the present senior generation of physical educators received their doctorates in education, it is understandable that their orientation has been toward the profession of education rather than the development of a subject field of knowledge.

In fact physical education has the doubtful do not recognize as a subject field, since the typical physical education department is unique in being under the jurisdiction of or closely related to the school or department of eduction. Some schools or colleges of physical education do exists in large universities and are patterned after the schools or colleges of education. When a young person planning a high school teaching career begins his college or university degree work with a major in, for example, chemistry, he starts out with freshman chemistry, which has as a prerequisite a course in high school chemistry. He then takes other lower division chemistry courses, to which the first course is prerequisite. In his junior and senior years, he completes an upper division major in chemistry, in order to qualify for the bachelor's degree. This major consists entirely of course content for more advanced than anything he will teach in a high school. Similarly, the student who majors in mathematics must have an upper division major in advanced mathematics, and even his most elementary freshman course in mathematics will be at an advanced level in comparison with the usual high school mathematics courses. In marked contrast, the student who obtains a bachelor's degree in physical education typically has a major that is evaluated and oriented with respect to what he is to teach in the secondary schools, and how he is to do the teaching or how he is administer the program. Many physical education major programs, for example, do not even require a course in exercise physiology. Actually, it is both possible and practical to offer a degree with an academic major in the subject field of physical education, and several universities have such a degree.

If the person obtaining this degree plans to teach in the schools, he supplements the academic major with the necessary courses in methods and other professional topics. Academic vs. professional is not an issue of having either the one or the other, since the two are not mutually exclusive. However, the present discussion is not concerned with the merits of one or the other or the nature of the best combination. Rather, it is concerned with defining at least in a general way, the field of knowledge that constitutes the academic discipline of physical education in the college degree program. An academic discipline is an organized body of knowledge collectively embraced in a formal course of learning.

The acquisition of such knowledge is assumed to be an adequate and worthy objective as such, without any demonstration or requirement of practical application. The content is theoretical and scholarly as distinguished from technical and professional. There is indeed a scholarly field of knowledge basic to physical education. It is constituted of certain portions of such diverse fields as anatomy, physics and physiology, cultural anthropology, history and sociology, as well as psychology. The focus of attention is on the study of man as an individual engaging in the motor performances required by his daily life and in other motor performances yielding aesthetic values or serving as expressions of his physical and competitive nature, accepting challenges of his capability in pitting himself against a hostile environment and participating in the leisure time activities that have become of increasing importance in our culture.

However, a person could be by ordinary standards well educated in the traditional fields listed above, and yet be quite ignorant with respect to comprehensive and integrated knowledge of the motor behaviour and capabilities of man. The areas within these fields that are vital to physical education receive haphazard and peripheral treatment, rather than systematic development, since the focus of attention is directed elsewhere. Thus, the academic discipline under consideration cannot be synthesized by a curriculum composed of carefully selected courses from departments listed under A, H and P and S in a university catalogue. True, the student who could master the field of knowledge must first be grounded in general courses in anatomy, physiology, physics and certain of the behavioural and social sciences. But upper division course need to be specialized, or else the development of the subject field will be haphazard, incomplete, and ineffective.

Twenty-four semester units, in fact, may well be insufficient to cover adequately the available body of knowledge. The areas to be covered include kinesiology and body mechanics; the physiology of exercise, training and environment; neuromotor coordination, the kinesthetic senses, motor learning and transfer; emotional and personality factors in physical performance; and the relation of all these to human development, the functional status of the individual, and his ability to engage in motor activity. They also include the role of athletics, dance and other physical activities in the culture and in primitive as well as advanced societies.

Consideration of the relation of these activities to the emotional and physical health and aesthetic development of the individual constitutes an application of the field of knowledge, but may well be presented and integrated with it, provided that priority is given to the basic knowledge rather than its application to health. This field of study, considered as an academic discipline, does not consist of the application of the disciplines of anthropology, physiology, psychology and the like to the study of physical activity. On the contrary, it has to do with the study as a discipline, of certain aspects of anatomy, anthropology, physiology, psychology and other appropriate fields. The student who majors in this cross-disciplinary field of knowledge will not be a physiologist or a psychologist or an anthropologist, since there has necessarily been a restriction in breadth of study within each of the traditional fields.

Moreover, the emphasis must frequently be placed on special areas within each of these fields—areas that receive the little attention in the existing courses. Any one of these disciplines encompasses far more material than can be included in the usual course of study for a major in the subject. This is comparable to the situation in a number of the discipline. A biochemist, for example, is necessarily deficient in his breadth of training as a chemist, and he is also necessarily narrow as a biologist. Nevertheless, he is a more competent biomechanist than is a chemist or a biologist. Special hazards and special responsibilities attach to the introduction of any new field of study. In a major that is made up of courses in a cross-disciplinary department, there is a danger that normal academic standards of depth may be relaxed. For example, an upper division course in exercise physiology will not be respected, and in fact will not ordinarily be authorized in a college of exceptionally high standards, unless a thorough elementary course in human or mammalian physiology is required as a prerequisite. This reasoning holds for all upper division courses in any major that is accepted as a discipline in such a college. Problems certainly occur in delimiting the field of knowledge outlined above.

The development of personal skill in motor performance is without question a worthy objective in itself. But it should not be confused with the academic field of knowledge. Similarly, technical competence in measuring a chemical reaction, or computational skill in mathematics, are not components of the corresponding fields of knowledge. Learning the rules and strategy of sports may well be intellectual, but it is highly doubtful if a course on rules and strategy of sports may well be intellectual, but it is highly doubtful of an academic field of knowledge at the upper division college or university level. One may well raise such a question as where is the borderline between a field such as physiology and the field of physical education? No simple definitive statement is possible, but it is not difficult to show examples that illustrate the region of demarcation. The existence of oxygen debt is physiology; the role of oxygen debt in various physical performances is physical education. We do not know why a muscle becomes stronger when it is exercised repeatedly. The ferreting out of the causal mechanism of this phenomenon can be considered a problem in physiology, although of explanation, when available, will be appropriate for inclusion in a physical education course.

On the other hand, the derivation of laws governing the quantitative relation between an increased in strength and the amount, duration and frequency of muscle forces exerted in training is surely more physical education than physiology. Determination of the intimate biochemical changes in a muscle during fatigue would seem to be a problem in physiology, although a muscle during fatigue would seem to be a problem in physiology, although of direct interest to physical education. Here again, the quantification of relationships and the theoretical explanation of their pattern as observed in the intact human organism is more physical education than physiology. This is not mere application—it only becomes application when such laws are related to practical problems.

The physiology of athletic training is not really application of physiology—rather it is physiology, of the sort that is part of the academic discipline of physical education, and only becomes applied when it is actually applied to practical problems. Unfortunately, in this particular area, what is called "physiology of training" consists to a large extent of over-generalized and speculative attempts to apply the incomplete and fragmentary fundamental knowledge currently available. It is to be hoped that this is but a temporary situation. The study of the heart as an organ is physiology, whereas determining the quantitative role of heart action as a limiting factor in physical performance in normal individuals is perhaps more physical education than physiology.

Thus the study of variables which cause individual differences in performance in the normal range of individuals is of particular concern to physical education but evidently of little interest to physiology. Textbooks on exercise physiology are written for physical education courses. Much of the research they describe was done by physiologists. On the other hand, a standard textbook on physiology written for physiologists may not even have a chapter on exercise, and if it does, the treatment is notably incomplete. Similar examples are to be found in the field of anatomy. Textbooks on psychology have at best a sparse treatment of such topics as reaction time, the kinesthetic sense, and motor performance. These are not matters of fundamental interest to present-day psychologists, although they did occupy a position of importance in the first two decades of the present century. Even though anthropologists have long been aware of the role of physical games and sports in all cultures, one cannot find any comprehensive treatment of the topic in anthropology textbooks. It would be unfair to say that scholars in various fields such as those mentioned above feel that it is unimportant to study man as an individual engaging in physical activity.

Rather, the neglect is because this aspect is of peripheral rather than central interest to the scholar in that field. To borrow a figure of speech, anthropology and other fields mentioned approach the study of man longitudinally, whereas physical education proposes a cross-sectional look at man as he engages in physical activity. There is an increasing need for the organization and study of the academic discipline herein called physical education. As each of the traditional fields of knowledge concerning man becomes more specialized, complex and detailed, it becomes more differentiated from physical education.

Physiology of the first half of the century, for example, had a major interest in the total individual as a unit, whereas present-day physiology focuses attention on the biochemistry of cells and subcellular structures. While the importance of mitochondria in exercise cannot be denied, there is still need to study and understand the aspects and implications of exercise as a whole. Furthermore, the purely motor aspects of human behaviour and for more attention than they currently receive in traditional fields of anthropology and psychology. If the academic discipline of physical education did not already exist, it would need to be invented.

The Domain of Physical Education as a Discipline

Man's curiosity about the unknown is probably as old as man himself. Yet it is only in a relatively recent times that man has been able to offer plausible explanations of what he observed in nature. True, scholars in some ancient civilizations sought logical explanations of what they observed. They noted that there was order in the universe. They observed relationships and were concerned with causes and predictions. But it was not until well after the Dark Ages that science as we knot it today began to flourish. Systematic observation provided data against which hypotheses could be tested.

Theories were developed and scientific laws established. The scientific method was born. With the advent of the scientific method, knowledge accumulated rapidly. From the very beginning, scientists classified like things together for systematic and detailed study. Thus separate fields of knowledge began to emerge on which scholars concentrated their attention. Some probed the mysteries of the universe, others examined the nature of matter, some studied living things. Each in his own field sought to extend the scope of knowledge. Knowledge thus gained has become part of our cultural heritage, passed from generation to generation in formal courses of study, each dealing with a closely related body of knowledge. Thus we have come to recognize segments of knowledge as disciplines. As knowledge and technical skill advanced, new disciplines began to emerge.

Today and first-class American university will offer an imposing list of courses in from seventy-five to a hundred fields of study. The last two decades have witnessed a marked increase in the number of fields of study, each with its own courses. What, then, does constitute the domain of a discipline? Fifty years ago the answer would have been relatively simple. Today it is highly complex except for the long-standing disciplines. We have come to realize that even though we live in an age of specialization, it is difficult to isolate one branch of knowledge from another. This is true even for such well-established disciplines as physics and chemistry. On the surface it would see that the lines here are neatly drawn. Yet there is some overlap, for the chemist must be informed about the intimate structure of matter, and the physicist must be informed about the transformations which matter undergoes.

In fact today every self-respecting chemistry department offers at least one course in physical chemistry. How have new disciplines emerged, and how have they been able to stake out their respective domains? Most often this has been done to developing a clearly defined segment of knowledge from an already existing discipline. Such, for example, occurred in microbiology molecular biology, and, in the early days, botany and zoology.

Each owed its origin to biology—the parent. Some disciplines of relatively long standing came into being without any apparent break from a parent discipline, such as astronomy, anthropology, psychology, and physiology. Other fields have the dubious distinction of just now being on the threshold of becoming disciplines. For example, a brief commentary in a recent issue of Science points out that professors of computer science are sometimes asked whether there is a computer science, and if so, what it is. According to these professors, it is a science which studies computers, investigating them with the same intensity that others have studied natural phenomena, using the intellectual curiosity which is characteristic of all scientific inquiry. It is pointed out that while computers themselves belong to engineering and hence have a professional orientation, there is a difference between the study of computers and the application of the resulting knowledge.

In a sense this is the problem facing physical education today: the professional as against the disciplinary orientation. In many quarters there has been a genuine concern about overspecialization and a recognition of the need for a synthesis of knowledge. Proponents of this viewpoint hold that students and scientists must view natural phenomena not in isolation, but in relation to other areas of inquiry and to the world at large. This has resulted not infrequently in a merger of disciplines, a breakdown of traditional disciplinary boundaries. We now see broad areas of study, such as geophysics, biochemistry, medical genetics, and medical physics. Similarly, the trend toward interdisciplinary research is gaining momentum rapidly. With this trend, the traditional concept of a discipline may have to be abandoned. Physical education today is generally identified as a profession in much the same way as engineering, law and medicine are.

Just as Webster defines medicine as "the science or art concerned with the prevention, cure or alleviation of disease", physical education is defined as "education in its application to the development and care of the body, especially with reference to instruction in hygiene and systematic exercise". In both, the major emphasis is on application of knowledge rather than on scholarship. How the knowledge is used is of little concern to a discipline.

As Henry points out, the content of a discipline is "theoretical and scholarly as distinguished from technical and professional". Over the years this has not been our orientation in physical education. We have for the most part been doers, not thinkers. It is nevertheless evident that physical education has within its scope a body of knowledge which is not the concern of any other academic discipline. It is equally clear that there is much that is borderline. Most certainly human movement is a legitimate field of study and research. We have only just begun to explore it. There is need for a well-recognized body of knowledge about how and why the human body moves, how simple and complex motor skills are acquired and executed, and how the effects of physical activity may be immediate or lasting. The question is sometimes raised: Is one justified in including the execution of a motor skill in and of itself as an integral part of a discipline?

The mechanics of the skill can be observed and studied, the physiological responses monitored, the feeling states noted. These are areas of legitimate study and research. On the other hand, do we need to clarify for ourselves the level of cognition that is required in learning and executing semi-automatic the level of cognition that is required in learning and executing semi-automatic motor skill? Perhaps we need to ask what level of insight and of understanding is required in a behavioural response in order for it to quality as a part of an academic discipline.

Can we justify as a part of our discipline behavioural

responses which are for the most part automatically controlled even though there is conscious direction of certain aspects of the movement and interpretative and affective controls which give to the movement refinement, meaning and beauty? All would agree that physical education is concerned essentially with exercise, active games, sports, athletics, gymnastics, and dance. Yet one would be hard pressed to build a case to support this categorization as a logical framework within which to develop concepts, hypotheses, theories and laws.

Reference to the organizational framework of a long-established discipline might be useful here. The classical organizational pattern of physics is straightforward and logical. Its focus is on matter and energy. It is developed around core ideas, theories and laws, neatly categorized into five different areas: namely, mechanics, heat, light, sound and electricity. This provides a systematic approach in the search for orderliness in nature. Physical education needs to come of age. As yet there is no agreement as to its focus. Nor does it have a clearly defined body of knowledge or scope of inquiry.

Physical education does, however, have a focus: namely, human movement and its correlates. This aspect of man's experience is our domain. No other discipline explores it. Thus we may say the following:

i. Physical education as a discipline is concerned with the mechanics of human movement, with the mode of acquisition and control of movement patterns, and with the psychological factors affecting movement responses.

ii. Physical education is concerned with the physiology of man under the stresses of exercise, sports and dance and with the immediate and lasting effects of physical activity.

iii. The historical and cultural aspects of physical education and dance occupy a prominent place in our discipline. The roles of sports and dance in the cultures which have preceded ours and in our own culture needs to be fully explored.

iv. Lastly, in physical education we are aware that man does not function alone. Individual and group interactions in games, sports, and dance are an important area, one which needs our attention. As yet we have no rationale for explaining the diversified behaviour patterns of individuals and groups as either participants or spectators.

We have a considerably body of knowledge to draw upon. However, it is widely scattered and at the moment not well-structured. An immediate need is to bring order out of chaos. If, in fact, we are serious in our belief that there is an identifiable body of knowledge which belongs to what we call physical education, we need to begin at once to build the general framework for structuring this body of knowledge. With this accomplished, we can perhaps more clearly pinpoint the future direction of our research and other scholarly efforts.

8

SIGNIFICANCE OF IDEALISM IN FITNESS, HEALTH AND PHYSICAL EDUCATION

The powerful force of a realism that is strongly materialistic has threatened America's idealistic superstructure to such an extent that it has been said that "traditional philosophic idealism, in all of its numerous variants, is probably obsolescent if not already obsolete". As disturbing as the above statement might be to an idealist, he would probably concur in the belief that it is necessary for America to build its spiritual core to meet the challenge of the second half of the twentieth century. The idealistic outlook and its implications for physical, health and recreation education is, according to Brubacher, part of the over-all essentialistic position.

Idealism is much more complex to analyse, since it cannot be said that it stands completely either for education of the physical or education through the physical. Brubacher places it somewhat on the border line between progressivism and essentialism, but he does state further that there is a measure of absolutism in idealistic philosophy of education which seems more properly to align it with essentialism. This writer believes that the individual professional should find his place on a spectrum through careful self-examination.

Aims and Objectives

Horne's stated that "education is the eternal process of superior adjustment of the physically and mentally developed, free, conscious, human being to God, as manifested in the intellectual, emotional and volitional environment of man". According to this approach it is necessary to determine what the highest good in life is, based on a particular view of human nature. In this hierarchy of educational values, the highest, or absolute, aim is the establishment of man's likeness to the spiritual order. Thus the most important educational objective would be an understanding of worship which brings man into a conscious relation with the infinite spirit of the universe.

The other educational objectives of the perfectly integrated individual may then be listed in a fairly straightforward descending order of importance. Ii education, then, is idea centred, and if these ideas, eternal and unchanging, shape the pattern of world, they necessarily become educational essentials. This does not mean, however, that physical education and vocational education are unimportant, but it does mean that they will undoubtedly occupy lower lungs on the educational ladder.

Physical Education as a Term

It was explained earlier that the experimentalist is most dissatisfied with the name physical education, whereas the realist would have no objection at all to the use of this term to describe this specialized area's function within the total educational pattern. If the idealistic physical educator were to examine himself and this philosophical tendency, he would probably be forced to admit that the term physical education is at least partially acceptable to him. Idealists speak of the organic unity of an individual and refer to man as a unitary being. They find themselves in a most difficult position, if they accept a dualistic theory of the nature of man which divides him into mind and body. They have therefore accepted a monastic approach, because the believe that it is necessary for mind to be active ceaselessly as it attempts to comprehend the world. They marvel at the growth and development of the physical organism as well and realize how necessary a healthy body is for the acquisition of life's higher values.

Hence, from one standpoint, the name physical education is quite acceptable and descriptive of the role that physical, health and recreation education fills within the educational pattern. From another standpoint, however, this term is not acceptable at all. According to the idealistic view, personality has ultimate worth, and the growth of this personality is paramount. The achievement of a cultivated personality is dependent partly on our inherited disposition, partly on the training and experiences we have had, and partly upon our choices, based upon reflection, of ideals to follow. Many physical educators, raised in the idealistic tradition, believe fervently that physical, health and recreation education has a truly significant role to play in the development of personality and character. For this reason, many are, and should be, dissatisfied with the term physical education as being descriptive of the function of the area within education.

Plato on Physical Education

A discussion of the implications of idealism for physical, health and recreation education that did not return to a consideration of the contributions of Plato to thought on this matter would be seriously lacking. Burke points out that "the definitive element of Idealism is its viewpoint that reality lies essentially in the realm of mind and spirit."

The field of physical, health and recreation education owes much to a major work written by Cahn in 1941. In great detail he presented that contributions of Plato to thought in our specialized area. He believed that a system of physical education was closely related to the sociological influences of that period in the history of ancient Athens. Plato's beliefs concerning physical education were seemingly determined by his conception of the answer to the purpose of life. Man's function is to live as closely as possible with the divine laws which govern the universe. A reasonable man would use physical education activities to assist him in the development of a good life. Such a physical-education program was vitally concerned with the individual's goals in life: moreover, any program of education which neglected it was markedly deficient.

Plato's aesthetic ideal envisioned the harmony of a beautiful form—a some what different concept than the Roman men sana in corporate sano. As Cahn saw it, "the Platonic ideal is more subtle and graceful; it suggests a keener intellect, combined with a poised power capable of acting quickly with the dignity of ease and beauty". An individual who endeavoured to approximate this ideal would certainly agree with Socrates when he "what a disgrace it is for man to grow old without ever seeing the beauty and strength of which his body is capable".

Christianity Influenced Physical Education Adversely

It is not our purpose at this point to trace idealistic influence on physical education in any detail historically, but it may be said that early Christian idealism furthered the dualism of mind and body—a concept which has had detrimental effects on physical education ever since. Furthermore, the doctrine of original sin, with the possibility of ultimate salvation if asceticism were practised, negated the fostering of the Greek ideal for well over a thousand years. It was not until the period of the Renaissance and the advent of certain humanistic educators that a rebirth of the Graco-Roman ideal to any extent became apparent. Despite the tremendous negative influence which Christianity has exerted on physical education in the past, there is considerable evidence that this situation has been improving gradually in the United States in the past hundred years.

Leaders in the Young Men's Christian Association movement just after the middle of the nineteenth century realized that physical education and athletics were very attractive to young men. Their objectives mentioned the improvement of physical status. An idealistic concept of physical education became apparent as man was viewed as an organic unity. Athletic activity in YMCA gymnasia was believed to exert a definite influence on the development of Christian character.

Idealism in American Physical Education

Early physical-education leaders such as Dudley Allen Sargent and William Gilbert Anderson may be said to have developed the thread of idealism present in American physical education as well. Sarget with his various resting devices whereby the individual might assess his own ability and development, had a great influence on physical education in the United States. He fostered the concept of self-realization through diligent application to the necessary prerequisites.

Burke Assesses Idealism in the Twentieth Century

Idealism in the twentieth century is assessed very cogently by Burke when he enumerates some of the characteristics of this philosophical tendency as: (i) reaffirmation of the principle of dualism between body and mind; (ii) the belief that values and moral standards are enduring and unchangeable; (iii) the concept that a liberal education is paramount because through it a man learns to appreciate life's true values as well as the ability to reason correctly; and (iv) the realization that man, actually a part of the Divine, is much more than an animal or some sort of a mechanism.

Burke explains further that idealism would definitely favour physical education to a considerable degree because of the status accorded it in Greek idealism; because of the transfer of training theory which implies that attitudes of sportsmanship and fair play learned through desirable athletic competition can and do transfer to life situations; and because idealistic emphasis on striving for perfection through achievement of the values of truth, beauty and goodness does not completely negate physical fitness and sound health—merely places them somewhat lower in a hierarchy of desirable aims and objectives in life. Now that we have discussed the purpose of this chapter generally, and also somewhat specifically in regard to some of the historical implications of idealism for physical education, it is time to consider some of the viewpoints on this matter as it has appeared in fairly recent literature and research.

Work of Margaret Clark Gannett

Special mention should be made again of the truly significant contribution made by Margaret Clark Gannett in 1943 when she attempted the philosophical interpretation of a program of physical education in a state teachers college. This appears to have been the first philosophical research of its type in the history of American physical education. Mrs. Gannett realized that physical education needed philosophical treatment, and, furthermore, she dared to treat physical education philosophically. As is so often the case with pioneering ventures, her complex analysis received little recognition by the field of health, physical education and recreation. She would probably the one of the first to recognize the limitation of her study. This writer wishes, however, to pay tribute to her effort and to those from whom she received guidance.

Voices for Idealism

Those who feel that idealism is on the wane and that consequently its influence on physical, health and recreation education is not worthy of much attention may be reflecting their own opinions, but they are obviously not fully aware of the many voices that are being raised in its behalf recently. For example, it may be pointed out that during World War II every effort was made to continue a competitive athletic program for as many young men as possible. It is true that pragmatism can take some credit for this retention. Because of its value pragmatically, it is probably also true, as Bair indicates, that "the retention of competition as a persistent value indeed an idealistic measure of stability relating to programs of physical education". When the Korean conflict came along so soon, physical educators apparently did not see the need to revert to an emergency fitness program that would of necessity sacrifice program enrichment.

In the 1951 report of the National Conference for the Mobilization of Education stress was placed on physical-education opportunities which would bring about organic and moral development of the individual. The importance of successful experience in a variety of motor activities was considered highly desirable. Such statements undoubtedly show idealism's continuing influence on our educational programs.

A Dual Influence and Eclecticism

Bair's study, in which he made an effort to identify some of the philosophical beliefs held by influential professional leaders in American physical education, was completed in 1956. Although there would be a division of opinion regarding his grouping of the four philosophies included two what he defines as naturalism and spiritualism, his findings have significance for us as we consider idealistic influence. The evidence clearly points to the persistent, pervading influence of idealism. A careful examination of Bair's findings, however, does show an eclecticism which would be considered by many to be philosophically indefensible. This writer hastens to say again that we should not expect our leaders to be purely anything—that is, wholly and purely idealistic, or realistic, or experimentalistic. But in the second half of the twentieth century we will need increasingly logical, consistent and sequential philosophical positions on the part of individuals and segments of our field. As professional educators, we can settle for no less.

Influence of the YMCA

The Young Men's Christian Association has exerted a significant influence throughout the world on health, physical education, and recreation. This influence has emanated from an idealistic base. In 1960 the theme of the World YMCA Consultation on Health and Physical Education, held at Rome in connection with the Olympic games, was Health and Physical Education—YMCA Practice and Purpose. At this important meeting, delegates from twenty-one national YMCA's in all five continents heard discussions from outstanding leaders of the movement concerning purpose and practice.

Steinhaus explained that "the concept of the mind-body-spirit unity of man is today a basic tenet of all sciences dealing with man, and also of education." Because of this, he stated his belief that "every impact of man on man or of programme on man invariably does influence in some way man's body, man's mind, man's spirit." Steinhaus means in this statement that a physical activity leaves its influence on the whole man, and there is a strong inference that the leader has a great deal to do with whether this influence is for good or for bad.

Friermood Lists Five Objectives

In another important paper presented at Rome, Harold T. Friermood, U.S. national YMCA secretary for physical education, assessed the role of physical education as an integral part of the YMCA program. He listed the five objectives for physical education which appeared in a publication resulting from a two-year study in the United States:

i. Development of health and physical fitness

ii. Education for leisure

iii. Personality adjustment

iv. Development of responsible citizenship and group participation

v. Development of a philosophy of life based on Christian ideals.

Pointing out that people are more important than the program tools, he explained that "things can happen in the life of a person that are just as significant for him in gymnasium, in the locker room, or on a hike as in a bible class." R.W. Jones of the United Kingdom, director of the

UNESCO Youth Institute, sounded a warning at Rome concerning "growing specialization" in sport.

The Fellowship of Christian Athletes

Organized Christianity has taken the role of sport much more seriously in recent years as well. One important indication of this interest has been the recent establishment and rapid development of the Fellowship of Christian Athletes. This organization was an idea in the mind of a sophomore physical-education major at Oklahoma State University in 1947. Subsequently, Don McLanen and a Presbyterian minister, Dr. Louis H. Evans, formed an advisory board in May of 1955. From this small beginning, and with the help of Branch Rickey of baseball fame, this group has made remarkable gains.

The main office of the Fellowship of Christian Athletes, Inc. is located in Kansas City, Missouri. It "exists to serve Christ and the Church. Its concern is to draw athletes in particular and youth in general into the realm and experience of vital Christian commitment within the Church". It is interesting to note the ecumenical nature of this movement. Dr. Samuel Shoemaker stresses that "loyalty to one's own church is stressed in the movements, but one is exposed to a great many who belong to other households of faith". Vance Morris, assistant football coach, Excelsor Springs, Missouri, writing in the FCA publication The Christian Athlete, states a fundamental idealistic tenant in a recent article, when he encourages athletes to strive for that same perfection that we seek on our athletic teams in our individual lives.

Jaarsma Sounds a Warning

Although athletics are recommended as a source from which good can come, there are many Christian educators who are most concerned about the ever-present possibility of overemphasis. Professor Cornelius Jaarsma, Grand Rapids, Michigan, states that "in selecting a physical education program the teacher must remember not to overemphasize competitive games". His first concern in this matter is that a certain percentage of the student body will be left out of an activity that is important in their overall development, whereas "others may become demoralized by repeated failure". Secondly, he stresses that interscholastic athletics may become a real stumbling block as we work toward the aim of a fine physical-education program for all.

Physical Education Does Have a Place

Jaarsma, of course, is concerned primarily with the Christian school as a setting for learning. He explains how "in Christian education the learner is viewed as a child in Christ, the goal is a formed personality as a son of God, and the body of subject matter is the learning material appropriate to the subject and the goal". Now what about the role of physical education? Although Jaarsma has been careful to restate that "subject matter is the principal medium for development in the school", he does believe that physical education falls within its legitimate scope.

Steen Stresses Values

Steen, director of physical education at Calvin College, bears out this idealistic philosophy of physical education as he describes the program at this institution. Emphasizing the concept of the unitary nature of man, he states his belief that physical education offers physical values, mental values, guidance toward ethical standards, and desirable recreational skills and attitudes. These beliefs appears to be borne out, with some exception, in a study conducted by Lozes in which she discovered that "the philosophy of physical education, as proposed by the eleven church-related institutions visited, stressed the integration, recreation and physical purposes of physical education, and gave less emphasis to the social and mental purposes".

Moral and Spiritual Values in Education

The whole question of moral and spiritual values in education has been a persistent problem in America.

Because of differences in religious belief, and the seeming impossibility of achieving any consensus as to what might be included in a course on comparative religion, public schools have remained almost completely secularized in this important matter insofar as direct teaching is concerned. It is generally understood, however, that the school does attempt to teach morals indirectly in a definitely incidental manner. Those who do not believe this matter can be handled effectively in such a seemingly haphazard fashion have found other means to meet this need. Those of us concerned with public education, and in this case especially with physical, health and recreation education, should understand how some educators believe this problem can be solved to a degree through the medium of our specialized area.

Physical Education Contributes

As far back as 1929, several important educational leaders expressed themselves in an idealistic manner on this subject. Henry S. Pritchett, a former president of the Carnegie Foundation for the Advancement of Learning stated that "for the sake of every youth whom school and college sport touches, the desired moral and social values that it can yield must be made realities". In the same year Professor Matthias of the University of Munich explained that we should "consider Physical Education as it affects the body, and then consider the effects as they manifest themselves upon the soul experiences of man".

General Respect for Religious Beliefs

Despite the many materialistic influences of the twentieth century, a strong idealistic current has persisted in the United States—a country which is largely Christian, although sprinkled with members of other faiths. Traditionally, the American public school has shown a respect for religious beliefs. Our Constitution and Bill of Rights are stated in such a way that religious ideals are recognized as a part of the culture, although it should be stated quickly that each person may worship God as he sees fit. The fact that there are more than 240 different religious groups in ample evidence that this right is generally recognized.

Yet, conversely, although a person does have a right to be agnostic or avowedly atheistic, he had better not be a presidential candidate once having declared such a position.

A National Report on Values

In a country such as this with such a strong religious base, it is little wonder that the question of moral and spiritual values would be such a recurrent theme when educational policy is being considered. This is true despite the fact that global warfare tends to lessen ethical sensitivity and that moral and spiritual values must be inculcated indirectly in our public schools because of misunderstanding and distrust. It was no accident that the Educational Policies Commission of the National Education Association and the American Association of School Administrators published a report on moral and spiritual values in the public schools. Classroom teachers were concerned about their role in this matter and asked that a study be made to develop ways of improving the teaching of such values.

The commission listed a number of values on which the American people are agreed. Idealists will rejoice in the assertion that the basic value of human personality is fundamental to all that follow. As the report states, "the basic moral and spiritual value in American life is the supreme importance of the individual personality". A complete listing of these values follows:

i. The supreme importance of the individual personality.

ii. Each person should feel responsible for the consequences of his own conduct.

iii. Institutional arrangements are the servants of mankind.

iv. Mutual consent is better than violence.

v. The human mind should be liberated by access to information and opinion.

vi. Excellence in mind, character and creative ability should be fostered.

vii. All persons should be judged by the same moral standards.

viii. The concept of brotherhood should take precedence over selfish interests.

ix. Each person should have the greatest possible opportunity for the pursuit of happiness, provided only that such activities do not substantially interfere with the similar opportunities of others.

x. Each person should be offered the emotional and spiritual experiences which transcend the materialistic aspects of life.

Sport has a Place

This report of the Educational Policies Commission goes on to say that all of the resources of the school should be used whenever possible to teach the above-mentioned moral and spiritual values. Of interest to us in physical, health and recreation education is that the members of the Commission believe that sports have a vital role to play in such instruction, and that the teacher of sports is usually one of the most influential members of the school community in the shaping of moral and spiritual values.

A Continuing Emphasis on Values

That there has been a continuing emphasis on the moral and spiritual values that may be gained by the individual through participation in physical-education activities is readily noticeable from an examination of the literature in recent years. Of course, idealists cannot take all the credit for this; the experimentalist would argue that values are man made in an effort to serve man's own ends. They are derived from experience and represent instruments which make possible effective functioning within our environment. An idealistic value system comes into the picture only when the individuals concerned believe that their value system is grounded on objective values of truth, goodness, and beauty that are embedded in reality itself.

The man who seeks diligently to apprehend these values is leading a good life insofar as his own quest for these values succeeds, and presumably insofar as he helps others to realize these values for themselves.

Resick on Values

Resick appears to be following in the idealistic tradition when he explained how physical education activities could conceivably contribute to each of the ten values listed in the report of the Educational Policies Commission. A particularly idealistic strain is evident when he writes about spiritual enrichment. He explains that "the word spiritual here denotes the highest level of the capacity of the human spirit". And then he gives his approval to a statement that "the prime value of the game is the spiritual life it affords through the liberation of powers and its secondary value is the feeling of physical well-being that ensues."

Wiston's Status Survey

In 1956, Wilton completed a most significant study in which he made a comparative analysis of certain statements made by important leaders in American physical education in relation to the moral and spiritual values which they felt their subject afforded. He accepted the listing of moral and spiritual values offered by the Educational Policies Commission and subsequently made comparisons between these values and the statements attributed to the outstanding physical educators. Because youth is interested in play and sport proficiency, Wilton reasoned that the play leader has a unique opportunity to encourage proper moral and spiritual growth. His hypothesis was that statements discovered would show that physical educators agree that their subject should be charged with the responsibility of improving young people and that teaching for the improvement of moral and spiritual values should be a planned part of physical education. It may well be argued by some that these values described could be considered experimentalistic ethical values as well.

The term moral values would probably satisfy the experimentalist and at the same time not offend the idealist. But spiritual values as defined by Wilton definitely coincide with idealistic philosophy of education. Idealists may gather strength from Wilton's summary and conclusions that the seventeen leaders picked a jury of experts ratified his hypothesis that physical education experiences are of real value in the development of moral and spiritual values. Under the pursuit of happiness the leaders believed that creative experience, noble achievement, true friendship, and spiritual satisfaction are encouraged by physical education. He found further that spiritual enrichment a term not associated with physical education typically, was enhanced greatly according to the opinions of the outstanding leaders.

Oberteuffer Explains Idealism

Writing on the subject of idealism in physical eduction, Oberteuffer emphasized many of the tenets of this position heretofore mentioned. Stressing initially that man is real but is really only when the mind and soul are included, and that he should be perceived as a whole, as an organic unity, Oberteuffer pointed out that this unity is the most powerful concept ever to bear upon what we do in physical education. It traps us completely denies us forever the doubtful privilege of not caring what happens to our charges as long as they grow strong, or perform well.

Starting from such a base he stated that the idealistic curriculum will not be child-centred, or subject-matter centred—but ideal-centred. Then he criticized certain modern trends and emphases in physical education. For example, he questioned the wisdom of testing a million children with a dynamometer without at the same time developing a solid program of total development to orient the test scores with some kind of relationship to things which are really important. He discussed the matter of the individual's interests and the moral imperative which is part of idealistic philosophy. Decrying twentieth century exploitation of the college athlete, he indicated that we cannot be satisfied with scores instead of character, and that we should leave competitive sport to a large degree in the hands of the boys.

It is sportsmanship and ethical choice that are important Bodily development is a means to an end leading to truth, beauty and goodness. Creative expression on the part of the individual is a worthy means whereby the idealist hopes to achieve his educational goals. As Oberteuffer concludes, "self-activity leading to self-development involving the total self is to the idealist the important thing".

Mabel Lee's Position

Before concluding this section treating the implications of idealism for physical education, the views of one more physical educator should be considered—the venerable Mable Lee, former director of physical education for women at the University of Nebraska. Morland has classified Miss Lee as an essentialist—of this there appears to be little doubt. Our premise here is that many of her beliefs were indeed idealistic. It is for this reason that she herself might say, "so most probably I am an essentialist in some respects and a progressivist about others". Let us consider some of her statements briefly.

In speaking about "fitness and the good life", she says that the "physically inadequate" will never receive the spiritual uplift from outdoor living. She stresses the need for physical reserve in life when she states, "whether of the body or of the spirit, burdens are more easily borne if there is a physical reserve. Build the more stately mansions, O my soul, is meant for both the body and the spirit". We need fitness to enjoy life to its fullest, physically, emotionally or spiritually. She and her co-author concur with a list of values which includes the value of spiritual and ethical character. In speaking about public relations, Morland summarizes her belief that it will take the combined efforts of the entire profession if the deeper meaning of physical education is to be realized by those who have such a large voice in determining the success of future programs.

Morland's Analysis of Lee

Stressing the importance of disciplined work, Lee criticizes those who advocate false philosophies such as physical education that is purely recreational in nature. The best type of teacher, she asserts, will insist upon disciplined training of the body. Such training has a spiritual as well as a physical value. Morland points out Lee's belief that good posture for instance, is considered as having direct spiritual, social, economic and health value. On the question of the philosophy of awards, Lee believes that the Greeks had the right idea. She states that even parents are coming to realize that it is a poor training to motivate children to favourable action by the hope of reward other than the spiritual recompense that comes from the satisfaction of having acted favourably. Dr. Lee sums up her beliefs about herself when she says, "I know I am an idealist, or I would not feel as strongly as I do against women teachers drinking and smoking but I also know I am a realist or I would not all these years in my professional work have seized upon every opportunity to present my idealistic views on the subject to young women in our profession".

From her many statements it is not possible to classify Dr. Lee as a pure idealist by any means. Her self-avowed eclecticism seems to hit the mark, but the balance is shifted very definitely to the side of essentialism. In the statement above she appears to equate idealism with high ideals and realism with practical common sense. Only in the past few years have any of our outstanding leaders begun to consider philosophy in a formal sense. Hence it appears that Morland's study is most helpful in that it arrived at philosophical classification from the delineation of practices.

Implications for Health Education

And now what about the implications of idealistic philosophy of education for health education? This is quite difficult to analyse, and there has been very little philosophical interpretation in this area which is rooted in medicine, public health, and education. There have been many disagreements by various leaders in regard to aims and objectives, curriculum content, and teaching methodology.

Cahn on Plato

Cahn, in delineating the thought of Plato on health, refers to health as a "dynamic equilibrium" between all inner and outer forces with the object of having an individual at harmony with himself and society. Any program designed to maintain and improve health should result from the application of a logical approach to everyday health problems—a continuous, never-ending process both for individual man and the community in which he lives. We should never think of a man and society as separate; a program of health education must be continually aware of this union.

A Seeming Contradiction

A very helpful statement of the idealist's position in the matter of health and health education comes from Horne. He begins by omitting it under a discussion of the essential studies except where it might be included incidentally under biology but then mentions health first in a list of nine basic values of human living. In another work, he mentions health by his first three answers to the question, "Are we educated?" He states that the truly educated individual should be physically fit, should live near the maximum of his efficiency and should have a body which is the ready servant of his will. How can we explain this seeming contradiction? The answer is that we must reconsider the idealist's aim of education.

Idealistic Stresses

In Margaret Clark Gannett's philosophical interpretation of a program of health, physical education, and recreation, she concluded that certain idealistic stresses were noted and that these were the concept of building wholeness of mind and body, the development of strong, healthy bodies, good habits of mental and physical health, and the right start in the teaching of health, safety, and physical education to children.

Downey's 1956 study

In 1956 Downey completed a study in which he attempted to identify the philosophical beliefs of certain teacher educators in the field of health education. One of the questions he asked was, "What are the dominant emphases in the basic beliefs of these educators with special reference to idealism, pragmatism, and realism?" He devised a Teacher Education Beliefs Indicator for Health Education and used it as a tool. He validated his instrument for accuracy and then established criteria which would indicate influences and possible directions in the field.

Although the chief influence being exerted in teacher education was pragmatic, a lesser influence was connected with the idealistic view especially in relation to methods, directed teaching, field experiences, and facilities and equipment. It is notable that there seemed to be disagreements in regard to the objectives and values of health, as well as in the role of the teacher educator. This gives some credence to the belief that idealistic views still exert a certain amount of influence.

Limbert on Health

Paul Limbert, speaking at the Fifth World YMCA Consultation on Health and Physical Education in Rome, September 12-14, 1960, pointed out that "the YMCA emphasis on health and physical education is rooted in a Christian understanding of man and his world". He asked the question, "How could the objectives of health and physical education in the YMCA be rephrased to show more clearly how this programme is grounded in Christian faith?" He continued by asking YMCA leaders to work for a larger measure of integration in the individual by promoting more intensive study of the body, leading to scientific knowledge: anatomy, body chemistry, hygiene, physiology, etc.; and attention to sex characteristics and habits, leading to a greater understanding of the place of sex in human life, with implications for hygiene. Commenting at this consultation, Thomson stated that the contribution which physical exercise makes toward good health is recognized.

Writing about the physical values to be derived from a program of physical education, Steen speaks about the healthful gifts produced by large muscle activity and that exercise helps prevent bodily injury, aids in medical restoration, and promotes desirable emotional release. Furthermore, he states that adequate diet, rest, health habits, and emotional stability are part of healthful living, but they are not complete without exercise.

Bennett Describes Mormon Position

The Church of Jesus Christ of Latter-Day Saints, of all the various religions and denominations therein, appears to be taking the strongest position in regard to the care of the body.

The Service Program

Despite all these statements which emphasize the beliefs of idealists concerning the importance of a healthy body, it still appears evident that good health is at the bottom of the hierarchy of life's many values. Yet, as he also indicated, it is esteemed very highly by the idealist as a basic value. Could this perhaps be the reason why the required program of health and physical education in American schools and colleges has been known as the service program? In this conception it provides a service to man by its contribution to his health thereby enabling him to pursue higher educational goals.

The Role of School Recreation

Lastly under the aims and objectives of the educational philosophy of idealism, the role of recreation in the school will be considered. The position here is not clear-cut and decisive because of the somewhat borderline status on the spectrum which idealism occupies. However, idealistic philosophy of education does belong more correctly on the essentialitic side of the spectrûm because of its concern with educational essentials. The importance of recreation and play in idealistic philosophy of education has perhaps not been fully understood or appreciated in the past. Their role in the development of the personality and the perfectly integrated individual is looming larger with each passing year. It is for this reason that a person subscribing to idealistic philosophy of education should reassess the contributions that recreation and play can do make in the education of man. That there is a great need for educational research along these lines is self-evident.

The Public Image is Blurred

Another difficulty that we encounter at this point is that it is often difficult to differentiate between physical education and recreation. One reason for this is that the public in the early twentieth century, and today for that matter in many instances, still thinks of physical education as being synonymous with physical recreation and vice versa. This belief has caused untold hardship for the physical educator who attempts to explain that it is just as difficult to teach his subject well as almost any other subject in the curriculum. People think typically that his task is to give a few exercises and then roll out the ball. The recreator has experienced great hardship also because he has difficulty explaining that his program involves more than physical recreation—that it consists of meeting the child's social, communicative, aesthetic and creative, and learning interests as well.

We are considering the role of physical, health, and recreation-education teacher in schools and colleges. Thus, we believe that this person should be responsible for physical recreation only in a direct way. In an indirect way, he should meet all the other recreational needs and interests of boys and girls by working cooperatively with the recreation administrator at all times.

A Compatible Theory of Play?

One other matter should perhaps be clarified at this point; however, it is extremely difficult to state that this or that theory of play seems to coincide identically with idealistic philosophy of education. We should be able to get some help in this connection by reviewing very briefly the idealistic view. In the first place, the ultimate worth of personality is paramount, and the highest virtue is respect for that personality. Idealists marvel at the growth of man's physical organism, but they are even more amazed by the growth of man's spirit. In the light of such a statement embodying man's uniqueness among all the creatures of the world—and because of his infinite possibilities for growth and for the acquisition of the ideal virtues, as well as the concept of the unity of the organism—it would seem that idealists might view very closely any theories of recreation and play which grant educational possibilities to these activities of man. This is not to say that instinct-based theories of play would be automatically eliminated.

The Self-Expression Theory of Play

Sapora and Mitchell devoted an entire chapter to the underlying theory of play and recreation. The five traditional theories of play described are the surplus energy theory, the recreation theory, the relaxation theory, the instinct-practice theory, and the catharsis theory. Each one considered individually seems to have merit, but none seems to provide the whole answer. It is quite possible that we will never have a completely satisfactory explanation. It is certain, however, that there will continue to be research conducted along these lines. The newer self-expression theory of play explained in detail in Sapora and Mitchell borrows from the traditional theories and yet combines, refines and clarifies. It begins by listing what appear to be facts which are basic to a modern theory of play. They are:

(i) that man is an active, dynamic creature;

(ii) that the physiological and anatomical structure of the organism predispose it to certain kinds of activity;

(iii) that the physical fitness of the organism has an effect upon the type of activity it engages in; and

(iv) that the psychological inclinations of the individual predispose him toward certain types of activity.

From this underlying reasoning the self-expression theory is developed, since this is postulated as the chief need in man's life—to achieve the satisfaction and accomplishment of self-expression of one's own personality. Here is an explanation that seems to consider quite fully the conception of man as an organic unity—a total organism. Many aspects of it seem compatible with idealistic philosophy of education, and yet it appears much more progressive than the dualistic theory of work and play of the strict essentialist which characterizes play only as a relief from work, as a means of using up surplus energy, and as a means of recreation, so that the individual may again be ready for the many types of work in which most men become involved.

Other Pertinent Factors

The preceding explanation is, of course, all very interesting. It gathers still further strength when other points of analysis are offered as follows: (i) the role of habit in play, which indicates that throughout the life the individual is inclined toward those activities which are habitual to him; (ii) the role of social contact in habit formation; (iii) the role of the physical environment as a limiting factor in the choice of recreational activity; and (iv) the role of universal wishes, which implies that all mankind may have universal motives or common desires such as the wishes for new experience, for security, for response, and for recognition, not to mention the wish for participation and for the aesthetic. We may ask at this point how these wishes differ from instincts. You may think that we are right back again where we started. It does appear that the naturalistic realist might regard these wishes as instinctive, and the pragmatic experimentalist would tend to view them as being determined as a result of experience.

The idealist, however, would probably revert to the theory of human nature which he holds and consequently look for those aspects of this self-expression theory which seem promising to him.

Recreation and the Eternal Values

You will recall that idealists believe generally that mind as experienced by all men is basic and real, and that the entire universe is mind essentially. Mind is the true reality. They believe further that man possesses a soul and is therefore of a higher order than all other creatures on earth. Without going again into the problem as to whether a particular idealist is a spiritual monist or pluralist, each of these various positions grants man freedom of will to determine which way his life shall go. Without reviewing again idealistic theories of knowledge acquisition and logic, we shall conclude this discussion by explaining that the idealist believes man is a propulsive being who is striving to achieve the values which are embedded in reality itself.

To the extent that the idealist can realize the eternal values through the choice of the right kinds of play and recreation without flouting the moral order in the world, he will be progressive enough to disregard a dualistic theory of work and play—a theory that has plagued us in the United States right down to the present day.

Plato on Play

As we now turn to some of the specific statements displaying idealistic beliefs regarding the values of play and recreation, we shall examine first, albeit very briefly, the essence of Plato's contribution to thought on this matter. In the first place, Plato had no intention of allowing play to be left to whim and fancy. Play or recreation of any sort, from children's games to behaviour at banquets, was a serious matter for the legislature. To make certain of this, he recommended that children should be under the very careful supervision of teachers at a very early age. He felt that the characters of future citizens are formed through their childhood games, and that play must be, therefore, most carefully utilized and supervised by the state. Cahn made one other extremely important point which Plato believed about recreation which coincides with certain present-day theories about its place in life as follows: "Recreation, the activity of leisure, is a necessary alternate with toil to balance the daily life to permit the growth of the integrated man within society".

Mixed Motives

Earlier in this chapter it was pointed out that early Christian idealism furthered the concept of the dualism of mind and body and that this has exerted a detrimental influence on physical education ever since. The same observation may be made about this influence on the development of physical and social-recreation interests at least, but it is very evident that attitudes toward all types of recreational activities, as well as sports and games, have been improving steadily with some exceptions throughout the twentieth century. It is not completely clear in some instances whether such affairs are being tolerated, are being exploited for the attraction that they hold for youth and adults, or whether their contribution to the achievement of integrated personality is being fully realized. Let us now examine some of the statements in the literature to help us make up our minds.

The Methodist Church and Recreation

Bennett describes briefly the history of the Methodist Church's attitude toward recreation. A specific list of sinful amusements was repealed in 1924, when the church reverted to Westley's original prohibition which is printed in the most recent Methodist Discipline. Members were urged to refrain from the taking of such diversions as cannot be used in the name of the Lord Jesus. Despite such prohibitions, Bennett does go on to say that such regulations were not actually carried out or even endorsed by all concerned.

Bennett on Recreation's Role

Bennett, himself a Presbyterian, believes strongly that recreation under religious sponsorship can serve to help the American people improve moral and ethical standards, but with the exception of the Church of Jesus Christ of Latter-Day Saints which does view the body as a non-evil component of the eternal soul of man and anticipates literal resurrection after death, he believes that Protestant churches are unsure of their role in this area and that the quality of recreational leadership and opportunity provided varies greatly within individual churches.

Lozes's Survey

There are distinct signs, however, that specific denominations are becoming increasingly aware of the role that recreation can play in the promulgation of the Christian idealistic way of life. In 1955, Lozes completed a study of the philosophy of certain religious denominations relative to physical education and the effect of this philosophy on physical education in certain church-related institutions. She visited and interviewed administrative personnel at eleven church-related institutions of higher learning and received additional information by written inquiry to thirteen other church-related institutions.

Interestingly enough, the purpose which the largest number of presidents, or their representatives, and also the largest number of physical education directors stated was to provide recreation for the students. In the main, also, it was felt that the religious denomination did have a definite influence on the physical-education program. Presidents tended to emphasize the physical, the integrational, and the recreational purposes of physical education, while the physical education department heads stressed the recreational purposes, integrational purposes, physical purposes, mental purposes and social purposes in that order. The majority of presidents and eight of the physical directors believed that physical education was equal in importance to other college subjects. Of interest, to our discussion at the moment was the statement by Lozes that "there did not seem to be a mind-body philosophy peculiar to a particular religious denomination unless it might be the lower hierarchy of the physical faculties mentioned by two Catholic institutions."

It was indicated further that the relatively lower status of physical education seemed to be due to academic influence more than to religious influence.

An Increased Awareness of Recreation's Role

In 1956, the Christian Education Commission of the Church of the Brethren published an entire volume entitled Recreation and the Local Church. A publication such as this shows an increased awareness of the role that recreation can play in the life of a Christian. Clemens, Tully and Crill make it very clear.

Wilton's analysis of Theories

Wilton's study completed in this same year made a comparative analysis of theories related to moral and spiritual values in physical education.

Christian Recreation

Body discussed the subject Recreation and the Faiths—The Southern Baptist Church Recreation Philosophy at Work at the 42nd National Recreation Congress held in Washington, D.C., September 25-29, 1960.

Divided Jewish Opinion

Bennett has indicated that "it seems apparent that physical education and sports are rather distant from the heart of Jewish religious life", and that the Jewish rabbis and synagogues have somewhat reluctantly recognized the need for the Jewish Centres which have largely supplanted the earlier Young Men's Hebrew Associations. Yet it would seem that there is a difference of opinion on this matter depending on whether the position is being stated by an Orthodox, Conservative or Reform Jew, Speaking at the AAHPER convention in Cincinnati, April 9, 1962, Rabbi D. J. Silver, a Reform Jew, spoke beautifully on the use of leisure in a truly idealistic vein. Explaining how the Jews had architected the Sabbath as a day of leisure, he emphasized that this should be pleasure with a purpose. He urged that we think of the whole man and his role in society. He asked the recreators assembled not to destroy the uniqueness of man; to put the whole of the world before the child and before the adult; and to fire the child with enthusiasm for life and learning. His message was a distinct challenge in that he pointed out how recreation could serve to carry out God's purpose for men on earth.

Historical Background

Turning aside from some of the statements of certain religious groups regarding the role of recreation in the educational process, we will now very briefly trace the development of the play and recreation movement in the United States with a cursory examination of some of the changing views of leisure down through the ages. It has been stated by Martin and Esther Neumeyer that no systematic theories of leisure or play developed until toward the end of the nineteenth century. Yet the views held, at lest by certain classes and individuals, affected both the amount and the uses of leisure. They continue by listing five of the changing views as follows:

i. Military Conception—gymnastics, sports, games and related activities were considered fundamentally as means to an end, because the focus of attention in the long run was upon the military objective rather than the activities themselves.

ii. Sports and Physical Training—there developed a special interest in sports and games among the Greeks and Romans that was somewhat divorced from the ultimate military value. The greatest achievement of the Greeks in athletics and sports was the development of the Olympic games, which eventually became international in scope.

iii. Cultural and Art View—the Athenian ideal of a citizen was that not only of a soldier and an athlete, but an artist, philosopher and statesman as well. But the physical side was not all. The Athenians utilized their leisure in philosophical disputations in cultivating the arts of painting, sculpture, drama, and music. The Greeks never completely got away from the notion that all activity had a purpose beyond itself.

iv. Puritanical Attitude—church leaders assumed a strong reactionary attitude toward recreation, but this hostile was by no means confined to the church intellectual and political leaders during the Middle Ages and years later joined hands with the religious forces to suppress sports, games and other forms of entertainments.

v. Recognition of the Values of Play—the recognition of its value began during the Middle Ages, but it was not until the modern era that the more favourable attitude became widespread. A series of inventions, reform movements in religion, politics and education, the spirit of scientific inquiry, intellectual interests, and the developments in social thought produced gradual but effective changes in attitudes and conduct.

In the United States recognition of the values of play and recreation has been largely a twentieth-century phenomenon. Playgrounds have developed to a point where they are an integral part of American urban life. The whole recreation movement catering to the needs and interests of all ages has been a fascinating chapter in developing leisure economy. A former mayor of Detroit, for example, played a backhanded compliment to this field when faced with a transportation strike by his remark that "transportation is an important to this city as water, sewage disposal and recreation".

Recreation programs are not in effect year round and

include activities designed to meet social, aesthetic and creative, communicative and learning interests, as well as physical-recreation interests. At present, recreation is clearly one of the major social institutions in American life.

Horne on Recreation

Our concern in this section of this chapter has been primarily how play and recreation fits in which idealistic philosophy of education. In conclusion we shall present a few more statements which show evidence of idealistic import. As stated previously, Herman Harrell Horne has been a leading figure in idealistic philosophy of education in this century. That he sees an important place for recreation in the education of man is obvious from a consideration of his stated beliefs. The ideal suggests the integrated individual in an integrated society growing in the image of the integrated universe.

Values in Recreation

Discussing values in recreation in his book Recreation in the American Community, Danford stated that "the development of a higher level of moral and ethical behaviour is the problem of every man, woman and child in this nation"

Jay B. Nash and Creative Recreation

Jay B. Nash, one of the America's great leaders in recreation and physical education, felt very strongly about the values of recreation and its place in our evolving democratic system of education. If we were asked to categorize him as to his philosophical position, we would have to call him a liberal or progressive idealist. His most recent book Philosophy of Recreation and Leisure abounds with his progressive and idealistic beliefs. One of the concluding chapters of this inspirational work is entitled Recreation: A Way of Life.

Spiritual Values in Outdoor Education

Outdoor education and school camping are gradually assuming an increasingly important role in the education of America's youth. In 1959 Moseley completed a study of the philosophies of camp directors and of the opinions of campers as related to the spiritual values derived in the field of camping. Some of her findings have definite implications for the promulgation of idealistic philosophy of education. She found that directors wanted a counsellor who is qualified to bestow upon the camper an intense desire to be the best type of person he or she knows how to be. The counsellor should set the example and encourage the camper to follow.

Campers however felt a need for improved religious services, a devotional period at the end of the day, and an opportunity to feel close to God. In conclusion, a statement of philosophy associated with the role of spiritual values in the role of spiritual values in the modern day camp was presented along with various methods by which these aims and objectives might be achieved.

Brightbill and Idealism

In concluding this section on the implications for recreation education from idealistic philosophy of education, one more fine contemporary statement of a philosophy of leisure must be mentioned. Brightbill's Man and Leisure: A Philosophy of Recreation explores the problem of man's new leisure and offers his beliefs about how man can have a personally satisfying and full existence through recreative living. An analysis of this work leads the present writer to the conviction that there is a definite kinship between Nash's progressive idealism and the philosophy of Professor Brigthtbill, although Brightbill offers much that will appeal to the realist and experimentalist as well. Brightbill, as a professor of recreation at the University of Illinois, is, of course, tremendously interested in the wise use of leisure.

He sees such a way of life as vital in the enveloping Western civilization of today's world. He defines this need as a social proposition that summons action. In concluding his philosophy of recreation he re-emphasizes the great and unique role that recreation can fulfil in the future and he warns that mankind is faced with amounts to a recreational imperative.

Methodology

What teaching methods shall be idealist employ? Now that we have discussed a number of idealistic aims and objectives carefully, the next step is to shift our focus and direct our attention to the means whereby these goals may be reached. It should be readily apparent that objectives and method must concur to the highest degree possible. As we indicated earlier, it is often possible to get a certain amount of consensus about long range objectives between conflicting educational positions. The truth of this statement appears obvious when we consider, for example, the seven cardinal aims of education published originally in 1918. The difficulty arises when any attempt is made to list them in order of importance, and when the necessary teaching methods, are discussed whereby specific objectives may be achieved.

Plato and Teaching Method

We can get considerable help on idealistic teaching method initially from Cahn's analysis of the contributions of Plato to thought on physical, health and recreation education. In the first place we are told that for Plato method was the tool used to carve out the good life. Furthermore, it should at all times be subordinate to the objectives of idealistic philosophy. The various activities of the physical education program and used as a means to an end—that end being the effort of the individual to achieve the good life. So, for Plato, the teacher should not concern himself necessarily with outlining the various aspects of the curriculum in great detail, nor should he be especially conscious of using one technique as opposed to another.

The teacher should use his reason and should base his selection of a particularly activity or teaching technique on the basis of sound scientific investigation which has demonstrated validity, and of course, proper psychological methodology. Although, for example, a play attitude is especially good with children, the instructor should not forget the time-proven proverb that the hard is the good. Life presents many problems to developing youth, and the teacher should be as logical as possible in devising the means whereby youth can be prepared for what lies ahead in maturity.

Idealistic Teaching Method

In her philosophical interpretation of a program of physical education in a state teachers college, Clark presented much both directly and indirectly which gives further insight into the problem of teaching method and technique as viewed by the idealist. She concurred that there are many ways of accomplishing the ends of education. This is borne out but Butler who stated that idealists are likely to insist that they are creators and determiners of method, not devotees of some one method. Whereas the experimentalist waxes ecstatically about the concept of learning by doing. Horne does not appear quite so upset about the spectator versus participant controversy that rages about the heads of those who sit in the stands watching interscholastic or intercollegiate contests.

Clark on the Teacher's Role

Clark believed further that the teacher has a most significant role to play in the education of youth and that this is especially true in idealistic philosophy of education. The word guidance was used a number of times in such ways as students, under guidance, choose objectives, activities, textbooks, topics, for reports, and the like; and that data about students, both objectively and subjectively derived, are used for individual guidance and group planning. She mentioned that the lives and works of great leaders are used to enrich the lives and works of a younger generation.

In physical, health and recreation education this would

apply to the lives and practices of great athletes and coaches, as well as to outstanding teachers and recreation leaders. Children are great imitators, and idealistic educators make full use of this teaching aid to encourage youngsters to strive for high attainment in athletic competition. As Horne pointed out "The child through imitating others, becomes aware of his own capacity for a wide variety of acts that he otherwise would have believed were beyond his powers."

Other Idealistic Stresses

A few remaining idealistic stresses according to Clark give still further insight into recommended teaching method. The idealist places great emphasis on the development of certain life values that stimulate desirable personality growth. One of these is a strong, healthy body. Such a body is developed and maintained only through vigorous exercise of a regular nature throughout life. Secondly, good habits of mental and physical health are necessary. It is essential to make the right start in the teaching of health, safety and physical education to children. Lastly, they should become skilful, have a reasonable amount of success, and get a lot of fund through physical activity. The idealistic physical educator, anxious to develop these life values, should give careful consideration to interest, effort and discipline as educational techniques. Interest is, of course, most important, but the idealist has discovered that it alone will not suffice to accomplish all the educational objectives necessary. It must often be supplemented by discipline in such a way that the student will respond with the effort needed to get the job done, whatever the responsibility may be.

Furthermore, when discipline is invoked to cause the student to respond with effort, he may well discover in a short while that his interest has been aroused. Approaching the task of education from the standpoint of interest only appears to be an extremely slow and costly method.

9

PLAY AND SPORTS—ALLIANCE WITH FITNESS & PHYSICAL EDUCATION

Why do you play? Is it for health, fun or social relationship? Are you satisfied with these answers? Are there other possibilities? Do these reasons accurately explain your presence in sport? Why do you play? Health, fun, and social contact, among other factors, are utilized by many as short but sufficient solutions to the question of "why I play". It is difficult to find individuals who do not have logical explanations for an activity, it seems that nearly everybody knows why he plays. Historically, play precedes any formalized teaching. It precedes compilation of a body of knowledge which might constitute a discipline.

Children play. Aboriginal tribesmen play. Animal play. And they all play without any sophisticated notions of why they should. Play is a more primary category than play for education, than play for health and fitness, than play for social acquaintances. Individually, the physical education professional person generally encounters the intrigue of play prior to coming to any decision to pursue a career in the field. Much of the fervour which is at times apparent in the actions of the teacher usually stems from an exciting encounter, either past at present, with some form of play. The instructor knows this enjoyment to be a part of his own history, and he often continues to recreate the actual engagement of sport or dance throughout his active life. Empirically, most of the research in physical education relates to play—how one can participate with greater skill or for a longer time, how one can train better and learn faster; or how can play more safely.

It seems then, that play is the cornerstone of the profession of the professional man, and of the field's scientific research. Play precedes all of the superstructure which develops around it. Given the significance of play and the number of statements which purport to describe this relationship between man, play and the profession, it is a curious fact that so little attention is now directed toward this issue. It is paradoxical that physical education, based on play, should house several scientific and humanistic branches which at this time seems to consider themselves self-sufficient, intellectual disciplines apart from ties with actual activity. It seems that the end of research—an understanding of play in all of its parameters, both scientific and humanistic—has been forgotten and the means have become a new goal. Statistics are exciting; scientific research is a challenge; philosophical and historical study command a compelling interest.

Yet the priority, play, remains forgotten in the background. Play, which initiated the profession, lies buried under mounds of research and academic discussion. It remains the victim of its own children. Is the issue of the relationship between man and play dead? But perhaps the question of demise is premature. Many of the traditional answers or solutions appear inadequate. Many physical educators begin their theorizing with two assumptions, that one can logically deduce ought statements from is descriptions and that man is rational. The discipline's philosophers articulate the various benefits which accrue to man through participation. They argue for the goals of increased longevity, safety, greater vigour, and increased opportunity for social interaction, among countless others. Both on scientific and sociological grounds the arguments for these objectives carry some weight, though they certainly lack verification. Let us assume that they are, in to, true.

It may be said these idealisms do occur in play. But it is the subsequent utilization of these facts which lead the theoreticians astray. From the fact that various goals are realized, they progress to the proposition that goals should be achieved and further, to the notion that man will work actively toward these objectives once he is convinced of the validity of the proposition. It is these latter two extensions of logic which place the rationale for play on tenuous ground. These difficulties can be clarified by means of examples. An instructor may lecture on the dangers of sky diving in an effort to discourage participation by any of his pupils. He begins with several statements of fact: (i) sky diving has a relatively high mortality rate and (ii) man does not search out situations in which he has a great chance of dying.

Given the fact that the student is a man, the teacher believes he is justified in concluding that the student should not sky dive. However, the instructor, when he initiates in that same mood. There are no grounds for his leap from an is description to an ought prescription. The theoretician cannot logically state:

a. All men who do not want to die do not sky dive.

b. Neeraj is a man who does not want to die.

Therefore: c. Neeraj should not sky dive.

All he is justified in stating is:

a. All men who do not want to die do not sky dive.

b. Neeraj is a man who does not want to die.

Therefore: c. Neeraj does not sky dive.

The physical educators, then, have many facts relative to the outcome or benefits of play. They incorrectly suggest that mere availability of the facts leads to valid conclusions concerning why man should play. Given the various facts of play, such as fitness, health, vigour and community, the instructors suggest that the student should play for these ends. What these instructors assume with such argumentation is that these entities are, in themselves, universal values. Fitness is not only a value but equally a necessity. Many should become fit. But common sense rebels against this reasoning.

An object can remain a good without any obligation to achieve it. Fitness can intellectually be recognized as a value without deciding it is necessary for oneself. It is clear then, that one who attempts to describe man's contact with play on logical grounds has major difficulties. For his account to be valid he must assume that the values of health, fitness and vigour carry with them their own command for action. But even if one could agree on the values of play, it would still not be this point, that man does and must make. It might be objected, at this point, that man does and must make value judgments, whether they be logical or not. In this light, all of the foregoing discussion becomes a wasted intellectual exercise. Who cares if a value judgment lies behind much of the profession's theory? Physical education is willing to stand behind its claims of value. It might be maintained, then, that the instructor has no difficulty convincing the student of a specific good. For example, a teacher may argue for the value of fitness, and the student may accept his discussion.

The student intellectually agrees to the proposition that fitness is a worthy value and that his subsequent actions should reflect that conviction. The student has complete knowledge of the connections between fitness and play and has no qualms in accepting the value of the former. However, it is not paradoxical that man, with some consistency, acts contrary to knowledge and commitment? Many people acknowledge the value of fitness while maintaining a sedentary existence. Many people who value their lives and who know that smoking may shorten the expected life span continue to smoke. Evidence shows that man often acts irrationally. Even the most disciplined individuals do inexplicably act against reason or the knowledge suggesting a singular mode of behaviour. The rationalists want to make play the result of consciously accepted goals and understandings.

Though play may be a result in isolated situations,

though an individual may initiate activity on rationalist grounds, he may continue to play in ignorance of benefits and in spite of potential detrimental effects. Perhaps man intuits that play is somehow an irrational activity. He often plays for no good reason, yet he cannot, it seems, let himself live with this fact. Play becomes acceptable when man can explain his activity on rational grounds. The rational is superimposed upon the irrational. The absurd is made to conform to the reasonable. Does one not hide behind the rational facade because he fears, as an academician, the indeterminate, the unpredictable? Is it not more comfortable to have the ready answer and finite reply for the interrogator? But does not this disposition restrict the search for answers to a predetermined arena, that of the rational? By limiting the range of the quest does one not presuppose the nature of the answer, that it must be logical? What if the truth were to fall outside of his realm? Clearly, it has been suggested that the solution does supersede the rational cause-and-effect motif.

Man's intrigue and persistent relationship with play cannot be sufficiently explained through a rationalist method. Health, fitness, strength, relaxation and other objectives probably accrue from play but to suggest that these explain man's presence in play seems unfounded. To propose that man is in sport because he should be, or that he participates as a result of knowledge of and commitment to a value, vastly oversimplifies the situation. Man is in sport or dance on grounds independent of the practical or rational. It was once asked what would happen to play if it were shown to have absolutely no beneficial results. Would play terminate? Once its useful ends were negated would its captivating effect on man likewise end? It is contended that play would not cease

It would, in fact, continue as before, perhaps with even more success because of its less artificial place in man's life. The riddle of why I play has no simple answer. Man plays before he asks the question. He plays while continually ignoring the question. He plays in spite of known detrimental effects. Play and man seem bound together with reason or without it. To explain the relationship between the phenomena of man and play on rational, cause-and-effect grounds is to render both man and play lifeless.

The problem of why I play is equal and related to the incredible complexity of man. Many plays for many reasons, yet he plays for no reason at all. Man cannot be given an input of reasons and be expected to produce consistent, mechanical behaviour. Man will act with spontaneity, irrationality, and abandon. The lived reality of this union between man and play defies all attempts to reduce it to a rationally explicable understanding.

Athletics in Education

Because athletics are of historical and social significance in our national culture. Because athletics provide a primary means through which may be developed and maintained the physical vigour and stamina required to defend successfully our concept of freedom; and to realize fully our potential as Americans. Because athletics provide a primary means through which may be developed the habits, and ideals requisite to ethical competition and effective cooperation in a free society. Because athletics provide a primary means through which may be utilized in a healthful and wholesome fashion the leisure of our citizens and youth. Because athletics have a powerful appeal for young people during their formative years and can be utilized to further the harmonious development of youth. We believe that participation in athletics should be included in the educational experiences offered to all students in the schools and the colleges of the United States We believe that these opportunities for all students to participate in athletics should be provided in the schools and the colleges through:

i. The basic physical education program for all students in which daily instruction and practice are provided in a variety of physical activities that are suited to the nature and needs of the students and that ensure the development of an adequate level of physical fitness.

ii. The physical recreation program in which opportunities are provided for all students to participate informally in a variety of physical activities.

iii. The intramural athletic program in which opportunities are provided for all students to utilize in organized competition with their schoolmates, the knowledge and skills acquired in the basic physical education program.

iv. The interscholastic or intercollegiate athletic program in which opportunities are provided in secondary schools and colleges for students with superior athletic ability fully to develop and utilize this talent through organized competition with students of similar ability from other schools and colleges.

We believe that the opportunities for participation in athletics that are offered in the schools and the colleges should be complemented by well-organized and well-conducted athletic programs sponsored by appropriate community agencies. Athletics, when utilized properly, serve as potential educational media through which the optimum growth—physical, mental, emotional, social and moral—of the participants may be fostered. During the many arduous practice sessions and in the variety of situations that arise during the heat of the contests, the players must repeatedly react to their own capabilities and limitations and to the behaviour of others. These repeated reactions, and the psychological conditioning that accompanies them, inevitably result in changes—mental, as well as physical—in the players. Because each contest is usually surrounded by an emotionally charged atmosphere and the players are vitally interested in the outcome of the game, the players are more pliable and, hence, more subject to change than in most educational endeavours. To ensure that these changes are educationally desirable, all phases of athletics should be expertly organized and conducted.

Physical Fitness

The desire to excel in athletics is one of the strongest forces available for motivating the American body to expend voluntarily the vigorous efforts required to develop a high degree of fitness. Because of his desire to excel in athletic competition, he will willingly and eagerly participate in strenuous conditioning programs and practice sessions to develop the strength, the endurance, and the skill requisite to excellent performance. He will submit to regular physical examinations by a physician, abide by rigid training rules, and adhere to recommend diets. Because his performance is evaluated regularly and decisively during each athletic contest, the relationship between his efforts and his success is readily apparent to him.

Thus, he learns how physical fitness is achieved and maintained. At the same time, he experiences the feeling of unbounded vigour and physical exuberance enjoyed only by those who are physically fit, and hammy form favourable and lasting attitudes toward exercise and toward physical fitness.

Skill in Movement

To attain success in athletics, the participant must train his mind and body to respond instantly and effectively to the multitude of situations that arise during the course of play. The resultant development of skill in movement enables him to accomplish the everyday physical requirements of his work efficiently and with ease and to respond quickly and effectively in emergencies that demand unusual strength, endurance, speed or coordination.

Social Development

Authorities on child growth and development agree that participation in competitive play provides the child with invaluable opportunities for expending effort that leads to success or failure, for judicious risks and thrills that build up his morale and his capacity to endure and to stand the gaff, and from which he gains his early concepts of sportsmanship. The competitive world—among children as well as adults—is neither gentle nor overly kind. In such a world, however, the youngster under wise direction begins to grow toward social maturity by learning to (i) suffer his mild hurts, mental or physical, in silence, (ii) control his emotional outbursts, (iii) disguise or hide his feelings of fear, (iv) restrain the outward expression of sudden impulses, (v) understand and endure delays in getting what he wants, and (vi) reject being babied. The intense and challenging situations in athletic competition provide the youth with socially acceptable channels through which he may express his aggressive tendencies and expend his excess energy.

Opportunities in which he may control many of his antisocial tendencies through sublimation—and in which he may compensate for real or imagined inadequacies—are abundant. In athletics, he can express his emotions vigorously in a socially acceptable manner. The growing boy earnestly desires recognition and prestige. He lacks self confidence and needs some means of gaining it. Athletics provide him an opportunity to take his place on a team and thereby gain group acceptance and group approval. Through success in athletics, his feelings of inferiority may be assuaged. By trying himself out in highly competitive situations in which he is emotionally aroused and experiences deep-seated feelings, he may learn to perform acceptably despite the intense emotional upheaval. Gradually, he may attain a mental poise and an emotional stability that will serve him well in moments of stress. In athletics, the boy may learn to work cooperatively as a member of a group that is striving for a common goal. He may learn to abide by the rules and to play fairly—not from fear of penalty, but because the success of his team and the enjoyment of all are thus enhanced.

He may experience the humbling lessons of defeat and so learn to readjust his value concepts. He may learn that he must discipline himself to meet his responsibilities if the group of which he is a member is to achieve success in which he may share. He may learn that in all successful group enterprises, some must lead and others must follow. He may learn the meaning and the value of group loyalty and group morale and may experience the emotional responses associated with the esprit de corpse that is developed as the members of the team practice together, suffer and endure together, and win and lose together. In athletics, the boy may learn to tolerate the weaknesses and shortcomings of others and to understand that all men have common desires and aspirations. Prejudices toward others tend to melt away during the gruelling practices and the trial by ordeal of the games. He may learn to judge his team-mates by their behaviour and their contribution to the success of the team and to disregard economic, racial or religious differences.

Recreation

Athletics can provide the youth and the adult with abundant opportunities for utilizing their leisure in activities that are both healthful and wholesome. The highly mechanized nature of American society and the consequent degeneration in the physical fitness of citizens and youth make mandatory an increased emphasis on the utilization of athletics as a means of recreation. Athletic games and contests are ideally suited to the leisure needs of youth. The normal body is bursting with energy. He restlessly searches for excitement, adventure and a cause for which to strive. Unless proper opportunities and proper direction are provided, he may find undesirable outlets for his boundless energy and his turbulent urges.

Athletics—sponsored by schools, churches, clubs, industries, communities and national organizations—offer him recreational pursuits that fulfil his immediate needs and provide a means through which he may develop qualities essential to living a useful and successful life. Dual and individual sports, together with the team games that do not demand of participants high levels of physical fitness and skill, offer the adult opportunities for healthful exercise and a release from the tensions and the worries that beset him as he struggles with the problems of living in a complex world. As spectators, both the youth and the adult can share vicariously in the spirit of the struggle, the despair of defeat, and the joy of victory experienced by teams and individual athletes performing in public contests. Such contests—between professionals as well as between amateurs—are common to the cultures of all modern nations and serve as a basis for world-wide communication and understanding between peoples of all nationalities and races. Because all students can benefit from regular participation in appropriate athletic activities, opportunities for such participation should be provided at all grade levels in schools and colleges.

The capacities, the needs, and the interests of the pupils differ markedly from grade level to grade level. Consequently, the nature of the athletic activities presented, the methods utilized in presenting them, and the emphasis given to each activity should differ in accordance with the characteristics of the students for whom the activities are intended.

Athletics in the Basic Physical Education Program

Under the guidance of a skilful teacher or coach, experiences in athletics provide unique opportunities in which the development of physical fitness and skill in movement, together with wholesome recreation and desirable social development, may be fostered. Hence, athletic activities should be a basic part of the physical education program for all students. In addition to instruction and practice in the fundamental skills of the athletics prominent in American culture, the students should receive instruction in the history, the rules, and the playing strategies associated with these sports.

Provisions should be made for appropriate sequence and progression in both skill and knowledge from grade level to grade level. Particular attention should be given to developing in the students a lasting interest in athletics and an appreciation of the role of athletics in American culture. In Elementary school the basic physical education program should include rhythmical activities, creative play, gymnastic stunts, self-testing activities, and athletics that are suited to the nature, the needs, and the interest of elementary school youngsters. Basic instruction and practice should be provided in climbing, throwing, catching, kicking, running, jumping, dodging, tumbling and similar skills, the mastery of which is requisite to skilful performance in athletics.

In the primary grades, simple relays and games of low organization that have but few rules and that come quickly to a climax should be utilized to orient youngsters to informal competitive situations. In the intermediate grades, modified team games, together with relays that involve the fundamental skills of athletics, should be emphasized. The development of desirable habits of behaviour in competitive situations should be stressed. In junior high schools, the basic physical education program should provide opportunities for increased emphasis on instruction and practice in athletics, particularly in team games.

The intense interest of adolescent boys in athletics, together with their urgent desire to gain status among their peers, causes team games to be especially effective vehicle through which the desirable social development of the participants may be fostered. Cooperation, loyalty, respect for others, conformity to the rules of play, and similar aspects of good sportsmanship should be stressed. In senior high schools, from 30 to 50 per cent of the basic physical education program for boys should be devoted to team sports. However, during the junior and senior years, individual and dual sports in which the students may continue to participate after they leave school should be given attention. Golf, tennis, archery, badminton, and bowling are examples of such activities. In colleges and universities the basic physical education program for men should provide opportunities for instruction and practice in all forms of athletics. Because the basic physical education programs in many high schools are inadequate, provisions should be made in college and university basic programs for all levels of instruction in athletics—beginning, intermediate and advanced.

Athletics in Physical Recreation and Intramural Programs

Because the physical education classes are utilized primarily for physical conditioning and for instructional purposes, the physical recreation program and the intramural program should provide for all students opportunities to put voluntarily into practice the knowledge and skills acquired in the basic physical education program. In the physical recreation program, facilities and equipment should be made readily available during specified hours to enable the students to participate informally during their fee time in athletic activities of their own choosing. In the intramural program, organized competition in the athletics presented in the basic physical education program should be provided. In elementary schools, particular emphasis in the primary grades should be placed on the physical recreation program.

In the intermediate grades, organized intramural competition in athletics should be introduced. Suitable activities for intramural competition for boys in grades 4-6 include modified forms of soccer, softball, touch football, basketball, volleyball and track and field athletics. Emphasis should be placed on participation rather than on the determination of championship teams. Under no circumstances should youngsters be denied the right to participate because of deficiencies in skill. In junior and senior high schools, organized intramural competition should be offered in all athletics in which instruction and practice are given in the basic physical education classes. Every effort should be extended to make the intramural program as attractive to the students as the interscholastic athletic program. Definite procedures for the organization of teams slowed from year to year.

Records of outstanding teams and of individual performances should be kept in an attempt to establish a tradition for the participation in intramural competition. In colleges and universities opportunities for organized intramural competition in many forms of athletics should be provided for all students. Because the academic class schedules vary markedly and students have free periods throughout the day, extensive opportunities in which facilities and equipment are made available for participation should be provided.

Interscholastic and Intercollegiate Athletic Programs

Interscholastic and intercollegiate athletic programs provide opportunities for students with superior talents to develop and utilize these talents fully in organized competition with students of similar ability from other schools and colleges. Rather than limiting interschool athletics to completion between varsity teams, competition between several levels of teams should be encouraged and fostered to provide opportunities for increased numbers of students to participate. Because the extreme interest of the spectators and players in the outcome of the contests often creates highly emotional situations, interscholastic and intercollegiate athletic rank among the most effective means in the total educational program through which the values described in the first part of this document may be realized.

However, the characteristics that cause well-organized and well-conducted programs of interscholastic and intercollegiate athletics to be usually potent tools for accomplishing educational objectives also cause poorly organized and poorly conducted programs to be equally potent in bringing about undesirable outcomes. Athletic programs in which the students are exploited to entertain the public, to advertise the school, to earn money for the school, or to enhance the professional reputation of the coach have no place in educational institution and should not be tolerated. To utilize fully the potential in athletics for educational experiences, interscholastic and intercollegiate athletic programs should be organized and conducted in accordance with these six basic principles.

i. Interscholastic and intercollegiate athletic programs should be regarded as integral parts of the total educational program and should be so conducted that they are worthy of such regard.

ii. Interscholastic and intercollegiate athletic programs should supplement rather than serve as substitutes for basic physical education programs, physical recreation programs, and intramural athletic programs.

iii. Interscholastic and intercollegiate athletic programs should be subject to the same administrative control as the total education program.

iv. Interscholastic and intercollegiate athletic programs should be conducted by men with adequate training in physical education.

v. Interscholastic and intercollegiate athletic programs should be so conducted that the physical welfare and safety of the participants are protected and fostered.

vi. Interscholastic and intercollegiate athletic programs should be conducted in accordance with the letter and the spirit of the rules and regulations of appropriate conference, state, and national athletic associations.

In elementary schools, athletics between schools should be limited to informal games between the teams from two or more schools and to occasional sports days when teams from several schools assemble for a day of friendly, informal competition. At such events, emphasis should be placed on participation by all students. The attendance of spectators should be discouraged. High-pressure programs of interscholastic athletics, in which varsity teams compete in regularly scheduled contests that are attended by partisan spectators, should not be allowed under any circumstances. In junior high schools, limited programs of interscholastic athletics that are adapted to the capacities and the needs of junior high school boys are desirable.

The physical and emotional immaturity of the junior high youngster requires that such programs be controlled with extreme care to ensure that participants rather than on producing winning teams and that the physical welfare of the participants is protected and fostered. In senior high schools, interscholastic athletic programs should include team and dual sports of a variety compatible with the enrolment, the equipment and facilities, and the professional personnel in the school. Every effort should be extended to provide opportunities for all interested boys to participate. In colleges and universities, intercollegiate athletic programs should include as many team, dual and individual sports as finances will permit. Such programs should be conducted in strict adherence to the rules and regulations of the appropriate governing body.

Professional Personnel

Athletics at every level should be conducted by professionally prepared personnel of unquestionable integrity who are dedicated to the task of developing their charges to the highest degree possible—mentally, physically, and morally. In addition to a knowledge of athletics, such personnel should have a knowledge of (i) the place and purpose of athletics in education, (ii) the growth and development of children and youth, (iii) the effects of exercise on the human organism, and (iv) first aid.

Certain basic competencies in physical education, specifically applicable to the welfare and success of participants in competitive sports, should be a minimum prerequisite for teaching or coaching athletics at any level.

A Philosophical Interpretation of the National Institute on Girls Sports

I propose to discuss with you what would be more correctly titled a fundamental or operational point of view regarding sports programs and sports competition for girls and women. The term operational is used here to indicate action or functions. It is important to outline steps that I believe must be taken to improve and expand sports programs for girls and women and to increase the benefits to be derived by the participants. Let us begin by setting the record straight. For many years many professional and nonprofessional sports personnel have believed that women have opposed competition for women. This belief is basically untrue.

Women have opposed those competitive events in which harmful practices and exploitation have minimized the benefit to the competitor. And yet, as recently as the September 30, 1963 issue of Sports Illustrated this statement was made: "After a squabble over U.S. team leadership, professional women physical education instructors were left off the U.S. team's staff. Scorned, the physical education teachers at most high schools and colleges immediately eliminated instruction in the techniques of running, jumping and throwing. Ladies should not perspire. This thinking still holds 35 years later, encouraging otherwise athletic young girls to retreat behind the pose of fragility when it comes to track and field". In 1922, the AAU sponsored a women's track and field team to the Olympic Games in Paris in 1923, Mrs. Herbert Hoover called a national meeting of women interested in athletics. As a result, the Women's Division of the National Amateur Athletic Federation was organized.

The platform statements of this group did a great deal to influence the attitude of women toward competition. Agnes Wayman, one of the members of the original group, wrote that "We have often heard it stated that the Women's Division does not believe in competition for women. As a matter of fact, the games on a nation wide basis. It is the intense, highly specialized type of competition of which the Women's Division was organized to promote participation in sports and games on a nation wide basis. It is the intense, highly specialized type of competition of which the Women's Division disapproves." (ii) The key words here are "participation in sports and games on a nationwide basis" versus "highly specialized type of competition".

Briefed even more, one might conclude that the issue

was participation versus competition, but this would be a misinterpretation of the Division's intent. It was not a question of one or the other; the issue was to preserve sports for all girls and women as evidenced by this statement quoted from the Platform: "Resolved, that for any given group we approve and recommend such selection and administration of athletic activities as makes participation possible for all, and strongly condemn the sacrifice of this objective for the intensive training of the few.

The misunderstanding and the misinterpretation of this philosophy has related in years of debate on the question, "Should we have competition for girls?" So far as the Women's Division was concerned, and so far as the Division for Girls and Women's Sports is concerned, the only issue is how can we best conduct competitive activities to benefit all girls. It is quite evident that these early women feared curtailment of participation in order to provide a few, highly specialized performers. Although these things happened 40 years ago, we could find ourselves engaged again in a needless battle of words that would be useless and wasteful of time, energy and talent. We could find ourselves embroiled in such arguments because of questions such as: "Will United States women do their share in Tokyo in 1964?" There is urgency in that question, and unless we keep our perspective, we could panic and turn our girl's programs into a search for championship talent. But let us pause a moment and take a closer look at the situations.

In the 20's when the issue of women in the Olympics was new, the only international competitions were the Olympic Games every four years. The world was still large and it took at least a week to get from New York to Europe. Now in the 60's sport and sports competition have become a major factor in international prestige. The Federal government and the State Department regard excellence in sports as an essential weapon in the cold war. The world is smaller now, and in the interim between Olympics there are numerous international contests. With the United States and Russia playing a home-and-home series in track and field, the American public eye is kept trained on abilities of our athletes as compared with athletes of other countries—especially athletes from Iron Curtain countries.

If we were to succumb to the pressures, we would concentrate all our efforts on the few talented prospects we could find. This is neither practical nor philosophically sound. We must do two things: train the best we have to perform to the best of their ability and at the same time promote all sports for all girls and women so that eventually we will have more prospects from which to choose the best. I am really proposing that we have more prospects from which to choose the best. I am really proposing that we have our cake and eat it too.

As an educator living in a democracy, my major concern is that every girl in this country benefit from participation in sports, that every girl who has the desire and the ability be provided with opportunities to excel in a sport and become a champion. The only sound philosophy that is operational in our world of today is one that promotes sport for the good of all who participate. A champion should benefit from participation; he or she learn many things of great value. The champion learns the satisfaction of achievement, the discipline and self-sacrifice necessary in the pursuit of excellence, the thrill of winning and the disappointment of losing; the champion gains personal confidence and may come to know the advantages of teamwork and combined effort. There are many other benefits to be listed, but the point is that the little kid from Podunk Hollow who wins the 25-yard dash at the local Fireman's Picnic can derive many of the same benefits as the gold medal winner at the Olympics.

There is a difference in degree and in the amount of prestige, but that is practically the only difference. We must be concerned that every participant benefit from participation in sports because, as we become better individuals, we become a stronger nation. This approach does not deny the development of champions, but it does emphasize the development of skill for many girls. Our great need is to raise the national average of performance by girls in all sports including gymnastics and track and field. I am not as concerned about our women champions as some people are, but if we had many more near-champions, we would be a better nation, and it is very likely that we would have better national champions too. Where shall we start? What steps shall we take? There are those who believe the best procedure is to increase the number of competitive events for girls and women—run more races, organize more meets, have more state, district, and national events.

Others, including the Olympic Development Committee, believe we must first provide more instruction, more coaching and practice. Some of our national champions whose techniques were criticized by the Russians are self-taught. To provide more instruction, we must train more leaders. It was this philosophy that prompted the Olympic Development Committee to approve this Institute, and it was this philosophy that influenced the Division for Girls and Women's Sports and the American Association for Health, Physical Education and Recreation to co-sponsor the institute. In an effort to extend the benefits of the institute, each state team had to pledge itself to conduct one workshop on the state level for the folks at home. There is little doubt that each of you has gained personally from the National Institute, but we are concerned that others gain, too.

Do you care about improving and extending sports programs for girls? Are you convinced we should provide more opportunities for girls to participate, to improve, to excel? If you do care, may I suggest that you plan your state event so that the results of this institute reverberate like ripples in a pool. For example, suppose your team arranged a state workshop for regional teams who would pledge themselves to at least one regional workshop for local teams. Or suppose you decide to do more than the one workshop to which you have pledged yourself. In any case, please do more than teach your local leaders how to teach gymnastics and track and field events—teach them the philosophy of more for everyone that goes with it. You have a unique opportunity to exert a positive influence for the betterment of sports programs for all participants at all levels of skill and in all degrees of competition.

The quality of the job done will be directly proportional to the quality of leadership you demonstrate. I would like to list several steps that I believe must be taken to provide vital and constructive leadership for all girls and women who wish to participate in sports:

i. We must keep the scope of our thinking and our influence as wide as possible to include all persons conductive all kinds of sport activities for girls and women. All persons means men and women, professional and non-professional. If they are willing to help, let us see to it they are taught how best to help. All kinds of sports activities means just that. The emphasis at this Institute has been track and gymnastics only because leadership is especially lacking in these two areas. We did not wish to imply that these two activities are more important than others.

2. We must strive for balance in our programs. Balance, as used here, has both a horizontal and a vertical connotation. The horizontal aspect implies a broad program that provides a variety of activities so that we provide an activity for every girl and have every girl active. The vertical aspect means depth of program—a program that provides for the girl who just wants to try as well as providing the extra training for the girl who wants to be a champion.

3. We must coordinate our efforts and cooperate with each other for one purpose; to provide better programs and more of them. Women physical education teachers have long been dedicated to providing activities for as many girls as possible. They now recognize the fact that too little has been done for the highly skilled girl. Few of our women are adequately trained to coach highly skilled performers so they need help preparing themselves to do a better job for girls at the top of the scale. Women need the help of qualified men. They need their cooperation. It should be remembered,

however, that women want to do the job themselves; they will accept help and cooperation but will resist having things taken out of their hands. Providing more opportunities for girls within the framework of the school program is extremely difficult because of the limitations of time, facilities and money.

Adding programs without curtailing already existing programs appears to be almost impossible. If we accept the fact that the schools are dedicated to education for all, school sports programs must serve the masses. But there is no good reason why we could not develop a cooperative plan whereby agencies and individuals outside the schools set up programs of extra opportunities for interested students and young adults, not in competition with school programs but coordinated with them, each with the purpose of complementing and supplementing school programs. Such programs should do more than provide competitive events; they should provide instruction and practice culminated by competitive events designed to stimulate more practice, more instruction, and to motivate participants to pursue excellence.

4. We must protect the health and welfare of the participants, and must judge program results in terms of benefits to the participants. This is obvious you say and you are correct. A recent letter printed in Sports Illustrated, however, illustrates a lack of understanding of the welfare about which I am speaking. The letter writer suggests the reason for the low level of participation and performance by our women in track and field is due to rules that (i) limit the number of events a woman may enter in one day—men, he said, are limited by stamina; (ii) require a woman travelling overnight to have a chaperone; and (iii) until 1963 prohibited women from running a race of more than 880 yards.

These rules were made to protect the social and/or physical welfare of the participants. There is very little research evidence on women in competition but we do know that what is done for and by men is not automatically the best design for women. It may be especially true if our best women competitors come from the 14 to 18 age bracket as they do in swimming. Our teachers, coaches and leaders have a great responsibility for providing sound, constructive and expert leadership. They must possess and be guided by a personal set of moral and ethical values and good, old-fashioned common sense. They must anticipate problems and be ready with sound solutions based on principles of integrity, dignity, justice, and self-sacrifice for the welfare of the participants.

5. We must, above all, maintain our perspective. If our leadership is strong enough, our programs will be balanced and every boy and girl who wants to run and jump and throw will be able to do so in any one of several different sports. At the same time, the boy or girl who has the desire, as well as the ability, can grow to be a champion. Our needs for better programs and expanded programs are critical. The time is now. Never has the challenge been so great.

Is the Program of High Secondary Athletics an Integral Part of Physical Education?

It is believed that the program of high school athletics is an integral part of physical education. In fact, athletics comprise a laboratory phase of physical education. Here, pupils are afforded an essential opportunity for the practice and perfection of personal and group skills which have been presented in the more formal physical education class instruction. It is during this laboratory experience that pupils become increasingly aware of the need for strength and stamina, so essential to full participation in many competitive sports. It is here, also, that they develop qualities with themselves essential to successful democratic living. They co-operate with team-mates, they observe the rules, they accept decisions, they quality performance.

It promotes in the performer some cultural appreciation of the genuine worth of these activities to his personal well-being and life satisfaction. The athletic program is, in my opinion, not only an integral part of physical education, but also an intrinsic phase of the educational curriculum. It may be extra-class, but as an educational enterprise it is never extra-curricular. It involves a great variety of courses of instruction which contribute generously toward meeting the educational objectives of physical education. Athletic activities comprise, for the most part, the games and sports phase of physical education. The element of competition is usually implied whenever we think of athletics. Such athletic competition is conducted with varying degrees of intensity and under a considerably variety of organizational patterns. Such terms as pick up team, informal game, scheduled game, league game, tournament game, invitation game, play day, sports day, intramural, interschool, and others are used to indicate the kind of event, the intensity of play, the organizational plan as well as to imply to many people the importance of the contest. If the emphasis is entirely on winning league or tournament play becomes very important to the people involved.

If, on the other hand, the emphasis is on the personal development of the boys or girls who play, the contest itself is but a vehicle which contributes worthwhile experiences toward their growth. The skills attained in athletic play are potent motivators to continued participation. They contribute greatly toward giving the pupil a sense of satisfaction and success. They encourage a constructive cycle of practice and play which encompasses a multitude of worthwhile activity experiences. These, in turn contribute to progress toward worthy educational objectives. This is one of the situations which, while not confined to athletics alone, justifies athletics as a vital part of a program of education. Movement, exercises and physical activity are not only adventures, which have great attraction for both children and adults, but are purposeful experiences in their education.

The natural activities such as running, jumping, climbing, throwing, catching, hitting, in various combinations, are included in every phase of physical education. They are used as simple games, rhythmic activities, highly organized athletic sports, stunts and exercises for normal children, as well as for development and fun in programs adapted for the atypical and the handicapped. It is through participation in these activities that man has consistently gained competence and confidence and developed the initiative essential to survival. They are the media through which physical education becomes a fundamental and essential phase of any educational program designed to serve the growth and development needs of people. As in the present program of physical education, the athletic phase of that program is composed also, in various combinations, of the natural, basic activities of running, jumping, throwing, catching and the like. However, in athletics there is a natural interest and motivation to perfect the skills of the activity.

Just as physical education activities must be modified and simplified for the slow learner or the handicapped so must they be accelerated and skilful, through the athletic phase of the program. For many years we have talked about meeting the needs of all the children through physical education adapted to meet and satisfy those needs. Actually our programs have tended toward regimentation and conformity rather than adaptation to individual needs. Program pace needs to be slowed down for some and accelerated for others. In the high school athletic offerings of intramurals, sports days, invitational games and interscholastics we have a program with excellent variety in which most pupils can find a satisfying place and a pace suited to their needs. In many high schools throughout the United States the athletic program serves only a few of the more mature and highly skilled. It is my candid opinion, after many years as a participant, teacher-coach and administrator of athletics from the elementary school to the college level, that athletic programs have fallen far short of their potential contribution.

They tend to serve the few at the expense of the many and there are glaring inequities in the allotment of time, facilities and expert teaching personnel to the development of a select few. The development of the child tends to be less important that the game score. Frequently athletic programs are directed more at spectator interest and the gate than at the developmental and educational benefits of the players. Thus players may become the medium to secure a victory to satisfy a partisan mob rather than the reasons for a game designed to secure for them lasting educational benefits such as physical fitness, and the qualities of initiative, honesty, cooperation, loyalty, courtesy and other elements of social fitness so essential to the development of individual human personality. The very freedom we enjoy in American Democracy are based upon the individual right of every person to achieve his highest potential in terms of human dignity and the ability to serve himself and his fellows.

Athletic games and sports, properly used, are very effective media for developing social fitness. They are practical educational laboratories for inculcating the kind of attitudes and habits so necessary for effective living with others. Yes, the athletic phase of physical education has great natural interest for both player and spectator. Perhaps, it is because of this interest that athletics has moved into the spotlight. This has tended to bring with it may problems. There is no phase of education with so many emotionally interested followers—followers with a deep sense of ownership and pseudo authority over the destinies of the team and especially the tenure of the teacher-coach. There is probably no area of education in which it is more difficult to develop a stable policy of administration. Athletics tend to be managed by incident rather than governed by policy.

Loud emotional protests are often generated over the ineligibility by one player who has had his chance and little if any thought given the younger boy who takes his place and begins to have a chance at competitive athletic play. Again the question might be raised: "Is the boy being used as a medium for winning, regardless or is the game to be a medium for developing the boy?" During the past two decades there have been a great many constructive efforts made to insure that high school athletics are being conducted as an integral phase of physical education. Nearly every state now has an association of high schools organized to conduct interscholastic athletics. Some states have regulated such programs under powers residing by law in their education departments. Local school officials and authorities have set up principles and policies for their own teams.

Studies have been made concerning the effect of athletic activities on people of different ages and organized bodies of educators have published reports for the guidance of school officials. Notable among such reports are the following:

i. Desirable Athletic Competition for Children;

ii. The Bulletin of the National Association of Secondary School Principals;

iii. School Athletics.

The first of these reports deals with athletic programs suited to the needs of elementary and junior high school children. The second deals with problems in physical education. The emphasis is on high school competition and its valuable contribution as an important phase of physical education. The report of the Educational Policies Commission constitutes recognition by this powerful group of educational representatives of the tremendous educational values inherent in athletics. The guiding purpose of the report is indicated by the Policies Commission in its introduction as follows: (a) to increase understanding of athletic problems and potentialities, and (b) to stimulate the fuller achievement of educational objectives in school athletics.

One of the paramount issues in this report is this: "Are we using athletics for educational purposes and for the growth and development of children?" The report faces squarely such issues as exploitation and the place of championships in an educational program. It discusses appropriate athletic activities of children of various developmental levels. Throughout the document athletics is considered as an integral part of physical education. The more physical domination and exploitation creeps in the more educational benefit seeps out. This is true whether such domination or exploitation is practised by education officials including teacher-coaches or by individual or groups having no official connection with the school.

As Oberteuffer says in his book Physical Education—"The more the adult control, the greater the depreciation of educational value to the students themselves". This is indeed a great loss to people when we sell the tremendous educational benefits to growing boys and girls which are inherent in the athletics of physical education for a few effervescent raucous cheers of a partisan mob which paid to money fee to watch the game. Some will recall an important experiment in New York State which took place under the leadership of Dr. Frederick Rand Rogers over a quarter century ago. It was called "Player Control" and its objective was to "give the game back to the players". I had the great privilege of being closely associated, in over 6000 school athletics contests, with this great effort to make athletics more beneficial to players, thus more truly educational.

The plan was to apply the principle of learning by doing. The coaches under this plan were required to do better teaching and the game itself became a demonstration of not only pupil learning and development but also the quality of teaching. During game time the coaches of the two teams sat in the stands where they had ample time to analyse the game in terms of both player improvement and their own teaching strengths and weaknesses. They were not permitted to give their students the answers while the examination was in process. They were permitted, in the interest of player protection, to withdraw a player from the game. Such withdrawn player could now, however, be returned to that contests.

In other words, the plan set up a practical learning situation in which players chose their own plays and made their own substitutions. In short, they made their own decisions and accepted responsibility for those decisions. In this situation the coach could not direct each play and thus dominate and exploit each player for the purpose of satisfying his own ego or to cover up his own shortcomings as a teacher. Player control was a noble effort, one that was and is, in my judgment, educationally sound and practical. It was not understood by most coaches and was violently opposed by them and by their allies, the local sports writers. They interpreted player control not as a worthy educational procedure but as a dangerous threat to their domination of school athletics which had become so popular with the general public. Athletics can exert a wholesome and powerful educational influence.

The selection of appropriate athletic activities for children of various ages and periods of development is a responsibility of great consequence. The manner in which they are conducted is even more important. The responsibilities should rest only on those whose prime interest is in the well-being of youngsters. It is a first responsibility of school authorities to provide facilities, staff and programs which will satisfy these needs. Frequently opportunities to participate in athletics are reserved for a few mature and highly skilled boys. Schools are responsible to provide athletics for all through physical education, including instructional classes, intramural and extramural athletic programs. What happens in many American communities when a trained physical educator or school administrators sets out to provide athletics for all and to conduct them as an integral part of the community's over-all educational enterprise? He bumps head on into special interest.

The ugly head of exploitation, with its many faces, shows itself clearly. Frequently, the high school coach wants the elementary and junior high school programs delimited to providing more material for his teams. He must protect his reputation as a winning coach. He therefore attempts to adapt the professional athletic Farm System to his purpose with vicious results to children. Well-meaning but misguided adults in the community promote teams of children to provide athletic spectacles to satisfy their own vicarious interest in sports, through what they think is worthwhile community promote teams of children to provide athletic spectacles to satisfy their own vicarious interest in sports, through what they think is worthwhile community service. Commercial interests scc advertising possibilities so they also cut rate their way into the act.

To make the situation more completely phoney, in terms of the child's educational needs, these self-appointed do-gooders often wrap the whole package in the shining tinsel of sweet charity. To climax the sorry mess the local press sees many good stories ahead so it plays up individuals and all possible angles of controversy. In view of these situations, which I assure you are not as unreal as they may sound to the naive, what does the teacher or school administrator do? He has at least two courses open: (i) He merely goes along and accepts exploitation of children as an inevitable evil about which he can do nothing; or (ii) he acts on the principle that the well-being of children must come first in any school athletic program and sets out to provide a sound program in his school to satisfy their interests and needs. He also must act concurrently to get better understanding of these needs by his community leaders.

Thus he may secure support for his program and insure its success. Boards of Education are slowly coming to realize that athletics are a part of the physical education which is required by law in most states, and that this means that they are integral parts of the school curriculum. Let me re-emphasize a previous statement—athletics may be conducted either in class or after class; they may be intramural or extramural, but as far as the school is concerned athletic programs are never extracurricular. It is the duty of the Board of Education to permit only qualified teachers to teach, coach or conduct school sponsored athletic activities. Coaching is teaching and teachers are licensed professionals who are trained to understand children and to conduct programs to meet their needs.

The physical educator-coach has a potentially great opportunity to provide, in the athletic program, a realistic, interesting purposeful and fruitful experience for boys and girls in democratic living, unmatched in all education—and which they will enjoy, profit from, remember, and support as citizens. The well-being of boys and girls must receive first consideration by Boards of Education in determining both the breadth and the adequacy of their athletic programs. This should occupy the position of primary importance to each board member as he seeks to discharge his duty to all the children of all the people. Furthermore, such boards must accept, for the citizens of the community, full responsibility for providing adequate financial support from tax moneys for its athletic program. In carrying on their duties to all children, state and local Boards of Education may properly formulate for the conduct of athletics, rules consistent with the best professional advice available to them.

The most important of such rules deals with the protection and well-being of participants. Each child should receive a thorough health examination by a qualified physician before engaging in strenuous competitive sports and periodically throughout the season as indicated. There should also be a follow-through to inform parents and help them understand that they should secure indicated treatment of all remediable defects. This determination of health status is very important to insure the child's gaining the best results from his school experience. It is also important in planning the athletic program to best serve his needs. In fact it is basic to his eligibility to engage in athletics. In my judgment, high school athletic officials have tended to promote eligibility rules on an expediency, incident-management basis rather than on a sound, continuing, policy-governed basis.

Frequently, much time is spent trying to legislate the retention of a star athlete who has had his chance rather than to encourage giving more and more boys an opportunity to play. Furthermore, the problem of equating competition on a scientific basis, so each team has a chance for success, has been all too frequently dodged by responsible school officials. We still seek, sometimes by questionable means, to secure advantage over our opponents before we enter the contest. The widespread use of such scientific devices as McCloy's classification index or Roger's strength index would do much to promote the acceptance and practice of the doctrine of equality between competitors in athletics.

It is my view that athletics will never be fully effective as a worthy phase of education until responsible educators accept the principles and practice effectively the doctrines of both equality of competition and player control. To accomplish this there are two other principles which I believe must be accepted and practice: (i) All school sponsored athletic activities should be conducted under the direct supervision of qualified school personnel; and (ii) all costs of such activities should be paid by the school district from public funds. How can we make progress in the use of athletics as an educational enterprise? We make progress pursuant to policies formulated from expert opinion.

We must use the results of scientific study to help us make policy and test its practical results in terms of the common good. In the high school athletic programs we have a great opportunity to lead the way in making athletic experiences wholesome and worthwhile parts of childhood education. We must insist on school officials governing the school athletic program. Boards of Education must accept full responsibility for adequate financial support of this program. I venture to prophesy that if we provide an equal chance for success in competition and permit athletes to take more responsibility for playing their own games eligibility difficulties will tend to disappear. It is my view that the hope of athletics becoming truly an educational enterprise rests in the high school program. At this time there is too much special interest involved in college athletics. Intercollegiate sports have in the main become commercial enterprises and public spectacles.

The time may come when this Frankenstein will destroy itself. But until that time we professional physical educators must concentrate our energies on providing the best possible educational experiences through athletics for elementary, junior high school and senior high school pupils. In my opinion, this is the suggest way to establish the principle that athletic activity is an integral part of physical education. The athletic phase of physical education should, of course, be directed to the same general educational objectives as the total program. The two objectives we hear most about are physical fitness and social fitness. We must keep in mind, however, that when we concentrate specifically on one of these objectives we contribute at the same time to the other—at least in general. Man is a total being and what affects one part of him affects all of him. Man is mind and body together.

In other words, mind is body and body is mind. Man, to live effectively and satisfactorily and fully must efficiently combine his mental and physical fitness. Man must have both intelligence and physical fitness. Intelligence is somewhat static but physical fitness may be improved. It is the prime responsibility of physical education to improve it. How important to man is physical fitness? Do they, in right combination, improve man's general potential to learn, to serve, to live? What is that right combination? How may the athletic phase of physical education contribute to man's capacity to learn, to serve, to live? Is this phase of physical education being used for purposes that are in man's best interest? Are athletics legitimate parts of physical education? I believe that they are but the answers to many of these random questions must be scientifically worked out and put into a practice before athletics can take their rightful place as an integral part of a program so fundamental to education as is physical education.

Prevention of Sports Injury

Sports medicine is now undergoing a period of growth in interest which has begun a few decades later than the interest in other medical specialists but which will in the end show the same remarkable progress. This modern period can be traced back to the founding of the International Federation of Sports Medicine in 1928. In this country the two significant landmarks are the founding of the American College of Sports Medicine and the establishment in 1955 of the American Medical Association's Committee on Injuries in Sport. Although European writers have been describing and classifying the injuries of sport and discussing their special treatment for many years, the impetus for the development of techniques and equipment for the prevention of sports injuries has developed largely in the United States. The advances which have been made in improving conditioning and equipment have resulted until recently almost entirely from the work of coaches, trainers and sporting good manufacturers rather than from that of physicians. The beginning of the prevention of injury in sports comes with an understanding of what makes an injury in sports different from other injuries.

The age and degree of physical fitness of the injured person are important factors in establishing this difference. The necessity for an early return to functional activity certainly makes a difference in the way in which the injury will be treated and in the individual's response to that injury. The serious consequences which may result from sustaining any residual, and particularly any permanent, disability again emphasizing the difference in the entire management of sports injuries from other injuries. The practical approach to the prevention of injuries requires an intimate knowledge of the techniques of all sports which are to be considered together with the particular hazards which are to be encountered by the competitors. Factors inherent in the performance of these techniques which may pose dangers to the body of the athlete either by acute or chronic trauma must be closely analysed. External conditions including all those of the environment in which the sport is practised must be taken into consideration.

The rules and regulations of these sports must become thoroughly familiar to the person interested in injury prevention. The investigator must further possess a detailed knowledge of the anatomy and physiology of the human body which will inform him of the physical and physiological limits which may not be exceeded without danger to the competitor.

He must be aware of the effects which can be produced by the alliterating of diet, climate, training schedules and even psychological factors, which may influence the injury potential. The student of injury prevention must have sufficient knowledge and experience of methods and analysis of statistical studies in order to be able to determine where the greatest emphasis must be placed, and whether this emphasis must be along certain lines only, must take a broad approach, or whether in fact, preventable factors are involved. He will soon discover that certain types of injury are common to many sports. This is true with regard to certain commonly involved parts of the body such as the head, fingers, knees and ankles. It is also true with regard to certain varieties of trauma which occur commonly in sports such as those caused by a small mass moving at a high velocity. It is true with regard to certain broad classifications of traumatic effects, such as lacerations and fractures.

And finally, he will find it is true with regard to conditions which are the effects of chronic trauma acting in a specific tissue, such as enthusiasts. All of this knowledge will eventually bring him to focus on certain areas of the body where, in order to enable it to stand special stresses, he may wish to apply some sort of protective device. He must then learn what can be done with simple and readily available materials such as adhesive tape. He must become familiar with the properties of other materials which can be built into reusable protective equipment. He must find out how the applications of this equipment can be made effective without impairing the efficiency of the athlete. Not least important he must be assured that the fitting is correct and that the athlete will wear the equipment as it was designed to be worn. The commencement of injury prevention in the actual sports situation is at the time of the pre-season physical examination.

The physician who examines the athlete must realize by his careful evaluation of the whole individual from the standpoint of his structural and functional capabilities he may be preventing an injury by not allowing the occasion for it. Estimation of muscle strength, range of motion of joints, and appraisal of the skeletal structure must be considered an integral part of this examination. A search must be conducted for evidence of previous injuries. Potential hazards of the sport for which the examinee is a candidate must be kept in mind. Psychological factors, which might predispose to injury, may become apparent during the course of the examination. The next steps in injury prevention fall in the planning and execution of the program of pre-season conditions and with the follow through during the season to maintain the peak of conditioning. Not only is the strengthening of muscles important, but also the balancing of strength in antagonistic muscle groups.

Full ranges of motion in all joints essential to the sports action must be established without weakening the ligaments which protect these joints. Resistance to fatigue, which favours injury, is developed by endurance training. When it comes to the consideration of protective equipment, there are many factors to be taken into consideration. Until every recently very little real research has gone into the development of this equipment. Custom, style and guesswork have played a big part in its design. How to make it efficient without being too cumbersome has been a big problem. The advent of new materials has begun to solve some of these questions. The proper wearing and fitting of equipment is not being stressed as it should be. The traditional reluctance of the athlete to be encumbered in any way is being overcome by practical demonstration of the value of the newer equipment. In view of publicity given during the past few months to the 47 fatalities observed during the 1961 football season, a few remarks regarding the football headgear might be in order here.

First, it should be noted that only 20 of these fatalities could be classified as direct, that is they could be directly attributed to an injury sustained while playing or practising football. Of these, 15 were apparently due to injuries to the brain, 3 to the neck, 1 to the spleen and 1 to the kidney. It has been alleged that the plastic helmet as presently designed can be forced back into the neck as it is hyperextended, causing a serious if not fatal compression of the spinal cord. In two of this year's fatalities due to cervical fracture, the mechanism is known to have been hyperflexion, and in other the mechanism is unknown. The rigid shell plastic helmet presently in use with various types of internal suspension is felt by most persons familiar with the problems of athletic headgear to provide the best protection so far available. That this protection is not perfect is evidenced by the fatalities which continue to occur.

Other factors are operative, however, notably the increased height and weight of today's players which greatly increases the impact with which they meet in tackling or blocking. Changes in football tactics, such as the practice of using the helmet for spearing the opponent are bound to have an effect in producing injury. At least one fatality occurred in a boy who had already suffered a severe head injury earlier in the season. The desire of many persons, including quite a few college football coaches, to return to the old leather helmet prompted me to undertake a historical consideration of the subject of helmets generally. The interesting conclusion is that there is a parallel between the development of the war helmet and the football helmet, and that the clock cannot be turned back for one any more than the other. The face guard has come in for some criticism this year. It offers an inviting target to the opponent as currently designed. It has been inevitably grabbed and twisted, sometimes with unpleasant results to the neck. The number of facial and dental injuries has been greatly reduced, however.

With modifications in design the face guard will continue. The use of a mouth or tooth protector has now also become mandatory in the National Football Alliance. Injury prevention also implies control of the physical environment. Properly lighted, surfaced and sized playing fields and courts free of obstructions, defects and foreign objects are essential to safety in sports. Control and restraint of spectators is equally important. Where the climate cannot be controlled, its effect in favouring injuries or pathological states must be acknowledged by cancelling practices or games when conditions are extremely unfavourable. Good officiating, which means strict observance of the rules, is essential since many rules of sports are designed to minimize the possibility of injury. Good coaching aims at teaching these rules to the athletes until their observance becomes second nature.

10

DIETARY SOURCE OF ENERGY IN HUMAN BEINGS

A dietary source of energy must occupy a central place in any nutrition scheme, since energy requirements must even at the expense of protein requirements. However, dietary energy requirements are difficult to define in any species, and particularly so in human bcings. The nutritional objective of livestock farmers is clear: they have to raise their animals as profitably as possible. For a given strain of pig, for example, a certain ration can be shown to be optimum to yield the most meat at least cost, but such criteria do not apply in human nutrition. The human nutritionist cannot play safe and recommend a minimum of energy in the diet.

It is possible to define 'enough' vitamin C, and if the requirement is exceeded not much harm is done, but the same latitude does not apply to energy intake. Grossly excessive and grossly efficient energy intakes are both damaging to health. At least in the short team, there is no need for energy intake to match expenditure, since a temporary excess or deficit can be met by adjustment of the energy stores of the body, chiefly in the form of fat. In the long term, of course, intake must match output, but alterations in the energy stores of the body are themselves associated with alterations in metabolic rate, and hence in energy requirements. Therefore, to discuss energy requirements it is necessary to consider in turn energy expenditure, energy stores, and then the adaptive responses which tend to stabilize energy balance.

Energy units

Until the change to SI units, human energy intake and expenditure was usually expressed as kilogramme. The SI unit is the joule, and the conversion: 1 kcal = 4.18 kJ Since direct calorimeters are usually calibrated with respect to electrical standards, the rate of heat output by direct colorimetry is expressed as watts: 1 watt= 1 J/s, So 1 kcal/min=70 watts. When energy expenditure is measured by indirect colorimetry, the heat equivalent of the respiratory exchange can be calculated using the Weir formula.

However, a fundamental limitation of the accuracy of indirect colorimetry is that the mixture of expired gases does not necessarily reflect the metabolic mixture being produced in the tissues. CO_2 may be stored in the tissues, so the apparent RQ may not equal the metabolic RQ. For this reason it is prudent to report the results obtained in indirect colorimetry in terms of oxygen uptake, rather than converting to heat production using an assumed value for the heat equivalent of oxygen which may not be correct. However, to provide the reader with an easy conversion of oxygen uptake to energy expenditure the following equation will suffice: Oxygen uptake × 7 = kcal/day.

TECHNIQUES FOR MEASURING ENERGY STORES

If energy intake exactly matches requirements, the energy stores of the body will remain constant. It is easier to make accurate measurements of energy intake than of energy expenditure, especially under field conditions. Therefore, it would be convenient for those who try to estimate energy requirements if the energy stores of the body could be relied upon to remain constant or alternatively if the magnitude of the change in the stores could be accurately measured. In practice, neither of these helpful situations prevails. The components of body weight which are relevant to energy storage are fat, protein and glycogen.

None of the other components has any significant energy value. Body weight is not a very reliable index of the state of the energy stores, since change in body water affects weight but not energy stores. If this man is starved for 24 hours much of this glycogen store will be used up, and body weight will fall sharply, because each gram of glycogen binds about 3-4g water. However, if the period of starvation continues the rate of weight loss will decrease, for when the glycogen stores are exhausted the energy deficit must be met from fat or protein. Lean tissue has a similar energy density to the glycogen: water pool, since the energy value of a gram of protein and a gram of glycogen are similar, and each is associated with 3–4 g water.

However, adipose tissue consists of about 83% fat, 15% water and 2% protein, so each gram of adipose tissue stores about 7.5 kcal.

Fat soluble gases

Several gases, such as xenon, krypton and cyclopropane, are much more soluble in fat than in water, so if a person breathes an atmosphere containing a known concentration of one of these gases the amount taken up in the tissues at equilibrium should provide a measure of the amount of fat in the body. This technique has been used to measure total body fat, and it has great theoretical attractions. However, it is not generally used because the gas is slowly transported in the blood to the fat depots, which are not used at a uniform rate, this attaining equilibrium is a slow and uncertain process.

Body density

It is known that the density of human fat is close to 0.90 g cm. If it is assumed that the average density of all fat-free tissue in the body is 1.10 g cm, then it is evident that a determination of total body density will permit a calculation of the ratio of fat to fat-free tissue in the body. Of the available methods for measuring body composition in living subjects, densitometry is probably the best, but it has both practical and theoretical difficulties. A practical difficulty is that, although it is easy to weight a person with an accuracy of about 50 g, it is very difficult to determine the volume of the tissues with commensurate accuracy.

If the true fat content of a man who weighed 70 kg was 14 kg, and if the volume of his tissues was overestimated by 500 ml, the calculated fat content would be 16.8 kg. Thus to provide a reliable estimate of fat content it is necessary to measure tissue volume very accurately. It is not simply a matter of submerging the subject in water and observing the displacement, or apparent weight loss, because the air in lungs and gut also displaces water, thus falsely increasing the apparent fat content. Another practical difficulty is that many people are unable, or unwilling, to submerge completely and calmly in water.

Many attempts have been made to overcome these problems, and the most satisfactory solution so far has been to use a chamber in which the subject is submerged only up to the neck with the head enclosed in a clear plastic dome. It is possible to measure the volume of air around the head, and in lungs and gut, by observing the pressure change for a given volume change within the dome. By this method replicate readings on individual subjects yield estimates of fat content which agree within about 0.3 kg. However, even with technically accurate measurements a theoretical difficulty remains. The method depends on the assumption that fat-free tissue has a density of 1.10 g cm, this is not necessarily true, and certainly it is not true that the density of fat-free tissue lose or gained by subjects who are not in energy balance has a density of 1.10g cm.

Skinfolds

Most of the fat in a normal, or obese, person is situated in a layer under the skin. If the skin at sites such as the front or back aspect of the upper arm, at the angle of the scapula, or between the umbilicus and the iliac crest, is pinched up between the fingers, the thickness of the fold indicates the thickness of the layer of subcutaneous fat. Extensive studies, notably by Durnin and Womersley, have related the fat content of subjects, determined by density, to the thickness of the skinfolds at these four sites. This method is very convenient for subjects of average build, but it requires considerable skill to obtain reproducible readings of skin-fold thickness, and on very obese subjects it may be impossible to obtain a reading at all.

Total Body Potassium

The naturally occurring radioactive isotope of potassium, K, is uniformly distributed with the stable element, so potassium in human tissues can be measured by the characteristic high-energy gamma radiation coming from this endogenous label. If the assumption is made that fat-free tissue contains a constant amount of potassium then a measurement of total body potassium by gamma spectrometry of K radiation provides an estimate of fat-free mass, and hence of fat. This method has the limitations that the assumed constant ratio of potassium to fat-free mass is not quite valid. To this must be added the disadvantage that measurement of potassium is less accurate than measurement of water. Instead of achieving analytical accuracy of 0.5%, it is reasonable to expect something around 3-5%, depending on the design of the counter used. The effect of these limitations is that, using the same basis for comparison as that used for total body water, the error in fat content of obese patients, based on measurements of total potassium, is about 3.5 kg.

Total body water

Recent advances in isotope mass spectrometry have made it possible to make very accurate measurements of the deuterium content of body fluids. It is very accurate measurements of the deuterium content of the serum of a subject, administer a known does of deuterium oxide and, after allowing about 4 hours for equilibration, take another serum sample and measure the enrichment of deuterium. In this way estimation of the exchangeable deuterium pool can be made with an error of about 0.5%. The measurement of water in itself throws no light on the energy stores of the body, but if the assumption is made that fat-free tissue contains 73% water, and that all water is in fat-free tissue, it is easy to calculate the total mass of fat-free tissue, and hence of fat, from an estimate of total body water.

The limitations of this approach are in the assumptions involved. It is obvious that although 73% is a reasonable estimate of the water content of the fat-free component of most tissues, it is plainly incorrect for skin and for heart, kidney and adipose tissue. Furthermore, some of the water in the body is extracellular, and this compartment may increase without proportional increase in cell mass, thus causing clinical oedema and upsetting the assumed water to fat-free mass relationship. Out own studies suggest that estimates of the fat content of obese patients, based on measurements of total body water, are likely to be in error by about 2 kg fat.

ENERGY EXPENDITURE

Components of energy expenditure

Physical activity—There is considerable confusion about the magnitude of the contribution made by physical activity to total energy expenditure, and hence to energy requirements. The National Academy of Sciences and National Research Council Report on Dietary Allowances says 'Although physical activity is the major variable affecting calorie requirements, no simple procedures has been derived for estimating calorie allowances in relation to expenditure of physical energy'. Report, which indicates the energy expenditure of the 'reference' man and woman, who are deemed to spend 8 hours per day lying, 6 hours sitting, 6 hours standing, 2 hours walking, and 2 hours in others in other activities requiring an expenditure at 4.5 kcal/min for men or 3.0 kcal/min for women.

On the other hand if they were employed in a heavy manual occupation, so 8 hours a day was spent at the highest rate, the extra energy expended would be about 840 and 588 kcal for the reference man and woman respectively. These differences agree fairly well with the observed difference in energy expenditure between people in very sedentary, or very strenuous, occupations. However, as the quotation above indicates, there is no simple procedure for relating energy allowances to physical activity. This is an improbable assumption. They very sedentary person would almost certainly lack the physique to perform very heavy work, so the difference in energy output depends partly on the actual pattern of activity, and partly on the body composition which goes with that pattern of activity.

Basal metabolism—When indirect colorimetry was introduced into clinical medicine it was mainly for the purpose of diagnosing thyroid disease. At the Mayo Clinic by 1929 some 60000 individuals had their 'basal metabolic rate' measured: that is energy output while physically and mentally at rest, at least 12 hours after taking food, and in a thermoneutral environment. These conditions were used to try to obtain a standardized test, in which a change in metabolic rate due to thyroid disease would be most likely to be detected. Basal metabolism is usually measured in the early morning, after an overnight fast. In fact, conditions at this time of day are not very standard.

The change from a sleeping rate of about 60 watts to the average daytime rate of about 90 watts takes place rather unsteadily between the hours of 0700 and 0900, which is the time at which 'BMR' is usually measured. The fall from daytime rate back to the sleeping level occurred in these women between 2300 and 0100. This diurnal rhythm is to some extent influenced by patterns of sleep and activity, but the changes cannot be abolished however rigorously the environmental factors are controlled. However, it is obviously dangerous to attach too much significance to any measurement of BMR at one time of day, since a measurement on the same subject, under the same conditions but at a different time of day, would probably give an answer which differed by some 20%

Energy cost of growth, pregnancy and lactation—Infants, and children during the adolescent growth spurt, have surprisingly high energy requirements. This is related to the energy cost of growth, which cannot easily be measured. The effect is seen most clearly in severely malnourished children who have been prevented by undernutrition from growing in the first year of life, and who are then fed at a level which permits catch-up growth. The metabolic rate of a severely malnourished child, aged 1 year, is quite low until it is refer, but when very high growth velocities are attained energy requirements may double. During pregnancy energy requirements increase by about 200 kcal per day.

During the early stages of pregnancy the extra energy is laid down as fat, and this subsidizes the greatly increased energy demands during the last few weeks of pregnancy. The lactating woman, who is supplying the energy requirements of her infant with breast milk, obviously has to cover this extra route of energy loss either by sacrificing some of her fat stores, or by additional dietary energy. The energy requirement of a lactating woman cannot be defined in general terms: it must be calculated in light of her output of breast milk, and the state of her fat stores.

Thermogenesis—It is implicit in the definition that 'basal' metabolism is a minimum value, so any change must be an increase. This is not necessarily true in special cases, e.g. during hypothermia, but for practical purposes the generalization is true. Metabolic rate will, of course, increase during physical activity, which is considered in the next section. The present heading, 'thermogenesis', is used to cover all those situations in which metabolic rate is raised above basal levels in the resting subject. One of the commonest and most important stimuli for thermogenesis is food. After a meal resting metabolic rate increases, and reaches a maximum about 1 hour after the meal.

The effect then decreases, and is no longer detectable

about 5 hours after a meal supplying 1000 kcal. The total extra energy expended as a result of dietary-induced thermogenesis is about 10% of the energy value of the meal. This is an approximate figure, because it is difficult to make an accurate measurement of the effect in man. Some workers make the mistake of obtaining a 'baseline' measurement of metabolic rate before the meal, and then observing the increase above this baseline when the meal has been consumed.

Therefore, to make an accurate estimate of the thermogenesis caused by a meal, it is necessary to perform at least two studies on the same subject over the same period of the day, but to include the meal on one occasion and omit it on the other. It was taught by Rubner and his pupils that dietary protein had a 'specific dynamic action', not possessed by other dietary energy sources such as carbohydrate, fat or alcohol. This teaching was based on observations of dogs, and it was suggested that the metabolism of protein as an energy source necessarily involved loss of metabolic energy in the oxidation of amino acids and formation of urea. In man dietary manoeuvres can greatly alter the rate of diminish and urea production: e.g. a meal containing a large amount of gelatine will increase urea production, since the amino acid composition of gelatine is such that it cannot be used for protein synthesis.

If it were the case that urea production was an important determinant of 'specific dynamic action' then the effect should be much more marked after a meal of gelatine than after an iso-energetic meal of glucose, but this is not so. An extreme case of dietary-induced thermogenesis would be the 'luxus consumption' postulated by Neumann. He reported that he had increased his energy intake by some 100 000 kcal over a period of one year, but did not show the expected steady weight gain: it seemed, therefore, that the excess energy was being burned off by some thermogenic process. Twenty years later Gulick repeated the experiment on himself with similar results. Over the ensuing half-century many attempts have been made to prove or refute the idea that a 'luxus consumption' mechanism exists, and there had been no clear victory for either side. At present, the best that can be said is that during long periods of over-feeding or underfeeding changes in energy expenditure occur which tend to minimize the extent of energy imbalance.

The nature of these adaptive mechanisms is discussed later in this review. Other factors which may affect resting metabolic rate are the environmental temperature, emotional stress, certain drugs and hormones—notably thyroid hormones and the catecholamines. The effects of severe heat and cold stress are of more interest to those studying thermoregulation than those who are concerned with nutritional requirements. Severe cold stress can indeed increase metabolic rate, and hence energy requirements, but the changes in micro-climate around the average person who has normal clothing and shelter are too small to make a significant contribution to energy expenditure. People living in extreme climates may incur extra energy costs if, for example, they have to move about in very heavy insulating clothing, but this is a special case of physical activity, not of resting thermogenesis. Drugs such as salicylates, caffeine and dinitrophenol cause an increase in metabolic rate, but there is no circumstance in which the normal use of these drugs would affect energy requirements in the long term.

Thyroid hormones will certainly increase resting metabolic rate by some 30%, and this increase can be sustained for many months if necessary. Noradrenalin infused intravenously at a rate sufficient to cause a five-fold increase in the basal level will cause an increase in metabolic rate of some 20% while the infusion continues, and it is likely that both catecholamines and thyroid hormones are involved in thermogenic reactions in general. The effects of anxiety on metabolic rate are very difficult to investigate, since the effect, if any, is small.

Therefore, it is necessary to study the subject in a relaxed and steady state, and then cause a high level of anxiety without otherwise affecting the experimental conditions. Apart from any ethical considerations, this is a very difficult task. Landis made a heroic study of his own, and his colleagues', reactions to severe sleep deprivation, gastric intubation and electric shocks, and there was little to show for all this bravery in terms of metabolic response.

Replication of results in individuals

There is little value in making very accurate measurements of energy expenditure by direct colorimetry if the energy output of individuals changes capriciously. Fortunately, replication of results is good on individuals measured under standard conditions. For example the six women whose daily energy losses are measured twice, and the mean difference between duplicate measurements was 2%.

Techniques for measurement of energy expenditure

Direct colorimetry—The classical studies on human energy expenditure were performed by Atwater and Benedict with a direct calorimeter. This was a copper box 2.15 m long, 1.22 m wide, and 1.93 m high. The subject entered through an aperture 49 cm wide and 79 cm high; the aperture was then sealed with a sheet of plate glass embedded in molten beeswax. Great care was taken to ensure that there was no heat gradient across the walls of the calorimeter, and the heat produced but the imprisoned subject was exactly removed by careful regulation of the flow of cold water through pipes inside the chamber.

In the ensuing 70 years there have been considerable advances making colorimetry less arduous for both the subject and the investigators, but the accuracy of the original apparatus has not been surpassed. The great advantage of direct colorimetry is its accuracy and case of calibration. An electrical heat source, or a lamp burning ethyl alcohol or butane, can be used as a reference standard, and the burning ethyl alcohol or butane, can be used as a reference standard, and the observed heat production should agree with the theoretical value within 1%. The disadvantages of direct colorimetry are that it is expensive, laborious and slow.

The design of a relatively simple direct calorimeter, which was constructed by the Division of Bioengineering at the Clinical Research Centre in 1976. The calorimeter chamber is constructed of slabs of expanded polystyrene 20 cm thick, faced on the inner and outer surfaces with sheet aluminium. Access to the chamber is by a door in which there is a pass-through hatch, with clear plastic panels hinged in the inner and outer faces; this also provides a window. The chamber is furnished with a bed, chair, table, small television set and radio-tape recorder. The great majority of patients admitted to our metabolic unit are quite willing to spend a period of 26 hours in this chamber on several occasions. The air inside the chamber is circulated by an axial fan along a duct into a plenum chamber 10 cm deep covering the whole area of the right-hand wall of the chamber.

The inner wall of this chamber is made from

perforated hardboard, so the air escapes into the chamber and flows in a laminar fashion from right to left across the chamber and enters a similar plenum chamber on the left-hand wall. From here it is sucked down to the duct, where part of the stream of air passes through a heat exchanger, and part bypasses the heat exchanger. The proportion of the position of the shutter, which is driven by a servo motor which is sensitive to the temperature gradient across the walls of the chamber. Thus, if the thermistors mounted on the inner and outer aluminium skins of the chamber detect a new outward flow of heat across the walls, the servo motor is instructed to move the shutter so a larger proportion of the circulating air is cooled, and if the net movement of heat through the walls is inward the shutter moves in the opposite direction to reduce the amount of heat extracted from the circulating air.

In this way the heat flow across the walls is kept close to zero over any long period, so any heat produced by the subject in the calorimeter is quantitatively extracted in the heat exchanger. Heat loss by convection and evaporation is not separately measured, since evaporative heat loss is recovered by the heat exchanger as the water vapour is condensed on the cold metal surface. In order to supply fresh air to the subject, without affecting the heat transfer, about 501/min of air is taken into the calorimeter from the shell space through a small heat exchanger, and an equal volume of calorimeter air is extracted through a similar heat exchanger.

Air passing through these heat exchangers is cooled to 6°C, so the change of water vapour is negligible. The supply of cold water for the cooling system is fed from a reservoir in an adjacent room, water is maintained at 4° C by a commercial refrigeration unit. The main flow of water passes from this reservoir to the outgoing fresh-air cooler, then through a reference heat which introduces exactly 100 watts into the stream of water, them through the main heat exchanger, and so back to the reservoir. A second stream separately supplies the incoming fresh-air cooler. The temperature of the water is measured by thermistors at points a, b, c and d. The heat loss of the subject in the calorimeter is calculated by comparing the temperature rise across the reference heater with that which occurs in the same stream of water across heat exchangers. Since the rise across is known to represent a heat uptake of 100 watts, the heat uptake from the calorimeter is easily calculated and displayed on a recorder. The cost of this apparatus at 1976 prices was about £15000.

Other methods—Alternative methods for measuring human energy expenditure have been discussed in some detail elsewhere: the main conclusions are summarized. The direct calorimeter is the most expensive and most accurate. All forms of indirect colorimetry share an error of 2–5%, since this is the error in analysing respiratory gases and converting the results to equipment heat analysing respiratory gases and converting the results to equivalent heat production. The one respect in which respiration chambers are better than direct calorimeters is that they are cheaper, and therefore it is practicable to make them larger and more luxurious, and hence to hope that subjects will tolerate a longer period of continuous measurements.

However, large chambers carry a heavy penalty in having a slow response time, so it may not be possible to observe, for example, in increase in metabolic rate following a meal because the effect of one meal merges into that of the next. Estimates of energy expenditure based on observations of heart rate are inaccurate, especially in relatively sedentary subjects in whom heart rate is determined more by posture and emotional influences than by metabolic requirements.

Variation between individuals

The task of assigning energy requirements to groups of individuals is very much easier than that of defining the requirements of an individual. Reports on dietary allowances, and national rationing policies in time of war, need only guess correctly the average requirement of a large groups. In the case of most nutrients it does not matter if the guess is rather high, so long as most people get enough. The problem of a clinician facing an individual patient is more exacting, especially if he is responsible for treating a condition of energy imbalance in this patient.

The fact that the patient is not in energy balance may indicate that the requirements of this individual are not 'average', so it is important to recognise the range of individual variation. As a first approximation, energy requirements can be adjusted for differences in body weight. Activities involving large body movements are harder work for bigger people, but this factor is trivial. The effect of this calculation is to add or subtract 300 kcal/day for each 10 kg by which a man differs from the reference weight of 70 kg, and 250 kcal/day for each 10 kg by which a woman differs from the reference weight of 58 kg. However, a 'correction' of this sort does very little to reduce the scatter among individuals. More sophisticated correction standards have been proposed, of which the best known is that based on the observations of Booth by and his colleagues at the Mayo Clinic.

This involves a monogram in which the subject's age, sex, weight and height are entered, to obtain an 'expected' basal metabolic rate. When the observed basal metabolic rate of 22 women was compared with the Mayo 'expected' metabolic rate, the correlation coefficient was.

0.791, which was exactly the same as the correlation with simple body weight. Thus corrections for age, sex and surface area do little to explain individual variation. It is not only among obese patients well matched for age, sex and body weight that there are large differences in metabolic rate.

A striking example of individual variation was given by Warwick who studied two normal young women, both aged 23 years, both weighing 54 kg, and both with a surface area of 1.5 m. On direct colorimetry these two women showed differences in energy expenditure of 633 kcal/day, although each gave reproducible results on replicate measurements, and the difference could not be explained by any difference in the level or pattern of physical activity.

CONSEQUENCES OF ENERGY IMBALANCE

Major excess-obesity

In the affluent countries of the would obesity is the most common and important nutritional problem. The essential feature of obesity is an excessive fat store, and this cannot arise unless energy intake exceeds requirements. It has already been pointed out that transient errors of energy balance occur in almost everyone, so the factor which characterizes the obese person is that the cumulative error in energy balance is large and positive, and not automatically corrected by whatever mechanism maintains energy balance in 'normal' people. Many attempts have been made to show that obese people eat more than normal, and although some do, many do not.

This is not surprising in view of the very large range of individual variation in energy requirements. In the United Kingdom, the record for positive energy imbalance is held by one William Campbell who diet in

1878 at the age of 22 years. In his short life he achieved a weight of 340 kg, which implies a storage of about 1 750 000 kcal in the form of excess adipose tissue. If this is expressed as an average daily positive imbalance it comes to 218 kcal per day for 22 years. This imbalance, which produced record-breaking obesity, is small compared with the variations in energy expenditure which are observed between individuals of similar weight and body composition.

Thus it is likely that some obsess people, even while they are increasing in weight, must be eating less than some lean people of constant weight. The disadvantages of being very obese are serious: life insurance companies know that overweight people die younger, and hence are less profitable to insure, surgeons and anaesthetists know that they present difficult problems if they require surgical operations, they and their babies are at greater risk during childbirth, they are more prone to degenerative disease of weight-bearing joints, and to develop adult diabetes mellitus, and they also have social problems. In general, the disadvantages of obesity are reversible on weight loss. With so much to gain from weight loss, it might be supposed the treatment of obese patients would present no problem: 'Since the immediate caused of obesity are overeating and under exercising, the remedies are available to all, but many patients require much help in using them'. In fact, the situation is less simple than the above statement suggests.

Probably, had William Campbell increased his energy expenditure by 219 kcal/day, and eaten the same as before, he would no have continued to gain weight. However, to lose weight it is necessary to generate a negative energy balance; typically about 800 kcal/day deficit will result in a rate of weight loss between 0.5 and 1 kg per week. If a diet is chosen which provides

800 kcal/day less than requirements, and it is strictly adhered to, the rate of weight loss will decrease as time goes on. In part this is due to a decrease in the mass of tissue on which energy requirements depend; it is obvious that a person who weight 100 kg will have lower energy requirements when his weight is reduced to 70 kg. However, it has been known since the day of Benedict that during undernutrition metabolic rate decreases more rapidly than can be explained merely by loss of weight.

The cause of this adaptation to a reduced energy intake is not clear, but it is established that the initial metabolic rate is most closely linked to the initial lean body mass. Among the 19 patients cited earlier metabolic rate was no more closely related to the value predicted by the Mayo standards than it was to body weight but thc best correlation was with lean body mass. Therefore, it is probable that weight loss associated with a large loss of lean tissue lowers energy requirements more than a similar weight loss in which there has been relative sparing of lean tissue, and loss predominantly of adipose tissue.

Minor imbalances

Minor and transient imbalances between energy intake and expenditure are of no consequence whatever. Man is a meal eating animal, so energy intake occurs sporadically throughout the day, whereas energy expenditure is continuous. Thus one can only consider energy balance, or energy requirements, over a period of a day or more. During a period of total starvation these could yield about 4000 kcal and 108 000 kcal respectively, so an energy imbalance of about 10 000 kcal spread over a few weeks would hardly be noticed.

This degree of imbalance probably occurs in most

people during holidays, special festivities, or times of stress such as examinations, when food intake may be unusually high or low. The effect on body weight would be a change of perhaps 2 kg. Longitudinal surveys show that most normal people show fluctuations of body weight of about 10 kg over a period of several years, but tend to revert to a habitual weight by some mechanism which is not yet clearly understood.

Major deficit–protein-energy malnutrition

Although obesity is the most important nutritional disease in affluent countries, in the would in general the main nutritional problem is undernutrition. Since young children have relatively high nutritional requirements, they are the section of the population which show most clearly the effects of nutritional deficit. At one stage the clinical syndrome of malnutrition in children was labelled either 'marasmus' if the child was grossly stunted in height and emaciated, or 'kwashiorkor' if the child had obvious oedema, depigmentation of the skin and hair, and sometimes fatty infiltration of the liver.

These terms have now given way to the more general term 'protein-energy malnutrition', since it was found that it was impossible to make any sharp distinction between the syndromes of marasmus and kwashiorkor: every shade of intermediate from of malnutrition has been found, and during the course of treatment a marasmic child may develop some of the features of kwashiorkor, and vice versa. It is difficult enough to determine the food intake of people in normal circumstances, and virtually impossible to find out accurately the diet on which protein-energy malnutrition develops. The energy requirements of affected children can be determined from their response to treatment, and it can be assumed that while they were developing the disease they were not receiving these requirements.

However, even this assumption is uncertain, because children on a marginal diet may be precipitated into malnutrition by infection, especially if it is associated with diarrhoea and vomiting. In the treatment of protein-energy malnutrition it is important to distinguish two states. In the severely ill child the first task is to restore fluid and electrolyte abnormalities towards normal, and to treat infections. In this early stage too vigorous attempts to re-feed the child may be fatal: the objective is to give enough food to prevent the malnutrition becoming worse. When this first phase is over the second stage is reached, in which the objective is to provide the child with enough food, and particularly energy, to enable it to catch up with the growth which was lost as a result of undernutrition.

11

NUTRITIONAL PROGRAMMES FOR CHILDREN

Teachers have the responsibility of helping students learn to the basic principles of nutrition so that they will understand the important relationship between nutrition and health and will increase skill in solving food and nutrition-related problems. The concept of nutrition is quite abstract to younger elementary school children, often seen as somehow connected with but divorced form eating. Your job in teaching nutrition is to make that concept more concrete and real to your students by presenting learning opportunities that relate nutritional information to daily life.

In other words, you must personalize the information so that students will internalize it and recognize its relevance to health. Avoid a rigid, by-the-rules approach, and do not reduce nutrition education to a set of rules. Not only will this approach make nutrition seem grim, it will also cause children to reject sound principles as unrealistic. Help students to understand the motivations for choosing and eating certain foods, and that some of these motivations have little to do with the amount of nutrients to be attained from a certain food. For example, a person might be choosing a certain mid afternoon snack because that snack was the one always offered by his or her parents, but that snack might not be as nutritious as another readily available snack. Children and adults will change their habits only when they personally recognize the importance of doing so. Do not expect changes overnight. Encourage introspection, and foster positive decision-making skills. Act as a role model for changes you with to bring about. Respect differences in tastes, likes, and dislikes. Slowly you will begin to see that your message getting through.

VALUE-BASED ACTIVITIES

Health Food Voting

Start by asking students what their favourite foods are. Make a list of these on the chalkboard. After making these lists, make two separate columns with the following, headlines: "Healthful" and "Un-healthful." Then call out the list of favourite foods, and have the students vote whether each of the foods should go in the "Healthful" of "Un-healthful" column.

Rank-Ordering Favourite Foods

Have each student prepare a list of three or four favourite foods or dishes from each of the four food groups. Then tell the students to rank-order each food or dish, with the most favourite being labelled "1." Now have the students compare their lists. What class preferences seem to emerge? What are some individual preferences? Follow with a discussion of personal likes and dislikes.

Nutrition Sentence Completion

Have students complete the following statements with phrases that come to mind immediately on hearing the key phrase beginning the statement:

a. Eating a good breakfast is —

b. The most important meal of the day for me is —

c. My favourite foods are —

d. I think that my present diet is —

e. Eating right means —

f. One problem about nutrition for me is —

g. Between-meal snacks should be —

Values Continuum

Pass out continuum sheets. One end of the continuum represents a lifestyle where every meal is eaten at home under relaxed conditions. The other end of the continuum represents a lifestyle where every meal is eaten outside the home under hurried or hectic conditions. Have each student place an X on the continuum representing his or her assessment of eating life-style. Follow with a general discussion of how eating lifestyle may affect growth and development as well as emotional state.

What's for Lunch?

Objective—The students will be able to analyse the nutritious quality of their school lunch.

Description of Strategy— Have the students write down and analyse the school lunch for three days. After three days, have the students share what thcy thought about the school lunch. Discuss which food groups were depleted and which food groups were given. Have the students give their own opinions about the school lunch. As an instructor, make sure good things are said as well as bad.

Materials Needed: none

Processing Questions:

• Did you enjoy these lunches?

• Were you able to eat the types of foods you enjoy?

• Did your analysis determine that your lunches were healthful? Un-healthful?

My favourite meal is....

Objective—The student will be able to describe his or her favourite meals.

Description of Strategy— Have the students write about their favourite breakfast. Then, have them write about their favourite lunch and supper. Have a group discussion about what they wrote. Ask them why this is their favourite meal. If it is non-nutritious, ask them how they can make it nutritious. Have the students rank their meals from 1–10 from most nutritious to least nutritious. Discuss the results.

Materials Needed— paper and pencils

Processing Questions:

• Are the foods you like generally healthful?

• Why do you think you like the foods you do?

DISCUSSION AND REPORT TECHNIQUES

Healthy Breakfasts

Objectives—The student will be able to explain why we need a good breakfast. The student will be able to choose healthy breakfast foods.

Description of Strategy—Give each child a magazine that they can cut pictures from. Have the students cut out enough pictures to create a balanced breakfast. Then have them glue these pictures onto a sheet of construction paper labelled "A Healthful Breakfast."

Materials Needed—magazines, glue, scissors,

construction paper, markers or crayons

Processing Questions

• What types of foods are good to eat at breakfast?

• Why is breakfast called the most important meal of the day?

Grocery Shopping

Objective—The student will be able to purchase foods efficiently from a "grocery store."

Description of Strategy—Give each student $20 in play money. Have a variety of food labels set up on a table with their prices. Make note cards for fruits and other products that you don't have labels for. Tell the students that they need to purchase food for two people for three days. Have them shop for the food they'll eat by writing down the food item and its cost. Discuss the results by asking a variety of questions. Who here has bought enough food for three meals a day? Who has bought something from all four food groups? And so on.

Materials Needed—food labels, note cards?

Processing Questions—

• What can you learn about a food form reading the labels

• Why is it important to plan a budget for buying food?

Classifying Healthful and Un-healthful Snacks

Objective—After completion of centres, the students will able to categorize healthful and un-healthful snacks.

Description of Strategy—Introduce each centre as follows: "Today, class, we are starting a new week, and the topic is nutrition. All our centres this week will be related to nutrition. "First we have the book Centre. There are many books to read and look at. There are also a couple of books that you can listen to. "Next we have the Block Centre. In here I encourage you to use your imagination and relate something you build to healthful and un-healthful snacks.

"Next we have the Writing Centre. Here you can make your own nutrition journal by typing some decorative paper together. Today's topic is to draw or tell about the snacks that you like to eat. "Next we have the Cooking Centre, where you can mix your own healthful snack. After you mix together the appropriate ingredients, you can take your mix to the eating area and enjoy it. You will be mixing things such as Chex cereal, pretzels, peanuts, raising, and popcorn in a little bag and shaking it all together. Then it is ready to eat.

"Next we have the Art Centre. In art today we are going to make a collage of healthful and un-healthful snacks. Look through the magazines and find pictures of either healthful or un-healthful snacks. Then glue them on your piece of paper. Try choosing only healthful or un-healthful snacks for your collage. "In the Math Centre, you will sort the snacks into two piles of healthful and un-healthful snacks. There will be a checklist on the back of the title card.

"In the Language Arts Centre, there is a work sheet and on the work sheet there are both healthful and un-healthful snacks. Colour the healthful snacks. "In the Science Centre, you will taste healthful and un-healthful snacks, and chart how well you liked each snack. Then as a class we will look at the results to seen who liked what the best. "In the Game Centre there will be several games to play, such as X's and O's from Cheerios, Hangman using the Alphabet cereal, and the usual games that are there."

Materials Needed—paper, nutrition books, building blocks, decorative paper, healthful and un-healthful snacks, sandwich bags, magazines, title cards, Cheerios

Processing Question—What types of food provide the most healthful snacks?

Eating for Healthy Teeth

Objective—The student will be able to identify foods that are good for the teeth.

Description of Strategy—Write Healthful and Un-healthful on the board. Write one or two words under each category as an example. Then divide the class into groups of three or four. Say, "Please work as a group. Copy the chart and words off the board. As a group, complete the chart by listing healthful foods for teeth under the 'healthful' side and the un-healthful foods under the 'un-healthful' side." Walk around the room to monitor for understanding. Allow time for them to complete the assignment.

When all groups have finished, have the class help you complete the chart on the board. Have them explain why they put certain foods under certain categories. Sum up the lesson by reviewing why sugar is un-healthful for our teeth—it ultimately leads to tooth decay. Ask the students questions regarding the lesson. Have students bring in at least 10 pictures—drawn or cut out of magazines—of healthful or un-healthful foods for the four teeth. Pictures cut out of magazines must be glued or taped on paper. Label pictures "healthful" or "un-healthful."

Materials Needed—magazines, glue or tape, paper

Processing Questions—

- What are the foods to avoid hurting our teeth?

• What are the most healthful foods to eat for out teeth?

School Cafeteria Menus

Objective—The student will be able to write sample menus incorporating a variety of foods from the school lunch program.

Description of Strategy—Have the school dietitian bring various cafeteria menus to class and show how variety is incorporated into them. Have students write sample menus incorporating a variety of food characteristics for the school lunch program.

Materials Needed—pen and paper

Processing Question—Does your school lunch menu have foods from each level of the food Pyramid?

Healthful Snacks

Objectives—The students will be able to describe the function and role of snacking in relation to their eating habits. The student will be able to identify healthful snacks.

Description of Strategy—Have students compare their eating habits with those needed for good nutrition by writing down their favourite snack foods. Ask students if these foods belong to the basic food groups. Compare favourite snack foods to nutritious snack foods. If favourite foods do not belong to basic food groups, what nutritious foods can be eaten instead?

Eat a smart snack with the class. Have the students plan the snack time based on their regularly scheduled lunch time. Have a simple snack or popcorn or cheese and crackers, or if students brought various items from home, have a tasting party. Challenge students to use their knowledge of good snacking to think of five smart snacks that would sell in a "snack store." Consider setting prices on items and having students work out some math problems on the bottom or back of the work sheet.

Materials Needed—healthful snack foods

Processing Questions—

• If you snack, are there healthful snacks will enhance your health?

• Is it good idea to include snacks as part of your diet?

Food Advertisements

Objective—The student will be able to identify merchandising methods used in making foods more appealing.

Description of Strategy—Assign students to observe food advertisements on television and in magazines and newspapers. Have them notice merchandising methods used to make foods more appealing and interesting. Have students report their observations to the class.

Materials Needed—magazines and newspapers

Processing Questions—

• Do you think food advertisements have enticed you to buy a food that you did not actually need?

• How are food advertisements produced to make you want to buy and eat that particular type of food?

Learning About the Food Pyramid

Objectives—The student will identify the levels in the Food Pyramid. The student will demonstrate the ability to select foods in each category.

Description of Strategy—Pass out some magazines

and have students cut out pictures of different foods. As you cut out these pictures, think about the food pyramid. Try to find a picture to represent each food category. If they find a picture of a food that represents more than one food category, have them try to identify the different groups represented by that food. After students appear to have each category well represented, list each food group on the board.

For food that have ingredients from different categories, list the food as a whole and then the ingredient in the category. Continue the list until it is long enough to indicate that students have a clear understanding, of what foods belong in what categories. Using the food pictures, set up a "cafeteria line" from which students will choose a meal to place on a tray. Have students take turns being cashiers—checking to see that choice include food from each food group.

Materials Needed—magazines with food pictures, scissors, tray borrowed from dafecteria

Processing Questions—

• What foods are in each category of the food pyramid?

• What categories are in the Food Pyramid?

Food Safety

Objective—The student will be able to identify food safety legislation.

Description of Strategy--Have students conduct library research to determine federal and state legislation that helps ensure food safety for the public. Have them present this information in written or oral reports.

Materials Needed—none

Processing Questions—

• What kinds of lows are in effect that make foods safer?

• What organizations protect our health by ensuring that the foods we eat are safe?

Food Label Activity

Objective—The student will be able to identify report on regulations concerning labelling food.

Description of Strategy—Have students research the regulations concerning labelling of packaged foods and present their reports either orally or in writing. Individualize the activity by having each student prepare a report on a specific food product. Then have the student discuss his or her findings in class, explaining what information is contained on the label of the package. Later, put all the packages on display so that students may examine them.

Materials Needed—various packaged foods

Processing Questions—

• How can such labels help us eat in more healthful ways?

• Why do packaged foods have labels?

Weight Management Programmes

Objective—The student will be able to learn healthy weight reduction methods.

Description of Strategy—Invite a leader of a weight reduction group that stresses balanced nutrition in its programme to discuss the effect and health implications of prolonged overeating and crash diets. Have students submit questions on cards in advance to be answered by the resource person.

Materials Needed—index cards

Processing Questions:

- Why are fad diets so popular?
- What are the dangers of dieting improperly?

Brainstorming About Nutrition

Objective—The student will be able to brainstorm concerns about the school food service programme.

Description of Strategy—Organize students into several groups. Have them identify students' the problems they have identified. Have them summarize their ideas and present them to the school dietitian.

Materials Needed—none

Processing Questions—

- What barriers to effectiveness do most school food serve programmes face?
- How would you rate your school food service program?

"Candy Machines in the Schools" Debate

Objective—The student will be able to debate whether candy machines should or should not be installed in the school cafeteria.

Description of Strategy—Should candy machines be placed in the school cafeteria? Have two debate teams argue the issue. Act as moderator, and keep the debate on track. Follow with a general class discussion.

Materials Needed—none

Processing Questions—

- Do the presence of some machines encourage poor eating habits on the part of some students?
- Why are candy machines present in some schools?

Diet Modification

Objective—The student will be able to compare different diet modifications.

Description of Strategy—Give students a problem such as modifying diets for athletes or planning inexpensive party menus. Have them consult at least three different sources of planning inexpensive party menus. Have them consult at least three different sources of information. Compare the conclusions that might be reached from the information derived from the three sources.

Materials Needed—none

Processing Questions—

• Why is it important to plan the meals for such events?

• How do professional nutritionists help us eat in a more healthful manner?

Pyramid Essay

Objective—The student will be able to identify foods from the Food Pyramid that he or she likes the least and the best.

Description of Strategy—After a discussion of the Food Pyramid, have the students write a short essay about the food group they like the best and the least, along with their favourite and least favourite foods in the groups.

Materials Needed—Food Pyramid chart

Processing Questions

• Which levels do you like the most? The least?

• What is the purpose of the Food Pyramid?

Food Patterns over the Years

Objective—The student will be able to list the changes over the years concerning food patterns.

Description of Strategy—Have students interview grandparents or others of that age to see how food patterns have changed over the years. Have them report on how and why the patterns have changed.

Materials Needed—none

Processing Questions—

• Do you eat more healthfully now as a child than your grandparents did when they were your age?

• How have the eating patterns changed since your grandparents' day?

DRAMATIZATIONS

Star Search

Objective—The student will bc able to describe various nutrition problems.

Description of Strategy—Divide the students in groups four to six students. Have the students make up a song, poem, dance, or skit about a nutritional problem. Examples of problems are: eating too much junk food and not eating foods the four food groups. Have the students try to guess what the problem is and then discuss it. At the end of the class, reward everyone with star stickers, cookies, or whatever.

Materials Needed—none

Processing Questions—

• How can such nutritional problems affect our overall health?

• Why do so many people in our country have

nutritional problems when we have such a plentiful supply of food?

Eating for Special Needs

Objective—The student will be able to plan meals for people with special needs.

Description of Strategy— Have a couple of students in the calls role-play patients in the hospital. Example: patient 1 is a sixty-seven-year-old man who has no teeth and an ulcer. Have each student think of breakfast, lunch, and dinner that will fit his needs. Patient 2 is a seven-year-old girl who has had her tonsils removed and has a sore throat. Patient 3 is a forty-five-year-old man who is overweight and has serious heart ailment. Make or plan a breakfast, lunch, and dinner for all the patients and then discuss the results.

Materials Needed—none

Processing Questions—

• What would happen to these patients if they eat or avoid certain foods?

• Why do some people need to avoid or have certain foods in their diets?

Foods That Keep the Body Healthy

Objective—The student will be able to identify certain foods that help keep the body healthy.

Description of Strategy—Draw an outline of three types of bodies: heavy, average, thin. Have students attach food pictures to the body type that might result from a diet of these foods. Discuss with the students why an excess of certain foods can have a negative affect on the body. To show the positive effect food have on the body, have children role-play a race. Let two children that are going to "run in a race" role-play different ways of eating in preparation for the event. For example, one eats very nutritious, light meals, whereas the other eats high-calorie junk food. Let the two students enact what they would feel like while "running in the race."

Materials Needed—drawing of the body types, pictures of food types

Processing Questions—

- What effect does food have on our energy level?
- What effect does food have on our body build?

Sanitary Habits

Objective—The student will be able to identify sanitary and unsanitary work habits with regard to meal preparation.

Description of Strategy—Have students dramatize sanitary and unsanitary work habits while preparing a meal, serving a meal, and eating a meal. The remainder of the class can observe the dramatizations and identify the errors.

Materials Needed—none

Processing Questions—

- What habits can you change to become more sanitary when preparing and eating a meal?
- Why is it important to practice sanitary habits when preparing and eating a meal?

Selling a product

Objective—The student will be able to simulate nutritional advertisements.

Description of Strategy—Divide up the students in groups of three to five students. Give each group a "product." Have the group members work together to think of a way to sell the product. Ask each group to come up in front of the class and try to "sell" its products. Choose nutritious foods and non-nutritious foods as products. Discuss the product and the food group it belongs to.

Materials Needed—boxes, bags, and other packaging of different kinds of food

Processing Questions—

• How should we evaluate such advertisements to make sure we make wise nutritional decisions?

Why do companies use advertisements to sell their products?

Role-Playing Nutrients

Objective—The student will be able to describe the significance of nutrients, vitamins, and minerals through role-playing.

Description of Strategy—The students assemble into their cooperative groups. The teacher assigns each group a category–either nutrient, vitamin, or mineral. The group then researches its category and dramatizes characteristics of its category. The nutrient category students may its category and dramatizes characteristics of its category. The nutrient category students may use food representations to dramatize characteristics, such as drawing a tomato with a face or a banana with legs. Each group presents its dramatization to the class and explains why it chose to dramatize it the way it did. The students explain the significance of their nutrient, vitamin, or mineral, and its relationship to a healthful diet.

Materials Needed—none

Processing Questions—What are the important

characteristics of each category of nutrients?

Proper Manners

Objective—The student will be able to identify appropriate and inappropriate eating behaviours in various settings.

Description of Strategy—Assign groups of students the task of role-playing eating in various settings. For each setting, have some students exhibit behaviours that would be appropriate and have other students exhibit inappropriate behaviours

Materials Needed—none

Processing Questions—What are appropriate behaviours when eating in public places?

Food and Energy

Objective—The student will be able to role-play eating various foods in preparation for a race.

Description of Strategy—Let two students who are going to "run in a race" role-play different ways of eating in preparation for the event; for example, one eats very nutritious and light while the other eats high-calorie junk food. Let the two students enact what they would feel like while "running the race."

Materials Needed—none

Processing Questions—

- What effect would poor food choices have on one's endurance?

- What food should you eat to prepare for a race or other or endurance activity?

Choosing from a Menu

Objective—The student will be able to select foods

from a restaurant menu.

Description of Strategy—Bring several actual menus from area restaurants or let students make "menus." Let several students enact a situation in which they are seated in a restaurant and make choices from the menu. Have others play the role of waiter or waitress to help guide the diner's choice.

Materials Needed—pan and paper

Processing Questions—Why is it important to know how to order form a menu in a restaurant?

Garden Puppet Show

Objective—The student will be able to demonstrate different foods that are grown in the garden, and be able to tell the benefit of each food for the body.

Description of Strategy—Let students make puppets of different foods that are grown in the garden. Let them enact a scene in a garden in which the various foods tell what they will do for the body when they are eaten.

Materials Needed—paper lunch bag or cloth for puppets, markers

Processing Questions—How do various garden-grown foods help our bodies function better?

Nutrients on Trial

Objective—The student will be able to determine essential functions of the nutrients of the body.

Description of Strategy—Have the students conduct of mock court, putting nutrients on trial. Give the students situations where the nutrients on trial have to be accused of not being useful to the body. The nutrients' defendants must defend their essential function in the body.

Materials Needed—none

Processing Questions—What are the useful functions provided by each food?

Which Nutrient Am I?

Objective—The student will be able to identify characteristics of various nutrients, vitamins, and minerals.

Description of Strategy—Assign various nutrients, vitamins, and minerals to individual students. Let them research the nutrient, then dramatize characteristics of the nutrient to the class. For example, for a fruit the student could simulate planting, growing, harvesting, shipping, buying, eating, and digesting the food. Let the observers guess from the dramatization which nutrient is being enacted.

Materials Needed—none

Processing Questions—

- Why is it important to know these characteristics?
- What are the characteristics of the individual nutrients, vitamins, and minerals?

Dieting Puppets

Objective—The student will be able to demonstrate the problems some individuals have in gaining weight and losing weight.

Description of Strategy—Prepare several puppets, some to represent thin people trying to gain weight and others overweight people trying to lose weight, and still others anorexic or bulimic. Have the puppets sitting at a table during a meal discussing why they are eating various foods.

Materials Needed—paper lunch bags or cloth for

making a puppet, telephone

Processing Questions—

How can such behaviour affect that person's health?

• Why do some thin people try to lose more weight?

Cafeteria Selection

Objective—The student will be able to select a meal by choosing foods each level of the Food Pyramid.

Description of Strategy—Using food pictures, set up a "cafeteria line" from which students will choose a meal to place on a tray. Have students take turns being the cashiers—checking to see that choices include food from each level of the Food Pyramid.

Materials Needed—food pictures from magazines, scissors, glue, paper

Processing Questions—Why do we need foods from each level of the pyramid?

Stranger in a Strange Land

Objective—The student will be able to discuss typical foods eaten in different countries.

Description of Strategy—Divide the class into small groups. Have each research the foods and dishes eaten in a different nation, such as Mexico, India, Malaysia, Germany, Japan, and Greece. Then have the students in each group prepare models or drawings of different typical dishes served in their assigned nation. You act the part of a traveller, just arrived in country and very hungry. Ask about teach dish the children have to offer. What is it made of? How does it taste? How does one actually eat it? Follow with a general discussion of different ethnic foods.

Materials Needed—paper, markers

Processing Questions—

• Why should we known about other cultures' dietary habits?

• How do other countries' eating habits differ from ours?

Food Puppets

Objective—The student will be able to select foods that provide a balanced diet.

Description of Strategy—After discussing the Food Pyramid and the nutrients food provide, have the class make puppets representing the various foods within the Food Pyramid. Prepare a skit that explains how the foods work together to provide a balanced diet containing all essential nutrients, including water.

Materials Needed—lunch bag or cloth for making a puppet

Processing Questions—How can combinations of foods help enhance our health?

DECISION STORIES

Ken's Problem

Ken was cut when he tried out for the gymnastics team because he had limited energy and was not muscular enough. His problems were not related to an illness, but a physician suggested Ken's diet might be the problem. Ken decided he needed to eat more, so he began to snack on high-calorie foods such as doughnuts, cakes, and candy. At regular meal times he was not very hungry, so he ate less than usual. He gained weight, but lost endurance.

What to Drink?

All has just come inside from playing a game of

football with his friends and is very thirsty. He opens the refrigerator and finds water, pop, and fruit juice.

Jane's Diet

Ten-year-old Jane decided that she needed to lose weight because her jeans were too tight. Jane's best friend also tried a new diet recently where she could eat as much tomato juice or pineapple as she wanted, but no her foods were allowed. Her friend claimed that the diet was wonderful. Jane decided to try her friend's diet, but after three days, she was bored with only two foods, and she lacked energy. Jane quit the diet and decided that she is doomed to be fat.

Fast Food

Tim doesn't like the food they serve in the school cafeteria. Some of his friends go to a fast-food restaurant near the school instead. He would like to go with them, but he knows that his parents want him to eat in the cafeteria.

Snack Time

John came home from school hungry. His mother told him that dinner would be late, so he could have a snack. She told him to go to the kitchen and get a piece of fruit to eat. But John remembered a candy bar that he had in his lunch box and thought of having that instead, even though he knew that the fruit would be better for him.

PUZZLES AND GAMES

Label Scavenger Hunt

Objective—The student will be able to identify certain foods just be reading the food labels.

Description of Strategy—Give several food labels to groups of students. Have them try to determine what food each of the ingredient labels are describing. Points can be awarded to the groups on the basis of guessing the correct food from the labels.

Materials Needed—food labels

Processing Questions—How can the information from food labels help us to identify foods?

Learning The Food Pyramid

Objective—The student will be able to describe the Food Pyramid.

Description of Strategy—Assign four to five students to each group. On each table there should be some magazines, paper bags, poster boards, scissors, and glue. Each student should have his or her own paper bag. Have the students cut out different foods from the magazines and place them in their bags. Then have the students exchange bags with each other. Tell the students to remove the different foods from the bag and paste it on the correct poster board according to the category in the food Pyramid it belongs to. Once the students finish, have each group show their poster boards. At the end of class, hang the posters around the classroom.

Materials Needed—magazines, paper bags, scissors, glue, poster boards

Processing Questions—

• Why is it important to know the various categories in the Food Pyramid?

• What are the categories in the Food Pyramid?

Food Scavenger Hunt

Objective—The student will be able to participate in a scavenger hunt, using cost as the criteria.

Description of Strategy—A variation on the

preceding game is the following: Ask parents to help students conduct a scavenger hunt in local groceries or kitchens at home. Have them look for the following: a food that costs more than $5 per pound, the least expensive from of milk per liquid ounce, the most expensive from of potatoes per pound, and the least expensive from of peaches per pound. After the hunt, have students compare results and discuss the factors involved in the cost of various foods.

Materials Needed—pen and paper

Processing Questions—

- If a food is more expensive, does that always mean that it is more nutritious?
- Why are some foods more expensive than others?

What Kind of Food Am I?

Objective—The student will be able to guess types of food from clues.

Description of Strategy—Say, "Now we are going to play the 'What kind of food am I? game." "No one is allowed to tell you what your food is, and you are not to tell them the name of their food." Once everyone has become a food, start the game. Call them up to the board one at a time. Have them turn around so the classmates can see the food. The classmates will start describing the food—which food group the student belongs to, the shape, colour, or size, or even other foods it might taste food with or be found in. After a student guesses his or her food, write it on the board under the correct category. Allow students to keep their food tags.

Materials Needed—tape, paper for food tags

Processing Questions—What types of clues about foods will help identify those foods?

Food Alphabet Game

Objective—The student will be able to list foods pertaining to the letters of the alphabet.

Description of Strategy—Divide the students into team and assign each team a number of letters of the alphabet. For example, one team can be assigned letters "A" through "E," the next team letters "F" through "J," and so on. Challenge each team to write down at least one food for each letter assigned to their team.

Materials Needed—pen and paper

Processing Questions—What are the names of foods that start with each letter of the alphabet?

Food Group Bingo

Objective—The student will be able to participate in being using food lists instead of numbers or letters.

Description of Strategy—Distribute bingo cards to the students. The cards will have several columns across, with each one labelled to represent a different category of the Food Pyramid. The spaces below each column will have the name of a food within that food category. Draw students place tokens over the names of the foods on their card. The first person to match four words across in the winner.

Materials Needed—bingo cards

Processing Questions—

• Why is it important to memorize foods within each category

• What are the different categories of foods within the Food Pyramid?

Brown Bag Contest

Objective—The student will be able to prepare and share a brown bag lunch where no refrigeration is available.

Description of Strategy—Have a contest to plan the most interesting and nutritious brown bag lunch for a situation where refrigeration is not available. Have the students prepare, display, and eat the lunches.

Materials Needed—lunch prepared by student

Processing Questions—

• What are some healthy choices that can be included in a brown bag lunch?

• Can a brown bag lunch be as nutritious as a school cafeteria-prepared meal?

EXPERIMENTS AND DEMONSTRATIONS

Complete Proteins

Objective—The student will be able to describe complete proteins.

Description of Strategy—Explain how complete proteins are ones that contain just the right amounts of all nine essential amino acids. Animal sources of protein contain incomplete protein. Plant sources of protein contain incomplete proteins. These are low in one or more essential amino acids. Have cards made that have the names of foods with incomplete proteins written on them. Take two balance cards and put them together. Label this as a complete protein. Then take one food that gives protein and add a food that gives another incomplete protein, to show how to make a complete protein, such as "Beans and Rice." Explain the fact that this is what most vegetarians do, because they don't eat meat.

Materials Needed—note cards

Processing Questions—

• What would happen to our bodies if we did not eat enough of the right kind of proteins?

• What role does protein play in our diet?

Fats and the Heart

Objective—The student will be able to describe the effects of a poor diet on the heart.

Description of Strategy—Put a picture of the heart on the wall. Point out the different valves. Explain how the blood enters and levels the heart. Ask a variety of questions about the heart. Show that if you eat too much junk food that contains fat, you can block one of the valves. When a valve is blocked, it can cause the heart to beat abnormally. If the heart doesn't beat normally, it can stop, and this can cause heart attack. Also bring in pieces of fat. Try to get a pound of fat so they can see what it looks like when one gains a pound of fat.

Materials Needed—picture of the heart

Processing Questions—

• How do un-healthful foods harm the functioning of the heart?

• How do healthful foods help heart function better?

Effects of Snacking on Teeth

Objective—The student will be able to describe the effects of healthful and un-healthful snacks on teeth.

Description of Strategy—Before class, prepare the following: Rice Krispies Treats and sliced apples for the class. Say, "I have prepared two types of snacks for you. One snack is healthful for our teeth and one is not. Please remember, just because food has sugar in it does not mean we shouldn't eat it. It just means we should limit the amount of that type of food. If we take good care of our teeth by brushing and flossing our teeth, going to the dentist regularly and eating plenty of healthful foods, it is OK to eat sweets once in a while. "Two snacks to be used in our experiment are sliced apples and Rice Krispies Treats. First, I want you each to come up and get one Rice Krispies Treat and return to your seat.

If you don't like it, then you don't have to eat it, but keep in mind we are doing a class experiment on healthful and un-healthful foods for our teeth. Your participation is important for our healthful teeth results." Once everyone has a treat, have them eat it: "These are sticky, aren't they? Do you like them? Do you think these are healthful or un-healthful snacks for our teeth? "All right, now let's get on with the next part of our experiment." Have each student come up and get an apple slice. "Go ahead and eat your apple slice. Does it taste good? Is it sticky like the first snack? What's different?" Give the students time to tell about each snack. "Did the sweet snack stick to your teeth? How about the fruit? While you were eating the apple, did it help clean some of the first snack off your teeth? Do your teeth feel cleaner after eating the apple than they did after eating the Rice Krispies Treat?"

Materials Needed—snacks

Processing Questions—What are the differences in un-healthful and healthful snacks with regard to consistency and how they affect the teeth?

Eating Fewer Fatty Foods

Objective—The student will be able to identify fatty and follow a plan to eat fewer fatty foods. The student will be able to identify sources of cholesterol-reducing fibre such as the fibre of apples—pectin—by reading cereal box labels and follow a plan to eat more fibre. The student will be able to identify different kinds of sugars and follow a plan to eat less sugar. The student will be able to determine salt content and follow a plan to eat less salt.

Description of Strategy—Use bacon and an apple for demonstration. Place the two foods on a section of grocery bag. Demonstrate how the bacon will leave a grease spot on the bag. Explain to the students that this same material can collect on artery walls. Use empty cereal boxes, and have the students read the cereal labels to determine which cereals contain sources of fibre.

Instruct the students to create a name for a cereal that tells the consumer that the cereal contains fibre. Write the following words on the chalkboard: sucrose, maltose, fructose, lactose, and corn syrup. Explain that these are words for different kinds of sugar. Add the word sodium, and explain that this word is used for salt. Have the students pretend they are sugar and salt detectives. They are to read labels at home to find what kinds of foods contain sugars and salt. The students should make a list of five foods that contain sugars and five foods that contain salt.

Materials Needed—slices of bacon, an apple, empty cereal boxes

Processing Questions—

- Why should you keep arteries clear of fat?
- Why should we eat more fibre? How does that make us healthier?
- Why is it important to read food labels?
- Shy should you use less salt?
- Why should you eat less sugar?

• Why is it important to eat foods with fibre?

Is It Healthful or Not?

Objective—The student will able to determine whether a meal is nutritious.

Description of Strategy—Set up a few meals on the table. Provide a really nutritious meal, a non-nutritious meal, half nutritious, and so on. Split the class up in groups. Have the groups go to each meal and look at them. Ask them to determine if the meal is nutritious or not. Give them five-seven minutes at each station. Tell them they are not to talk to any one. Have them write whatever comments they want to about the meal. Then have the groups get together and discuss what they wrote and why.

Materials Needed—food labels

Processing Questions—

• What combination of foods are needed to make a healthful meal?

• What happens to our bodies if we do not eat nutritious meals?

Using Disclosing Tablets

Objective—The students will be able to determine how well they brush their teeth after a meal.

Description of Strategy—Say, "We all just came back from lunch and none of us have hand time to brush our teeth yet. I'm going to give each of you a disclosing tablet. It is a chewable tablet that will show us what our teeth look like after we eat. It will show all the acid. Bacteria, and food build on our teeth that we can't see right now." The teacher will pass out the tablets. "Remember, for the tablet to work correctly, you must chew it up. After you have chewed the tablet, you may look in the mirror to see what your teeth look like."

After the students have had an opportunity to see their teeth and the effect of the tablets, the teacher will pass out the apple pieces. It's OK if the class is still standing around the mirror. "Now, eat the apple pieces and then look at your teeth. Apples taste good and work as a 'natural' toothbrush. Remember, it's better to use a real toothbrush but if it is not convenient, an apple will help make your teeth cleaner and healthier. "How did your teeth look after you ate the disclosing tablet? Why did they look like that? How did they look and feel after you ate the apple? What did you learn about you teeth today? Allow students time to answer questions after each one is asked. "Remember, apples not only taste good, they are healthy for our teeth."

Materials Needed—disclosing tablets, apple pieces, mirror

Processing Questions—

• How do disclosing tablets help us determine if we are brushing correctly?

• Why is it important to brush and floss after eating?

Food Diary

Objective—The student will be able to record foods eaten for two or three days and determine that status of the food in the Food Pyramid.

Description of Strategy—Have the students keep a food diary for themselves for two or three amount eaten. Have them look up each food in the Food Pyramid. Have them record the total of foods eaten in each of the food groups after the three days.

Materials Needed—Food Pyramid, food log

Processing Questions—How can the keeping of food diary enhance your nutrition decisions?

Preparing Cafeteria Food

Objective—The student will observe the cafeteria personnel preparing food to learn the steps involved in food preparation.

Description of Strategy— Take the class to cafeteria to observe a food being prepared, such as bread. To make the experience more interesting and informative, have the school dietitian explain each step in the process.

Materials Needed—none

Processing Questions—

• What sanitary activities did you observe in the food preparation?

• What did you learn from the preparation of the food in the cafeteria?

Make Egg Nog

Objective—The students will be able to make egg nog.

Description of Strategy—During the Christmas season, have children make egg nog from a recipe. Have the students beat eggs with a beater. Add 1/4 cup sugar, 1/4 teaspoon salt, 1/2 teaspoon vanilla, 1 quart milk, and a dash of nutmeg. Beat until thoroughly mixed, then serve.

Materials Needed—4 eggs, a beater, 1/4 cup sugar, 1/4 teaspoon salt, 1/2 teaspoon vanilla, 1 quart milk, and a dash of nutmeg

Processing Questions—

• Does your family have any such traditions centred around food?

• How do food traditions begin for special events such

as holidays?

Food Labels

Objective—The student will be able to identify the nutritional content from various food labels.

Description of Strategy—Distribute different food labels, and have students answer the following questions about each food: name, net weight, largest ingredient, additives, serving size, calories per serving, and percentage of RDA for the vitamins and minerals.

Materials Needed—food labels

Processing Questions—

• What important information can be found on food labels?

• Why do foods have labels?

Food Cleanliness

Objective—The student will be able to prepare and observe agar plates of certain contaminating bacteria.

Description of Strategy—Prepare agar plates to show the growth of bacteria resulting from lack of personal cleanliness. For each plate, have a student contaminate by coughing, sneezing, touching with dirty hands, touching with washed hands, or placing a hair in it. Have students view the plates the day prepared and several days later to determine how personal cleanliness affects the growth of bacteria.

Materials Needed—agar plates

Processing Questions—

• How can we prevent our food from being contaminated?

• How can germs be spread through unsanitary

behaviour around food?

Food and the Five Senses

Objective—The student will be able to use food to demonstrate the five senses.

Description of Strategy—Use a food, such as an apple, to teach about the senses. Cut the apple, and ask the students how the apple looks different on the outside and inside. Give everyone a chance to smell an apple that has been cut and one that is whole. Which has more odour? Ask the students to determine if the apple is warm or cool, soft or firm, light or heavy. Have students bite into an apple and describe the sound. Have the students describe whether the taste was sweet, bitter, or salty.

Materials Needed—apples

Processing Questions—How do the various senses work together to enhance our enjoyment of foods?

Food Preparation

Objective—The student will be able to prepare a food in a variety of ways.

Description of Strategy—Have students conduct a laboratory experiment in which they prepare one specific food in several different ways. Have them evaluate their perceptions of the food prepared in each way.

Materials Needed—a quantity of a specific type of food

Processing Questions—Whey is it important to know different ways to prepare the same type of food?

Microbe Growth

Objective—The student will be able to observe how heat inhibits the growth of microbes.

Description of Strategy—Have students do an experiment that illustrates how hot a food must be to keep microbes from growing. Heat water to 150° Fahrenheit. Use a meat thermometer to determine temperature. Have students take a few sips with plastic spoons to see how hot the water feels to the lips and tongue. Then cool it to 140°F, the point at which microbial growth of organisms begins, and have them taste again. Ask students to give examples of hot foods that also discuss measures that can be taken to prevent them.

Materials Needed—meat thermometer, water, hot plate

Processing Questions—

• How does the heating process enhance the quality of some foods?

• Why is it important to heat some foods before serving?

Foods Eaten in the Cafeteria

Objective—The student will observe various foods eaten by students in the school cafeteria to determine if healthy lunches are being eaten by the students.

Description of Strategy—Have students observe the kinds and amounts of foods eaten by students in the school cafeteria. Record the kinds and amounts of foods eaten by students at each grade level, if possible.

Materials Needed—observation from

Processing Questions—

• Does your school lunch program offer various alternatives of eating?

• Do most students in your school eat healthy

lunches in the cafeteria?

Energy Expenditure Versus Energy Intake

Objective—The student will be able to determine the energy expenditure of foods while engaging in certain activities.

Description of Strategy—Have students obtain a menu from the school cafeteria. Have the students compute how long they would have to engage in each of several kinds of activities to use the energy provided by one serving of each food.

Materials Needed—school cafeteria menu

Processing Questions—

- Why do we need more food when we exercise vigorously?
- How does food serve as an energy source?

Food Waste

Objective—The student will identify foods that are wasted by the students in the school cafeteria.

Description of Strategy—The previous experiment could be followed up with a food waste survey to determine which foods are not eaten from each food group. Have students make a graph of the information and present arguments to increase selection of the food groups that are not chosen or eaten often.

12

MEDICINAL CONCEPTS OF HEALTH EDUCATION

There has been a tremendous advancement pertaining the medicinal aspects of health education as in clinical setting it is growing and maturing practice. Federal efforts to contain costs are encouraging secondary prevention efforts such as screening and referral, compliance education, and general patient education activities.

The rise of the activated patient–one who takes an active role in the therapeutic process–forces medical providers to be more responsive to patients, and encourages more of a therapeutic alliance between providers and patients.

Health systems agencies and health maintenance organizations, which are community oriented, promote clinically based screening and referral, prepatient education, risk reduction activities, and life-style-education. health education in clunical setting is gaining popularity for good reasons. Patients are natural targets for health education.

They are ill, uncomfortable, and concerned about their health. They have a "need to know" about their health status and about how to take care of themselves. Regular contacts with providers give rise to "teachable moments"–those situations in which questions that arise for the patient or the provider can be answered readily by the other. Patient education, when properly applied, is effective in improving patient outcomes, encouraging early treatment, and reducing unnecessary hospital visits. In this chapter, the authors begin with a discussion of who is responsible for health education in clinical settings, examine the extent of professional preparation that those with responsibility for health education in clinical settings have, and then describe the type of health education activities prevalent in clinical settings. Finally, a hypothetical hospital-based health education program is presented.

Responsibility for health education in clinical settings

Traditionally, medical care professionals have been responsible for patient education. Today support for increases in clinically based education of patients and others comes from many quarters, including clinical, management, and education groups. Among clinical groups the American Academy of Family Physicians has taken a strong position on the need for increased and improved patient education by family practice physicians; and the American Academy of Pediatrics continues to promote public and patient education of children and youths.

According to the 1975 American Medical Association Statement on Patient Education: The provision of patient education services designed to assist the patient and his family in the effective management of individual health is a shared and continuous responsibility of both the physician and the patient. Educators, represented primarily by the Society for Public Health Education and the American Society for

Health Manpower Education of Training, have been equally supportive of patient education, and have taken the lead in encouraging planning and evaluation of patient education programs and health education training of clinicians and others with responsibility for patient education. Like other aspects of the health care system, health education is served in a pluralistic manner. Clinicians, educators, managers, and support groups all have some responsibility. There appears to be uniform enthusiasm among these groups for greater efforts to provide health education to patients and others.

Professional Preparation for Clinical Health Educators

It is probably safe to say that most health education in clinical settings is done by health or ducation practitioners who have not taken a single course in patient education. A recent survey reported by Pigg indicated that less than 20 percent of the institutions offering specialization in health education offered at least one course in patient education. Only 14 of these schools ofered a minor or major degree option in patient education, ten at the graduate level and four at teh undergraduate lelvel. The other 25 schools offered a single course or other coursework option such as fieldwork. In general this coursework in patient education was oriented toward a combination of (1) planning and coordination of patient education activities and (2) direct patient education services. There is a profound shortage of professionals trained to plan, implement, and/or provide patient education. Furthermore, with the exception of some recent graduates of some nursing schools, few medical care providers are fortunate to have received any instruction in patient education.

The professional preparation of health educators with

specialization in patient education is vitally needed, as are medical care providers with training in health education. As Pigg points out, most of the courses new offered in patient education were initiated since 1977. Perhapspatient education is becoming a better developed area of health education specialization than it has been up to now.

Health Education Activities in Clinical Settings

As hospitals have become more responsive to the needs of patients and potential patients they have incorporated more health education services into their routines. Adcock, Ettenheim, and D'Altroy provide an instructive glimpse into the everyday workings of health education in a metropolitan hospital. Increasingly hospitals are reaching out into the local community as well as offering a greater range of health education services internally. According to Lehman, the most prevalent health education, complicance education for inpatients and outpatients, expectant parent education, and community and hospital-based screening and either patient education or prepatient education.

Prepatient Education

Health education in clinical settings in increasingly directed at nonpatients or prepatients. This is especially true in prepaid group practices like Health Maintenance Organizations which are mandated to provide preventive health education to their subscribers. Health Systems Agencies' emphasis on local priority setting has encouraged much greater outreach health education on the part of many hospitals in many areas of disease prevention and health promotion. It has also led to an increases in the hiring of health educators to develop and carry out these outreach programs. HMOs are federally mandated to provide health education services to their subscribers. HMOs frequently hire health educators to write newsletters, develop smoking cessation programs, teach nutrition and diet, and establish CPR and screening referral programs. For the reader interested in more details, Mullen, Kukowski, and Mazelius provide a useful description of health education in HMOs.

Patient Education

Patients need education. They need information about their health problems, they need to participate with their providers in making decisions about their treatment, they need to understand their responsibilities for self-care. Also they need to know about clinic and hospital procedures, expenses associated with alternative treatments, inpatient and outpatient services available, and a host of related items and issues. Hospitals are complex and, for the most part, unfriendly places. Medical care providers generally are busy with many patients and therefore may resent the time it takes to teach their patients what they need to know to be truly informed. Furthermore, the responsibility for teaching patients is divided among a host of providers and other professionals. Generally, no one person is, in practice, responsible for all aspects of the patient's education. The need is great for coordinated patient education efforts. Also needed in increased training of medical care providers and others who work with patients. Patient education consists of three broad areas of responsibility: (1) compliance education, (2) Informed consent, and (3) pretreatment instruction.

Compliance Education

Compliance education has become increasingly important as therapeutic regimens have become more complex and complicated. For example, since insulin was introduced into regular practice in the 1920s, patients have been responsible for self-administration of injectable drugs. The current therapeutic regimen for diabetes patients may include inslulin, diet, regular exercise, and special hygienic practices. Some hypertensive patients take as many as four, five, or six different medicines, several times a day. Virtually all chronic disease patients have responsibility for at least some parts of their regimen, most notably medication taking. Unfortunately, many studies indicate that only about 50 percent of patients with various types of medical problems regularly comply with their medical regimens.

The need for compliance education to improve this situation is as great as its potential for improving health. In recent years there has been a dramatic increase in the number of patient compliance education programs initiated in clinical settings.

Informed Consent

Except in cases of emergency, before patients can be given operations, given medication, or treated in other ways, they or their guardian must give consent. Sometimes this consent is tacit or implied by the patient's nonrefusal; sometimes, consent in the form of a signed statement is required. In any case patients' consent can be informed only if they understand the implications of their consent–they should understand each alternative, the potential benefits, the possible risks, and the financial, psychological, and other costs. Since not all of this can be known for certain beforehand, no one can truly be fully informed. The issue, then, is one of being informed well enough. This issue of when a patient is informed well enough is of compelling interest to a growing number of scholars. Issues related to the process by which patients can become sufficiently informed are of equally compelling interest to educators, nurses, and other practitioners.

Pretreatment Instruction

Pretreatment instruction regarding the procedures to be undertaken, the likely effects of anaesthesia, expectations for postoperative recovery, and other information is now standard practice in many hospitals. One important study demonstrated that patients who received preoperative education required less medication for postoperative pain than patients who received no education.

AN EVALUATION OF THE STATE OF THE ART

To judge from the general enthusiasm for patient education and the incredible volume of recent publications on the subject, patient education would seem to be a highly developed health education specialization. In a recent review of the literature, Green et al. concluded that indeed there is cause for optimism. They noted in particular increasing scientific rigor, increasingly sophisticated educational methods, and many useful findings. In support of these conclusions they reviewed in depth several examplary studies that demonstrated these strengths.

They concluded that, on balance, the literature on the subject of patient education provides "..a scientific based for the planning of patient education that should enable practitioners to approach their task with greater confidence and with more testable hypotheses than were justified in earlier years." However, the literature also reflects some basic weaknesses that must be overcome. Green et al. note these typical shortcomings: (1) failure to assess the educational needed of patients sufficiently; (2) lack of theory-based program development and evaluation; and (3) incomplete analysis of program effects. These same shortcomings are probably all too typical of most areas of health education research and probably all too typical of most areas of health education research and practice. Part of the problem in patient education is that researchers have only recently become interested in patient education to any great extent.

Also, research funds in this area are not easiluy procured. Furthermore, evaluation of patient education is no easier than evaluation of any other kind of health education. It is a very difficult undertaking that requires a great deal of pallning, considerable institutional support, and highly supportive and well-trained staff. Finally, the lack of training in evaluation research methods of medical providers, and the naivete of most evaluation researchers vis-a-vis patient care greatly hinders research efforts in patient education.

Compliance Education and Research

Compliance with therapeutic regimens is a vastly popular area of health education activity. Blood pressure control is one of a great number of medical problems for which low compliance rates are documented problems; compliance rates as low as 50 percent have been reported for hypertensives. This is particularly disappointing in hypertension because the medication therapy is highly effective at controlling blood pressure and reducing the risk of more severe at controlling blood pressure and reducing the risk of more severe problems. Compliance education can be directed at improvements in pill taking, a relatively simple behavior with great potential for increasing blood pressure control. Until the inception of the Cardiovascular Program, compliance at Metropolitan was handled at the practitioner level.

Individual practitioners were responsible for encouraging their patients to keep their appointments, take their medicine, and follow their diets and recommended life-style changes. No formal program of compliance education existed. Indeed, there was hardly any recognition that a compliance problem even existed. To know if she was reducing dropouts, she first had to know how many patients were dropping out. Records on dropouts existed but they were not easily accessible.

With some help from individuals in the Office of Operations interested in the dropout problem, whe set up a reasonable system for detecting those who were dropping out. Those identified are contacted by letter or phone when possible and encouraged to return or seek treatment elsewhere. Literature that provides suggestions for improvements in clinic routines and medical team behavior to reduce dropouts was supplied to the hypertension clinic. Over time some of these practices were adopted. In order to reduce missed appointments, patients are called a few darys prior to their appointment and reminded. This, by itself, improves appointment keeping. Those who missed their appointments are telephoned to set up another appointment. There is a vast literature on compliance behavior and some literature on compliance interventions.

A few variables seem to be related to compliance regardless of the medical problem. They include patient locus of control, side effects and other barriers, prior compliance in medication taking, and patient–provider relationship. However, there isno generally applicable index of the compliant or noncompliant patient. There is no generally applicable theory to guide the development of programs to improve compliance. Edie's response to these startling facts was to teach providers who are interested what is known about compliance and how to improve it, and to encourage and support as much research on the subject as possible. Teaching providers about compliance turned out to be a very rewarding task. The nurses, doctors, pharmacists, and nutritionists were very anxious to improve the rate of patients who are taking their medicine.

They were well aware of the studies which demonstrate just how wrong providers' subjective estimates of patient compliance can be. They readily agreed to set up seminars, schedule guest speakers, hold conferences, and generally give the problem serious attention. Edie knew the literature and the people in the area who were experts on the subject. She worked tirelessly to set up conferences and perts on the subject. She worked tirelessly to set up conferences and lectures. She give presentations on the subject as often as she could find an audience.

But she knew that the real work of improving compliance must be done by the providers. Therefore, she alwasys treated compliance as part of the whole medical problem of high blood pressure–she presented the studies but she always asked the providers to interpret the results and make recommendations. She never tried to force her ideas on them.

A Hypothetical Health Education Program at a Metropolitan Hospital

In order to provide the reader with a general understanding of the kinds of health education that are practiced in hospitals, the remainder of this chapter is a hypothetical patient education program. There are two parts to this hypothetical example. The first is a survey of the major events of one day in the life of a professional patient educator. The second is a description of a major hospital program of which health education is an integral part. The two parts should enable the reader to gain some long-range perspective on the role of health education in hospitals.

Of course, the reader must keep in mind the fact that very few shopitals currently provide as supportive an atmosphere for healthy education activities as the hypothetical hospital presented here. The reader should also note that in this example most of the direct patient education is done by the health care providers, not by the health educator. The health educator is conceptualized as a trainer whose major responsibility is to encourage and prepare clinical professionals and others to conduct health education activities.

One Day in the Professional Life of Edie Programs

7 :30 a.m. Edie arrives at the office ahead of the traffic and early enough to get some work done before her first appointement at 830. She is working on a report on the one-year evaluation of a patient education training course which is regularly given to the nursing staff, residents, and other medical professionals who see patients. The popular course has been successful in increasing the amount and, hopefully, the quality of patient education aming the participating professionals compared with an established baseline. This is Edie's favorite program and she would to see it continued and to share it with other trainers across the country.

Working with her on the evaluation and the paper are an assistant professor of nursing and an assistant professor of health education, both at the local university. The hour slips away quickly and just before it does, Edie looks at her schedule for the day. To the appointments and program sessions she adds a small list of things to accomplish this day:

- Exercise.
- Read articles on prepared childbirth education.

• Make an appointment with the Childbirth Education director to discuss new arrangements for the classes held at the hospital.

• Outline a column on the importance of social support for the monthly newsletter.

8:30 A.M. Edie meets with Rea as is their routine on Monday mornings. They have coffee and discuss short-range and long-range plans and attempt to coordinate their efforts whenever possible. They often work together to make their work more efficient and effective or standing to help each other out. At the outset, Rea announces that she has a schedule conflict between a commitment in the community and her responsibilities as a parent. Edie offers to attend the evening meeting for her. This settled, they launch into a discussion of the student fieldwork training program. They have at least two and sometimes three or more fieldwork students every semester.

They are trying to formalize and coordinate some of the training they give the students to improve the organization of the experience, to prepare the students for more responsibility earlier, and to make more efficient use of staff time. They share a few ideas and agree on a working plan for the new students. Edie will write it up the Rea will review it before it is typed. 9:30 A.M. Edie must hurry to the sixth floor hypertension clinic to discuss a hypertension compliance project with a research team consisting of herself, the clinic director, a nurse specialist in hypertension, and a professor of preventive medicine.

They have recently completed a behavioral diagnosis the implications of the results for educational programs to improve compliance. One committee participant is late and the clinic director is paged three times during the meeting. It runs over and ends incomplete. Another meeting is hurridely scheduled for the next week. 10:30 A.M. Time for one phone call to set up an appointement with the Childbirth Education Association director. The director is out so Edie leaves a message with her secretary and plunges on. In a few minutes she will present to a group of recently hired nurses informaminutes she will present to a group of recently hired nurses information on the services and programs her division offers to staff and patients.

The nurses arrive a few minutes late and Edie now appears calm and composed as she makes a ten minute presentation and gives the twelve new nurses a handout with some of the same information she just gave them verbally. For another ten minutes she answers questions and encourages the nurses to enroll in the Patient Education Training Program scheduled for next month. 11:00 A.M. Relaxing at her dest Edie calls to arrange for a sitter for her two children for the evening. That arranged, she nobbles on an apple while she prepares an audiovisual presentation on vaccinations for school-age children main lobby of the hospital, starting today. The slide-tape machine is only available for those hours so that is when the program is run. 12:00 P.M. Satisfied with the final arrangements of slides to go with the audio cassette, Edie arrives in the main lobby with the slide carousel and cassette. In a few minutes a slidetape projector arrives from another part of the hospital.

Edie sets it up in a safe place at the information booth. She asks them to observe, when they can, how many people come over to see and hear the presentation, and to notice whether or not they stay with it through the whole three-and-a-half minutes. She observes for a few minutes longer before she heads for the gym and pool. 1:30 P.M. What good to educate about health all day if you do not practice your own advice? After a swim, stretching exercises, a shower, and a quick lunch Edie is back at her desk for her 1:30 P.M. appointment with Bee Ginning, a health education practicum student. Edie eats a peach for dessert as they talk about the project on which the student is currently working–a bulletin board display on the activated preoperative patient.

The objective of the display is to suggest to inpatients some of the general types of questions they might want to ask their providers before their operations. Edie has received administrative approval to place the display on the surgical service floor. However, it is now only an idea. When it is finished and approved at all levels, it will go to the audiovisual center for artist's work-up and silk screening. Edie makes a few suggestions and recommends that Bee also talk with Rea before putting the first draft together. This leads to a general discussion on how to get things done at the hospital. Finally, Edie breaks it off to answer the phone. 2:30 P.M. The call is from Bertha Nopain, director of the prepared childbirth program that operates out of the hospital.

They chat briefly and arrange a meeting for later in the week. Edie spends most of the next two hours reading articles, outlining the column on social support she is writing for the hospital newspaper, taking two phone calls, and making sure everything is ready for tomorrow. Tomorrow is the first session of the patient education training program for nurses and allied health professionals who work with cancer patients. She is facilitating a two-hour session in the morning and she is responsible for coordinating the four-day, 20-hour program. She makes a few calls to double-check that all the necessary equipment will be at the right place at the right time. She makes a few more calls to check with the presenters for Wednesday and Thursday. Satisfied that everything is as ready as she can make it, she checks with the secretary and heads for the bus stop

7:30 P.M. Home after an exhausting but rewarding day, Edie has half an hour with her children before she puts them to bed. She nibbles on last night's stir fried vegetables before she puts them to bed. She nibbles on last night's stir fried vegetables before calling Rea to report on the meeting she just attended. Her husband arrives home while she is still on the phone so she cuts her conversation short to have a little time with her spouse before going to bed. Tomorrow will also be a very busy and interesting day, but she will be home early, in time to spend the evening with her family.

The Office of Health Education

Edie Programs, a nurse health educator, has been the patient education coordinator at Metropolitan Hospital for 18 months. Her qualifications for the position include eight years' experience as a registered clinical nurse, the last three of which were increasingly.devoted to patient education activities, and a master's degree in health education which she completed at the local university by attending evening classes for three years. Patient education at Metropolitan Hospital is very decentralized. The clinical departments are responsible for educating their own patients. As patient education coordinator, Edie has the following responsibilities: (1) to assist and support patient education activities; (2) to develop and conduct patient education inservice workshops and training programs for nurses, residents, dieticians, and others; and (3) to design, implement, and evaluate patient and general health education programs.

Rea Chout, a community health educator who is the coordinator of outreach health education programs at

Metropolitan Hospital, is responsible for prepatient education. Rea has a bachelor's degree in health education and many hours of community experience. Her responsibilities include: (1) responding to the requested health education needs of community residents; (2) conducting health education programs such as CPR, smoking cessation, weight control, prepared childbirth, and parenting; and (3) organizing community health screening and referral activities. The two coordinators, puls the coordinator for continuing education of health professionals, make up the professional staff of the Office of Health Education, Which is located administratively under the Vice President for Professional and Patient Services.

The coordinator of continuing education, trained in educational administration, is responsible for organizing and coordinating conferences, presentations, and special education programs for professionals at the hospital. the support staff for Office of Health Education consists of one secretary and as many fieldwork students and volunteers as can be commandeered. The three coordinators share an office, a duplicating machine, and some supplies. Each of the coordinators operates on a separate budget.

The Cardiovascular Program

During the last five years, cardiovascular disease risk reduction, a national priority, has been one of the major areas of program development at Metropolitan Hospital. Stroke, Hypertension, myocardial infarction, and diabetes are very prevalent among the patient population at the hospital. Many patients entering the hospital for other causes are found to have hypertension or diabetes, and need to be referred to another clinic within the hospital for treatment. Treatment for these illnesses is most effective when administered early;

therefore, early diagnosis is important. Treatment requires the active participation of the patient for long-term management. Therefore, pativent education is an important component of cardiovascular disease prevention and treatment. Gradually, a program to impact on cardiovascular diseases evolved at the hospital.

The development of this program, or set of related programs, is a story of how programs are developed, but it also is a story about hospital politics–interdepartmental competition and interdisciplinary rivalry. It is in just such context that health education must compete for resources and responsibilities. When the decision was made by hospital officials to organize the various cardiovascular disease prevention and treatment efforts into a coordinated program, a task force was formed. This task force was initially composed of representatives from the Departments of Preventive Medicine, Nursing, Internal Medicine, and Family Practice. Later representatives from the Office of Health Education, the Hypertension Clinic, and the Departments of Community Medicine and Social Work were added.

It was the responsibility of the task force to develop a five-year plan for cardiovascular disease prevention and treatment at the hospital. This plan was to include a set of reasonable and measurable goals, a priority list of activities, a set of recommendations for administrative responsibilities, a budget, and a time line within which the activities could be carried out. Furthermore, all recommendations were to be supported by the best available information from the literature, and from hospital and community data sources. The proposal that emerged after many meetings, presentations, discussions, and draft proposals was as much a product of hospital politics as it was a response to the need for a risk reduction program. Predictably, Internal Medicine, the largest and strongest department in the hospital, became the administrative center for all activities of the program.

Nursing, Preventive Medicine, and Health Education would coordinate their activities with Internal Medicine. REsources for program development would be allocated through Internal Medicine. Decisions about program activities would be made by a group headed by the Director of the Hypertension Clinic and composed of representative departments and units, among which was the Office of Health Education. The proposal that was finally approved by the hospital board of directors included many activities. Some of these had been in existence at the hospital for some time. Others were developed to address the priorities established by the task force. One of the major new priority areas was research into cardiovascular disease treatment and prevention. To encourage research efforts, support for grant-writing activities was also included in the proposal.

The program, with its many facets, was officially known as the Cardiovascular Disease Prevention and Treatment Program. Popularly, it was referred to as the Cardiovascular Program. High blood pressure screening and referral activities, condlucted by the community outreach section of Health Education, were included in the Cardiovascular Program and Supported out of program funds at the same level as before. Inhospital screening and referral efforts, which in the past had been conducted spordically be the Office of Health Education, were now designated as the responsibility of nursing. Health education was to lend support services to this aspect of the program. Primary responsibility for developing and initiating activities to increase compliance with therapeutic regimen was assigned to Preventive Medicine.

Edie Programs was to share responsibility for the coordination of ongoing compliance activities with a staff person from the Department of Nursing. Ultimately, Office of Health Education had little administrative control but a lot of responsibility in each of the major program areas. The larger department units at the hospital had control of the funds and assumed the coordinating responsibility for the program. However, the importance of health education was recognized and Office of Health Education was rewarded with a lot of exciting work and program responsibility. In the following section we will look at some health education activities in each of the three program areas; (1) community outreach, screening, and referral, (2) inhospital screening and referral, and (3) compliance education and research.

Inhospital Screening and Referral

Blood pressure screening and compliance activities in hospital settings are at the same time easier and more difficultthan they are in the community. Blood pressure are routinely taken at almost every clinic visit on every patient. Long waiting times provide good opportunities for compliance efforts. This makes the task easier. However, in most hospitals, as at Metropolitan, little coordination exists between clinics and departments. Furthermore, there is seldom an organized program to encourage high blood pressure therapy. Therefore, the primary task at Metropolitan is to develop a useful system as it sounds; on the contrary, it is very difficult to achieve even minor changes in the day-to-day clinical operations of medical units. In the Cardiovascular Program a team of professionals is responsible for inhospital patient referral for high blood pressure.

The team is composed of Edie Programs, a hypertension clinic nurse, and a representative from the Office of the Vice President in charge of operations. They are trying to get every department to measure blood pressure in a standard way, record the measurements on a standard form, and report all elevated blood pressures. All patients with diastolic blood pressure over 90 mm Hg are encouraged to make an appointment with their medical provider or with a provider at the hypertension clinic. Those who do not seek treatment are followed up with phone calls and letters similar to those used in the community outreach, screening, and refferral program. Seminars and rounds for professionals are devoted to the problems of blood pressure measurement, health problems associated with blood pressure, risk factors for hypertension, referral procedures, and counseling for referral.

Administrators are made responsible for implementing referral procedures to encourage top-down change. It took six months before the system became fully operative, and another six months before its effectiveness could be assessed. One year from its inception the program could boast of a high rate of referral and a very low percentage lost to follow-up. Edie spent most of that year studying hypertension; developing the new referral procedures; working with the departments, clinics, and units in the hospital; and easing the transition. She was responsible for the compliance with referral program, with only a half-time secretary/ administrative assistant to help. She coordinated or conducted most of the 200 inservice program,s seminars, workshops, lectures, and rounds devoted to the subject at the hospital that year. This was only one of her many responsibilities.

Community Outreach, Screening, and Referral

There are several components to the program of community outreach, screening, and referral for cardiovascular disease risk factors as developed at Metropolitan Hospital. These include general community education about risk factors and programs, actual screening and referral activities, and compliance with referral follow-up activities. Rea Chout, as coordinator of outreach health education, is responsible for community screening and referral activities associated with the hospital and The Cardiovascular Program. Her first task in this capacity was to develop one-year and three-year activity plans to comply with the goals established by the program. Her plan includes a schedule of activities, target goals, required resources, personnel, and descriptions of activities.

A half-time administration assistant is employed to coordinate the various screening activities and to be a contact person for volunteers. High blood pressure is the highest priority for screening because of its prevalence in the population and its importance both as a disease and as a risk factor for other cardiovascular diseases. Several others local community groups were already screening for high blood pressure so one of Rea's first tasks was to form an ad hoc group to organize the various screening efforts of the local Heart Association, Red Cross, the hospital, and others. Community activists were included in the ad hoc group.

From many other shared professionl encounters, Rea had friends at these other institutions, so it was oly a matter of time before a smoothly operating system of comunity screenings was in effect. Solutions to the minor problems of equipment sharing, turf competition, and record sharing were worked out by representatives of the involved groups and presented for discussion in open meetings. Professionals involved in screening programs had suspected for a long screening were not entering treatment programs when referred. A major effort was expended to standardize screening procedures and referral information. A statewide, computer-assisted detection and follow-up program was just beginning. The screening groupadapted the statewide computer forms and gained access to the computer printout of who was screened, whether they sought medical care, and whether or not they were diagnosed and treated.

This information confirmed that many screened hypertensives came back again and again for blood pressure measurement but did not seek further diagnosis and treatment. The research literature on the subject indicated that the most costeffective method to increase compliance with referral was to counsel those with elevated blood pressure at the screening site, immediately after their blood pressure was taken. Therefore, this method was employed in the Cardiovascular Program outreach activities.

This fiveminute session conducted by trained volunteers included information about blood pressure, its risks to health, the need for further medical attention, and the efficacy of treatment. Subsequently, the screened person received (1) a telephone call urging him or her to comply with referral, and (2) a letter with additional information and an urgent note encouraging compliance. One year afte the system just described went into effect, the percentage of individuals rescreened was greatly reduced, the percentage of people who complied with referral increased, and the percentage of people lost to follow-up was reduced somewhat.

More peopel were entering treatment sooner, a good

indication of eventual improvements in morbidity and mortality from hypertension. Encouraged by this success, Rea is now in the process of evaluating the components of this program to assess their cost-effectiveness.

Current Trends

By any estimation patient education is a very important and promising health education specialization. The expanding picture of health education in clinical settings includes life-style education as part of the regular checkup. The increasing medicalization of social problems has led to special hospital for clinic-based programs for adolescent pregnancy, sex counseling, and alcohol and drug abuse education.

Many hospitals now offer death education and counseling for the terminally ill and their close relations. Also, hospitals are gradually moving out into their communities and assuming some responsibility for health as well as disease. At the same time some of the concerns and problems of patients are geing addressed as the relationships between patients and providers, and between patients and hospitals, gradually change. Breslow and Some envision patient education in the future to be part of family health care delivered by team of professionals that includes a health education specialist.

13

HEALTH FOR PHYSICAL FITNESS

Health can be defined as 'the ability of an individual to mobilise his resources, physical, mental and spiritual, to the preservation and advantage of himself, his dependants and the society to which he belongs'. Health is thus a state of preparedness for activity to ensure personal survival and achievement while at the same time safeguarding human relationships, especially in the family. The way in which a person uses this ability is not necessarily one which will be beneficial and is of course influenced by many personal and environmental factors.

However, such is man's 'make up' that continuing misuse of resources will result in their deterioration with failing health and ultimate destruction. The ability to mobilise resources advantageously is therefore dependent upon the extent and quality of those resources which accordingly reflect the degree of 'health'. Where resources are inadequate they cannot be successfully mobilised and ill-health results.

The Assessment of Health

Medicine has been more concerned with the treatment of the sick than the care of the healthy and the assessment of health has been more concerned with physical examination for fitness for specific activities, e.g. service in the Forces, strenuous games, hazardous occupations, routine examinations for life insurance. More recently regular screening for specific illness such as cancer and heart disease has gained popularity with executive personnel in industry and others with specific responsibility. In the field of sport, particularly the professional, assessment is important both in the maintenance of an ongoing standard of health and as a check on fitness immediately before competition.

Boxing provides us with a good example. Today, there is an increasing need for a wide acceptance and availability of health assessment, a need to divert some proportion of medical expertise away from the sick to the healthy as a more positive approach to preventive medicine. Any examination however will only reveal the health at the moment of investigation and follow-up is essential, i.e. assessment followed by regular monitoring. Screening, if presented as the sole object, may produce hypochondriacs. It should be no more than a bonus of the assessment and monitoring programme ensuring that where necessary a small proportion of those examined would be referred to conventional medicine for investigation and any necessary treatment. Full health evaluation must include a wide range of physical tests for all systems, motor, sensory, metabolic and coordination with considerable aptitude testing, i.e. practical tests of the ability to mobilise resources for a variety of realistic tasks.

Biochemical, haematological, radiological and other laboratory procedures are available to assist the examiner. Complete examination of the nervous system must be supplemented with investigation of mental aptitude, memory and decision making. Psychological probing can be valuable and revealing, particularly with a confident and confidential person-to person session. Finally, the spiritual resources must be considered with a frank assessment of the quality of life; affectionate regard for others; status, wealth, possessions and achievement; skill and knowledge, motivation and morale; attitudes to work, rest and recreation, and above all faith and philosophy. A simple scoring system could be adopted for the whole investigation and all the results used to form a basic profile for subsequent monitoring. Correlation and frequently be found and maintained between the profile and the continuing life style.

Resources

Resources are either inherited or acquired. At conception the fertilised ovum is provided with a genetic blueprint for its development embodying characteristic trends from both parents and their ancestors. The fertilised ovum is thus the investment for the survival of the species and a manifestation of the immortality of protoplasm. The genetic blueprint, it must be emphasised, is designed for living in a wholly natural environment in which survival is largely dependent on physical strength and swift reactions.

Physical resources, providing adequate nutrition is available, are programmed for activity. Without activity atrophy is inevitable. Thus, in an affluent society, the built-in drive, designed to maintain an adequate muscular growth, must, unless met by satisfying planned activity such as sport, lead to aggression and violence. Life itself is the ongoing manifestation of the continuing inflow of energy from the sun to the earth in biological evolution. Man absorbs an almost measurable amount of energy from food and oxygen whose intake is somewhat automatic. His metabolism demands the expenditure in positive activity of sufficient energy to balance the equation.

Man's physical resource thus provide an extensive and highly efficient locomotor system with groups of muscles in a highly mobile skeletal system crying out for regular and coordinate usage under the strict control of an equally advanced nervous system both reflex and conscious. Much activity is provided in everyday contact with the environment though this may be less demanding with mechanical alternatives to human effort. Thus if the physical resources are to be maintained at an optimal standard their continuing exercise must be assured. Unfortunately, health has been regarded as synonymous with physical or muscular development; 'physical fitness' being the key to good health. Equally important, however, are the sensory organs of the body whose care and exercise is essential to ensure the smooth and continuing acceptance of a summated sensory intake from the environment. Such a sensory input is necessary for the efficient working of both the mental and spiritual resources. Similarly, mental resources are programmed in the genetic blueprint for survival of the individual, to assess the promises and threats of the sensory intake, to secure food and shelter, to find a mat and to prcvide for children.

Experience from generations of trial and error and an ability to cooperate with other members of the species have produced exceptional development of mental resources. This has enabled man to exploit for his advantage the extensive potential of the natural environment. Storage and re-call of information, memory, is one of man's greatest asset enabling him to accumulate knowledge and use it is coordinating incoming data with outgoing motor activity. Muscular response, vocal communication, the use of equipment and technology are the direct results of mobilising his advanced mental resources. Mental resources are today becoming of greater personal importance than the physical ones. If the human race is to survive it must ensure that a reasoned use of motor energy is maintained by controlled activity to avoid outbursts of violence. Mental and physical resources are entirely complementary and must be exercised together. To maintain health each must be exposed to a minimum standard of usage. Finally the third resource, 'spiritual', is the most difficult to define and yet the most important.

However much mental resources may develop, each person maintains a unique individuality. To what extent spiritual resources are influenced by the genetic blueprint is not known but curiosity most certainly is an inherited human trait. The spiritual aspect of life is found in attachment to a creed or code of practice, in beliefs which are stepping stones to truth, and a faith that is some finite purpose in living. It is manifest in motivation and maturity, in affectionate regard for others, and an appreciation of the responsibility to use the more tangible resources not only for self-preservation but for the advantage of dependants and fellow human beings.

It is a commitment to competitive and abundant living sometimes described by sportsmen as "heart'. In an age where man is caught up in the turbulent wake of advancing technology he become increasingly dependent on the strength and integrity of his spiritual resources.

The Accident Equation

The use of the word 'accident' is perhaps unfortunate but it is nevertheless generally accepted as involving injury. In the sporting world 'injury' is a more formal and acceptable term as indeed it would be in any epidemiological investigation. The formula, equally applicable to injury and illness is:

$$I = CE \frac{p\,r\,f}{t\,m\,s}$$

Where 'I' represents the incident, injury, illness or even accident; 'C' represents chance and 'E' the environment, both of which may be favourable or unfavourable as far as the cause of the incident is concerned. Factors which are known to be contributory are p, r and f which respectively represent accident proneness, risk acceptance and personal failings which are usually temporary. Lessening the impact of the situation and helping towards prevention are t, m and s, signifying training, maturity and safety precautions.

This equation is more equation is more symbolic than mathematical but it can be modified to allow a scoring procedure for an incident research programme. The interpretation is made on the following lines and is particularly applicable to sporting activities.

Environment

The environment is natural or man made. The former includes all the hazards of land, sea, air and outer space. Some areas may not even sustain life. Animal and vegetable life is also an essential part of the natural environment and includes man himself. The man-made environment is of great significance including shelter, work place, sports arena and the many agents associated with modern life, weapons, vehicles, machines, clothing and so on. Man may come to terms with his environment and use its properties for safety and survival or on the other hand he may be caught by its hazards and succumb to injury or disaster. He may create a personal environment or 'with around' of protective clothing and life-support systems to improve his chances of survival. In sport the breathing apparatus and suit of the underwater swimmer is a good example.

Chance

Chance is the random coincidence of time and place. It plays a vital part in both physical and biological evolution and adds much to the interest and excitement of sport and recreation. Experience can help estimate the probability of events but the purely random factors cannot be forecast. If they could, life and evolution would come to a grinding halt! As far as injury is concerned in the United Kingdom the average person has, in any week, an 8000 to 1 chance against being seriously injured. Injury however gives no protection as far as chance is concerned and the odds remain the same for the survivor in subsequent weeks.

Personal factors

Accident proneness is currently a reality. Increased vulnerability to accident and injury is common in a society where the pace of life leads to frustration, anxiety, and instability. The normal reaction of a healthy man to an emergency, sudden threat or crisis is a natural call on reserves with adrenaline output, increase in heart rate and respiration, improved muscle tone and sensory awareness, i.e. an increased state of readiness with anxiousness and anticipation, which returns to normal after the crisis has passed. However, in conditions of continuing stress and harassment the reserves are already in demand. When the further crisis occurs there is little left to call upon and in extreme cases the result is panic, a common prelude to accident and injury. The acceptance of risk is a natural human characteristic.

In the crudest situation, risk are taken for survival, to obtain food, and for mating. In a more rational society they are taken for personal gain, for praise and adulation or simply for the thrill and enjoyment of the experience, i.e. for fortune, fame or fun. Risk taking is a very personal factor influenced largely by local opportunities and responsibilities. In sport it is available at all levels from gentle activities to dangerous highly competitive events such as car and motor-bike racing. High risk sports attract high rewards, glamour and real excitement. The dangers are accepted but codes of practice offer some protection. Many other human factors or personal failings increase vulnerability to injury. Most of these are temporary, such as illness, the incubation or post-febrile state of an infection, alcohol, drugs, hangover, hunger, fatigue, anger and the day-to-day physical and emotional upsets which are so common.

The performance of a sportsman can be greatly reduced by such occurrences and the likelihood of injury increased. Training is fundamental to any human activity and is possibly the most important single factor. It is closely associated with health. A person in good health is able to be trained for almost any activity. In the wide variety of sports, training may demand attention to selected muscle groups and reflexes but at all times this must be supported by a high standard of efficiency in all physical, mental and spiritual systems to achieve the best results. Maturity is not just the experience gained with age but a state of high motivation and understanding which ensures a coordinated and productive use of resources. Economy of effort aids endurance and emotional stability ensures success. Skills are more flexible and adapt with ease to changing circumstances and demands.

In sport, maturity may follow the physical triumphs of youthful endeavour to give help and example to the less experienced. Finally, the safety precautions or codes of practice are at the end of the list. Though essential for the protection of learners, the young and the elderly, they must be applied with care lest they interfere with production and enjoyment. All too often in a highly competitive commercial world they are used in place of training. Employers may also be pressed to take excessive precautions for fear of litigation.

In sport a compromise is needed and usually achieved by introducing rules which give equal opportunity to all competitors, fair play and a degree of personal safety to encourage adequate participation. Safety precautions are but one area in a side range of personal, environmental and chance factors. In the investigation of injuries in sport and elsewhere there is invariably evidence of the summation of many predisposing factors with one being responsible for the final nudge into catastrophe. Unfortunately many investigations seek to apportion blame and fail to look beyond the immediate cause to the background of events which gradually build up to the final critical pattern.

ILL-Health

When resources cannot be mobilised to maintain survival and they themselves deteriorate or are damaged, ill-health is assumed. Without therapeutic intervention this state will progressively worsen. The resources are, however, interdependent and failure in one area can be compensated by increased support from elsewhere. For example, gross physical deformities can be overcome by mental re-adjustment and spiritual strength so that a handicapped person can maintain good health. Man's diseases can similarly be compensated for, and life enjoyed with advantage. The maintenance of health throughout the normal life span can only be impaired by birth deformities, malnutrition, ageing, illness and injury.

In the developing and productive years of life it is

illness and injury which are largely responsible for ill-health and death. Prevention is therefore closely associated with health assessment and medical services might well re-orientate their activities to health maintenance with facilities for active intervention when things go wrong, i.e. a new and positive dimension in health care. For practical purposes illness and injury can be considered together. Each may produce distress, pain, disability and tissue damage. Each involves the whole person and each demands assessment, therapeutic intervention and appropriate rehabilitation.

Each involves personal and environmental factors and the influence of chance. Each invites an epidemiological approach to control and elimination. If man is to enjoy the health which gives him, his dependants and society continuing advantage he must find a compromise to his dual role. On the one hand he is a very private and unique individual with innate urges of aggressive selfishness seeking advantage for himself. On the other hand he is a member of a constantly changing and often hazardous environment of which is fellow men are also active participants. His health thus depends on the sympathetic interplay of three forces. This gives the pattern for epidemiological investigation, with the maintenance of health in mind, of illness or injury. Similarly, taking the individual as the starting point for management of illness or injury, i.e. ill-health, a similar pattern emerges.

A Formula for Health

Life is a an ongoing positive experience and too much attention to illness, injury and prevention may detract from enjoyment and achievement. In seeking better health and quality of life it is possible to apply the same factors with advantage. Only the simplest change in the formula is needed thus–with 'H' for health substituted for 'I':

$$H = CE \frac{t\,m\,s}{p\,r\,f}$$

The formula is applicable to any human activity and ideal for sporting and recreational occupations. If man's genetic blueprint demands a continuing state of good health, all system–physical, mental and spiritual–must be exercised in harmony. Where much of the physical activity associated with productive work is being replaced by machines and technology, rewarding alternatives must be found.

14

STRENGTH TRAINING FOR FITNESS

Strength Training

Principle of Overload

The principle of overload indicates that physiological systems improve in function when challenged to work at supra-normal levels. Muscle hypertrophies only when forced to operate beyond customary intensities. The stimulus threshold represents the work intensity below which no effect accrues. The ability to train muscle is greatest when strength training begins though some muscles may be in poorer condition than others and respond more readily. The load must be progressively increased to elicit further adaptive reactions as training develops and the training stimulus gradually raised. Gains become increasingly difficult to obtain as the muscle approaches its theoretical potential. Overload is accomplished by emphasising the duration or intensity of exercise. Many repetitions of low intensity work improve muscular endurance while few repetitions at high intensity develop strength. High intensity work at speed promotes muscular power as well as strength.

Many sportsmen wish to develop strength without accompanying hypertrophy. Boxers, wrestlers and oarsmen want to avoid excessive increases in muscle bulk which necessitate moving to a higher competitive weight category. Belated attempts to shed weight by dehydration are counter-productive since strength abates with fluid loss. Hurdlers and jumpers whose extra muscle constitutes an additional load to be lifted against gravity similarly seek to avoid undue weight gains. Alternatively throwers and rugby forwards can utilise beneficially the extra mass acquired. Though the demarcation line for non-hypertrophy is unclear, speed of contraction appears important in reducing the extent of hypertrophy.

Experience suggests that repeated sets of four to six repetitions at maximal intensity invokes hypertrophy while fewer sets of six to ten repetitions short of maximal effort promotes strength without concomitant muscle growth. Maximum can be conveniently determined by De Lorme's repetition maximum criterion which indicates the maximum load that can be lifted a given number of repetitions and varies with the number attempted. Mac Queen reported that when body builders employed less than RM intensity for considerably more than 10 repetitions and more than four or five sets hypertrophy did not result. Hypertrophy is regulated largely by testosterone which explains why pronounced muscle growth is not found when female athletes undertake severe strength training regimes.

Hypertrophy is observed when training is supplemented by synthetic sex hormones or anabolic steroids. Bouts of progressive exercise overload should be interspersed by regular rest periods to allow recovery. The common practice of weight training three or four times a week seems reasonable to avoid overuse but a minimum of twice-weekly strength sessions is recommended to provide adequate training stimulus. Ryan acknowledged insufficient rest as a factor contributing to injury and intermittent illness. De Lorme and Watkins found that five days per week was usually the heaviest schedule that could be employed without developing serious signs of delayed recovery. Clarke concluded that training at 6 RM for three sets, three times a week seemed an optimal combination. Progression involves an evolving upward spiral of overload-fatigue-recovery, with recovery improving as the individual gets fitter. Frequency and intensity may be reduced during the peak of the competitive season when the objective is to maintain the strength level already acquired and concentrate on speed and skill.

Evaluation and Measurement

Regular strength testing provides an objective basis for rescheduling regimes to apply progressive resistance. It serves also to evaluate the conditioning programme and give valuable feedback on the athlete's progress. It helps to identify weaknesses and devise individual schedules. Performance tests provide convenient criteria for strength measurement. Selected weight lifts can be used for 1RM, 6RM or 10RM. Tests involving moving a heavy load to exhaustion are also employed since muscular strength and absolute endurance are highly correlated. Strength measurement has typically employed instruments capable of recording the maximum force of an isometric contraction. These include cable tensiometers, dynamometers, spring balances and electrical strain gauges and administration is hardly feasible outside a sports science laboratory.

Peak force during dynamic movements may be recorded using isokinetic machinery. Static and dynamic measurement of rotational movements can be achieved by a dynamometer based on a rotary torque activator. The vertical and standing broad jumps conveniently indicate explosive strength and leg power. The softball throw or shot putt for distance have been used as indicants of muscle power in arm work. As power is a function of the rate of the rate of force application, strength is a major component. A power lever, based on wheel and axle lever system, permits direct measurement of the horsepower in a single explosive movement.

The stair run test of Margaria et al was designed to indicate the horsepower output of the phosphagens or maximum alactic anaerobic power. A comparable test for the bicycle ergometer has also been designed. Though these tests may be used for monitoring conditioning progress, the ultimate test of the validity of the training is the competitive performance.

The Principle of Reversibility

Reversibility indicates that a training effect subsides if training is discontinued. Strength gains are lost at about one-third their rate of acquisition. Athletes who abruptly terminate a crash course of pre-season strength training are likely to lose form in mid-season due to the relatively rapid strength loss. Isotonic training leads to greater retention than isometric. Strength loss after daily isometric training equalled the rate at which it was acquired in Muller's investigation. Hettinger and Morehouse claimed that strength gained can be retained with one high intensity session every two weeks.

At least a weekly work-out seems preferable for retention in top athletes through the competitive period through fortnightly sessions probably serve to retard strength loss. Strength gained is not entirely lost, a portion of it remaining indefinitely. Retraining, when commenced, is also considerably easier than initially. Special care is needed during the early weeks of retaining to avoid muscle pulls as athletes are often reluctant to accept their diminished function through inactivity.

Law of use and disuse

The organism habituates to the load placed on it indicating that structure is modified by function. Connective tissue and bone adapt as well as skeletal muscle. The muscle fibre and its surrounding sarcolemma thicken and the connective tissue of the muscle broadens and toughens. Primary cellular multiplication occurs in ligaments and tendons which grow and increase in tensile strength. Bones adapt to suit stresses and strains within their tolerance by forming new supportive trabeculae. Calcium phosphate and calcium carbonate in bone increase in response to training providing greater sturdiness. Severe repetitive strain may result in inflammation and osteoporosis as occurs in stress fractures. With prolonged rest, bones demineralise and weaken and muscles atrophy. The trainer's quandary is the recognition of the thin line separating harmful overload form the maximal stimulant for physiological accommodation. The triple principles of overload, reversibility and specificity contain a framework for regulating training regimes to permit continuous adaptation.

The Principle of Specificity

Specificity suggests that strength training effects may be limited to the pattern of muscular involvement in the conditioning exercise. Different types of motor units exist within muscle so that a give type of exercise units exist within muscle so that a given type of exercise recruits a specific combination of motor units best adapted to that demand. It is desirable that strength training routines should simulate closely the motor programme of the event and employ the specific muscle groups involved. This invites preliminary analysis of competitive skills. Specificity is also shown is isometric exercise in the strength gains may be restricted to the angle at which training occurred, so that isometrics should be undertaken at a series of joint angles.

Where great strength in needed only at the beginning of the movement, as in ballistic actions, exercises in that range may suffice. Specificity is further corroborated in that isometric programmes increase isometric strength more than they do isotonic strength, the reverse being also true. A strength training schedule should evidently be planned to suit individual needs. This must vary with the sport and be adjusted for age and sex. The curves showing average strength values in relation to age and sex can be altered by training which not only arrests the normal gradual decline after mid-20s but brings further improvement for another 10 to 15 years.

Though the difference between the sexes varies with muscle groups, it is common after adolescence to expect two-thirds of male strength in females. The difference is largely attributable to men's greater muscle mass though on average their bones, tendons and ligaments are also more robustly constructed. Female athletes are often unwilling to undertake strength regimes for social reasons and in consequence suffer more injuries in sports requiring explosive efforts.

Strength

Strength reflects the ability to apply force and overcome resistance. It is a function of the neuromusculo-skeletal system and closely related to muscle cross-sectional area. Its development is indispensable for success in sports performed against high power demands as shown by the muscular physique in top throwers, jumpers, sprinters and gymnasts. Muscularity and strength also favour performance in contact sports where the rigours of competition are more easily endured without injury. Manifestation of strength is found under various conditions.

Explosive strength

Explosive strength as defined by Fleishman denotes the ability to expend energy in one explosive act, as in jumping or projecting some object as far as possible. The force generated may be sub-maximal since force and velocity are interrelated. Muscle shortening velocity is greatest when externally unloaded while force is maximal at zero velocity or isometric conditions. In rapid contractions there is limited time for liberation of chemical energy and interconnections of myofibrilar filaments. Forces developed in eccentric contractions are greater at all velocities than those of concentric work.

Power output and mechanical efficiency are improved if muscle is pre-stretched allowing storage of elastic energy for immediate utilisation in concentric action. This is achieved in appropriate leg musculature by sinking the hips prior to jumping and in arm muscles by winding up before bowling. As explosive strength is applied rapidly under dynamic conditions it is imperative that technique is perfected to avoid injury. Absolute strength provides inadequate compensation for poor coordination when muscle or articulo-skeletal damage is promoted. In team games explosive strength must be allied to good timing. The rugby forward must strive to out jump his line-out opponent, win ball possession and avoid collisions at the same time.

Isometric Strength

Maximum isometric strength is defined operationally as the force of reaction achieved when the greatest possible effort is intentionally brought to bear in a static muscle contraction from two to six seconds duration. The muscle length stays constant and no movement occurs. Isometric strength is important when allied to the requisite sport skills where performance is periodically under static conditions or movement initiated by overcoming large resistance. This applies in rugby scrimmaging, tug-of-war, weightlifting and wrestling, for example. The hammer thrower needs to counter great centrifugal forces as he rotates and the soccer player balances statically on leg while place-kicking

Dynamic Strength

The strength of the limb muscles applied to moving or supporting body mass repeatedly over a given period of time was known as dynamic strength by Fleishman. It reflects the strength endurance of the organism or its ability to withstand fatigue under sustained strength expenditure exemplified in performing press-ups. Dynamic strength is especially important in maximal efforts of half-minute to three minutes duration. It is distinct from muscle endurance which indicates the ability of a muscle group to contract continually against a light load and which depends on the circulation. When muscle repeatedly contracts in a vigorous fashion fatigue is shown by its inability to continue delivering the same mechanical work. Maximal power output declines more rapidly due to a shift in the substrate subserving contraction.

Highest power is produced in the first few seconds of activity, values up to six horse power being found.

Fuel here is furnished by intramuscular phosphagens. When all-out effort is extended beyond these first seconds energy is supplied from glycogen within muscle anaerobically. This store increases the work capacity at a reduced power production. Eventually maximal effort is limited within a minute or so of onset by accumulation of metabolities and lowered pH within muscle, or lack of metabolic substrate due to retarded adenosine triphosphate synthesis. Under such fatigued conditions skill may become disjoined, judgement impaired and injury promoted.

Even in sustained activities where the organism operates with almost limitless though subdued power supply through oxidative phosphorylation, added strength facilitates both performance and individual safety since the relative strain on working muscles imposed by a fixed work load is now reduced. The poor strength and muscularity of endurance competitors leaves them vulnerable when responding to spurts from opponents or encountering steep uphill gradients.

Strength and muscle size

In general the larger the muscle the greater its strength, though the relationship has qualifications. Differences between muscles in strength capability arise from their pennation or manner of tendonous attachment. Muscles with parallel fibres, e.g. sartorius, have poor force production but great mobility compared to muscles whose fibres converge obliquely on the tendon. Surface area of contact is increased where muscle fibres approach the tendon from one side, e.g. soleus, both sides, e.g. rectus femoris, or multi-pennately, e.g. deltoid, rather than the end. Distributions of fibre types similarly account for variability between muscles and between individuals.

Thigh and calf muscles of top sprinters are endowed with high proportions of white or fast-twitch fibres compared with the abundance of red or slow-twitch fibres in endurance athletes. Responses of muscles and individuals to work-induced hypertrophy may very because of differences in fibre-type distributions. Finally, endurance training may reduce muscle size by decreasing intramuscular lipids or temporarily increase muscle diameter by combining exhaustive training and diet to boost muscular glycogen stores as done by marathon runners the week before racing.

Strength Training Methods

<u>Mechanical and Physical Resistances</u>

Weight training presents a convenient method of overloading muscle and is commonly employed in conditioning for competition. Loads are provided by dumb-bells or weights barbells and are easily adjustable for progressive resistance. Eccentric work can be incorporated by weight lowering in addition to the more usual lifting exercises so elastic as well as contractile elements in muscle are trained. Spring loaded devices allow eccentric arm work though they do not have inherent progressive resistance. Pulley systems permit alteration of the direction of force application and re frequently employed in land conditioning of swimmers. Hydraulics have been effectively incorporated in the design of rowing machines.

Isokinetic equipment allows constant speed of contraction and maximal force exertion throughout the complete range of movement. Multi-station apparatus affords an opportunity of training various muscle groups and engaging a squad of players on a single machine. Strength training can employ partner work if equipment is unavailable. Routines may involve pushing against an opponent's shoulder who reciprocates or performing half-squats with partner supported supine on the back. A whole team can be occupied in relay races, each member carrying a colleague on his back during his effort, adding variety to training. Resistance work using a partner is useful in sports where a partner or opponent is actually supported during performance as in ice-skating or wrestling.

Where facilities are improvised, a bench, box or chair is still easily obtained for step-ups. This can be useful where different strength requirements are juxtaposed. The long jumper, for instance, who needs great leg strength for take off and isometric back strength to stabilise his upper body in flight, can train both simultaneously by holding a medicine ball while stepping-up. Bench stepping has long been used for fitness testing as well as training as it permits calculation of mechanical work done. Other ergometric modes present suitable strength training methods under precisely controlled conditions. Cyclists might use friction braked bicycles which are also valuable in rehabilitation since bodyweight is not supported. Whole body and rowing ergometers are useful in conditioning oarsmen while motor driven treadmills can be modified for skiers. Flumes could be used for preparation of swimmers, canoeists and rowers under exact control. These facilities are expensive and could reasonably be made available only to the elite at centres of sporting excellence.

Isometrics

Isometrics implicate muscular tension without corresponding limb movement. Body segments or external objects may provide the resistance. Special isometric racks have been designed for use in diverse fashions in gymnasia. The scrummaging rack used by rugby forwards in training outdoors affords another example. Isometric programmes gained widespread appeal from the pioneer studies of Muller. The magnitude of the training effects reported initially were not replicated in later studies of fitter subjects. For these the work load had to be substantially elevated beyond the advocated daily contraction held for six seconds at 66 per cent of maximal isometric capacity to get similar results. Consequently the claims attributed earlier to isometrics were considerably qualified. Furthermore improvement may be restricted to the angle at which the contraction is held and this may not appreciably assist dynamic performance.

Thirdly, the concomitant compression of the vascular bed with occlusion of blood supply to the muscles under tension and the rise in blood pressure this precipitates make isometrics unsuitable for sedentary individuals undergoing exercise for prevention of coronary heart disease, particularly if they already possess predisposing factors. Isometric training is recommended where competition places specific demands for isometric strength It may be especially valuable to athletes desiring increased muscle strength without corresponding hypertrophy since isometrics do not provoke muscle growth. For the majority, isometrics can be judiciously incorporated into a broader conditioning programme.

Functional Overload

Strength can be improved by overloading the individual in practices closely related to competition requirements. Running in heavy boots, jumping with ankle weights or jackets weighted with lead are examples. The obvious advantage of this approach is the high likelihood of strength transfer to the event trained for. Functional overload can be applied to runners either by attachment of a harness held by a trainer at its ends, or drawing as led. The vigorous running action needed should not be greatly modified from normal for optimal effects. Wrist weights used by gymnasts are another example while weight throwers use excessively heavy implements or attempt explosive release of medicine balls. Various forms of rebounding and plyometric drills fall within this category.

These emphasise elasticproperties of muscle in their execution and tend to develop explosive strength. Drills include repetitive hopping on both legs together or separately, jumping decathlons or exaggerated bounding strides. In hopping, the hips should not sink below the level where the femur is parallel to the floor to safeguard the knee joint. Elevation onto or over a bench or box top on descent from a greater height. The quadriceps are stretched in lowering bodyweight prior to contracting powerfully and by storing elastic energy in the process increase the tension developed in positive work. Since the shock on landing is absorbed largely by the knee joints the complete drill must be smoothly controlled to avoid injury.

Strength training is considered an indispensable part of preparation for athletic competition and injury prevention. The programme should be geared to the individual's specific needs and be based on progressive resistance. General and specific conditioning should be developed and uneven strength gains avoided. Retraining during rehabilitation is important before returning to competition.

Natural Resistance

Muscles may be overloaded in working against supernormal resistance by carefully exploiting natural conditions. Running up sand dunes was vindicated in the performances of Australian middle-distance runners in the early 1960s. Flat soled shoes are recommended as barefoot athletes may tread on broken glass concealed in the sand. Weekly sessions are sufficient in incorporating sandhill training into the overall schedule in the early phase to avoid Achilles tendon trouble. Running along a flat beach or soft sand is another form of resistance training. In inland areas grassy hills provide a satisfactory alternative to sand dunes. Running on soft ground is also recommended provided conditions are not so slippery that hamstring tears are possible.

All these methods are eminently suitable for training dynamic strength. Other variations depending on climate and location include running on snow or ankle deep in water, as long as the normal running motion is not severely altered. Work in water may be especially useful for rehabilitation of leg muscles as the strain from lifting bodyweight against gravity is absent. Cyclists may take advantage of otherwise inclement windy conditions by repetitive short sprints against the wind. Man built environments may similarly be exploited. If conditions are too difficult for outdoor work, suitable indoor staircases can substitute for uphill gradients. Stadium terrace steps are frequently used by football coaches in the training of players.

Strength for Injury Prevention

Muscles act as agonists, antagonists and synergists to cause, permit and assist movement. Unwanted actions are prevented by muscles acting as stabilisers. The orderliness of patterned muscular involvement is regulated by the nervous system. Greater strength in stabilising musculature improves individual tolerance to those external exigencies promoting imbalance in various sports. The gymnast needs great leg strength to control landing from a vault as well as for the more explosive operations. In field-invasive games, greater leg strength assists the manifold manoeuvres such as turning, accelerating, decelerating, tackling and avoiding tackles without injury. In contact games great arborisation is needed and players with poor strength have greater difficulty in surviving prolonged competitive periods without being injured. Cahill and Griffith showed that pre-season total body conditioning significantly reduces the frequency and severity of knee injuries in American university footballers. Imperfect strength development in particular muscle groups may predispose to local injury.

This is because muscles may secure the integrity of joints by crossing the joint or having their tendons inserted around the capsule. Knee stability, for example, is considerably enhanced by strengthening the quadriceps which safeguard the joint in conjunction with the cruciate and collateral ligaments. Quadriceps exercises are especially recommended in rehabilitation of knee injuries as the joint is further unstable if their strength subsides. Return to contact games should be delayed until adequate knee strength is restored. Quadriceps development can allow professional athletes to make ligament or meniscus damage and osteoarthrosis. Similarly, shoulder stability is enhanced by training surrounding musculature and many back problems are avoided by developing the erector spinae. Improving the strength of abdominal and back muscles not only helps prevent lumbar pain but serves also to remedy low back pain conditions. Bodnar reported a relationship between the incidence of shoulder and neck injuries and weakness of the cervical muscles in American college footballers and recommended strengthening cervical and trunk muscles as protective measures. Uneven distribution of strength is likely to predispose to injury.

This may be manifested in disproportionate development in one of the agonist/antagonist pair. The hamstrings, antagonists to the quadriceps during the first 160 to 165° of leg extension, must equally be considered when devising training programmes for quadriceps. A greater susceptibility to hamstring strains is found when individuals have an inappropriate flexor-extensor strength ratio. The hamstring/quadriceps strength ratio recommended by Klein and Allman is 0.60. Uneven distribution is also evident in contralateral differences in strength acquisition. This inequality is seen in the girth of the serving arm in top tennis players compared with the non-playing limb and is a logical outcome of repetitive practice in throwing events and racket sports which impose unilateral demands. Imbalance can have serious consequences in the lower extremities as it is then likely to prompt asymmetrical locomotion. Liemohn found that all hamstring injuries in a group of track and field athletes were to the non-moniment leg, substantiating that the weaker side is the more susceptible.

Though specific unilateral demands are imposed in certain athletic performances, preparation should still involve bilateral strength training to avoid uneven gains. Some contra-lateral effects do occur in the non-exercised limb but are of insufficient magnitude to excuse not training both. Cross-training effects can however be exploited to reduce muscle atrophy and for reconditioning after immobilisation. Isotonic exercise has been found preferable to isometric for producing cross-training though both methods have shown equal effectiveness when equated for load and duration. Action potentials occur in contralateral musculature, demonstrating the irradiation of nerve impulses to extremities other than those directly engaged in activity. Seemingly, innervation of descending pyramidal fibres that cross sides before supplying muscles overflows to the smaller number of uncrossed fibres, so that movement occurs in an activated muscle and isometric contractions in its symmetrical partner.

Sufficient overflow occurs only under strong volition so high intensity is desirable for cross-education. The effect is supported by historilogical findings and underlines nervous system involvement in force application. Neural control of maximal voluntary effort results in a strength reserve not normally expressed. This reservoir may amount to 25 per cent and is released in exceptional circumstances and emergencies. It serves normally to protect the muscle, its tendon and bony attachment from over-exertion. This inhibition is eliminated under extreme motivational conditions. The effect is attributed to adrenaline release and reduced nervous inhibition which permit greater motor unit recruitment. This safety reserve is harnessed under strong motivation by athletes prior to strength events. It may also be tapped in training muscle by electrical stimulation though attendant risks make it inadvisable. Electrotherapy is valuable in rehabilitation to stimulate muscle which has temporarily lost its effective innervation since the motor pathways are minimally involved in electrical training.

Strength training reduces the effect of the inhibitory mechanism and permits greater tension to occur. This may be due to greater antagonist relaxation as the movement proceeds or to increased shielding of Golgi sensory organs by muscle connective tissue thickened from training, allowing innervation of the muscles to progress further uninhibited. A basic programme of general muscle conditioning is advocated to avoid leaving local weaknesses in the athlete' make-up.

A broad basis of general strength sets a foundation

on which specific strength can be safely developed. Improved arm and back strength allows the legs to be overloaded in power cleans and half-squats when leg strength in being specifically developed. An outstanding single benefit to a strengthened muscle is that greater stresses can be borne without training. Developed muscle also provides a fleshy shield to cushion the effect of blows on bone or abdominal organs, thereby affording some protection in combat sports.

The common definition of strength is the ability to exert a force against a resistance. The strength needed for a sprinter to explode from the blocks is different to the strength needed by a weight lifter to lift a 200kg barbell. This therefore implies that there are different types of strength.

What are the classifications of strength?

The classifications of strength are:

1. Elastic strength – the ability to overcome a resistance with a fast contraction

2. Maximum strength – the greatest force that is possible in a single maximum contraction

3. Strength endurance – the ability to express force many times over.

How do we develop each strength?

1. Elastic strength can be developed with:

- medicine ball exercises
- conditioning exercises
- complex training sessions
- weight training
- plyometric exercises

2. Strength endurance can be developed with:

- dumbbell exercises
- hill and harness running
- circuit training
- weight training

3. Maximum strength can be developed with:

- weight training

How do we get strong?

A muscle will only strengthen when it is worked beyond its normal operation, it is overloaded. Overload can be progressed by increasing the:

1. number of sets of the exercise
2. intensity reduced recover time
3. number of repetitions of an exercise

Medicine Ball

The ability to generate strength and power is a very important component for success in many sports, particularly in those involving explosive movements. Medicine ball training, in conjunction with a programme of weight training and circuit training, can be used to develop strength and power. Certain medicine ball exercises can also be used as part of a plyometric training programme to develop explosive movements. Medicine ball training is appropriate to all levels of ability, age, development and sport. To be most effective the programme should contain exercises that match the pattern of movements of the sport.

Technique and Safety

To ensure personal safety and good technique while doing medicine ball exercises the following points should be remembered:

1. On standing exercises plant feet before beginning to throw the ball

2. Maintain technique do not sacrifice control for distance

3. Inexperienced athletes should not take the ball too far back behind the head when carrying out overhead throws

4. Complete throws with full extension of the arms

5. When picking a ball, ensure the knees are bent and the back is kept straight

6. Always use the full joint range in the correct sequence in carrying out each exercise

7. When carrying out exercises lying on your back, ensure the lower back always remains in contact with the surface

8. Prior to a catch, ensure you:

- keep hands together
- keep arms extended
- keep eyes on the ball
- do not attempt to catch balls thrown wildly
- reach out to meet the ball prior to making contact

Planning a programme

The following are some guidelines in planning and running a medicine ball session:-

1. Before starting a session, explain the procedures for each exercise with your athletes

2. Medicine ball exercises must precede high intensity work

3. The programme should have exercises that match the pattern of movements of the sport

4. You will need to have a number of different weights of ball available-heavy, medium and light

5. Check there is sufficient space and that the structure of the walls are safe if any rebounding exercises are used

6. An effective work-out with medicine balls can be achieved in about 30 to 40 minutes, if the athlete works efficiently

7. Initial, athletes should use a light weight ball and gradually progress to heavier ones

8. Quality of movement is more beneficial than quantity of exercise repetitions or sets

9. Maintain good discipline as medicine balls can be dangerous if used incorrectly

10. Plan the programme to exercise alternate body parts

11. Always ensure the athletes carry out a thorough warm up and warm down

12. Partners who feed the medicine ball on certain exercises should be well drilled on what is required

13. Start sessions with lighter less dynamic exercises, then progress to heavier exercises

Example the following is an example of a programme of general medicine ball exercises.

Standing torso twist

1. Stand back to back 1 metre apart

2. Keep your hips facing forward and legs slightly relaxed

3. Keep your hips facing forward and legs slightly relaxed

How many – Two sets of ten reps

Chest push

1. Step forward and push ball upwards and towards your partner

2. Feet together

3. Hands behind ball and elbows out

Hamstring curls

1. Roll the ball along the back of legs

2. On reaching the heels the ball is filched up

3. Lie flat on the ground

Double leg kicks

1. Soles of feet facing partner

2. Partner throws ball in a looping path onto your feet

3. Lie on your back

4. Partner stands 3 metres away

5. Do not lower you legs to the ground

6. Bending your knees back to your chest the ball is then kicked back to your partner

Vertical extensions

1. Ball is returned between the knees

2. Stand back to back approx. 60cm apart

3. Ball is passed overhead

Straight arm standing throw

1. Place one foot 50 cm behind the other

2. Step forward and throw the ball to your partner, keeping the arms straight

3. Take the ball back, ensure hands are high, shoulders stretched and chest out

Lay back double arm throw

1. Throw another medicine ball to your partner
2. Partner returns ball to an overhead position
3. Support your back with a large medicine ball

Abdominal curl

1. knees bent
2. Draw knees up to the chest
3. Sitting up slightly, resting on your hands
4. Return to the starting position
5. Ball is held by the knees

Conditioning

One of the misconceptions in the sports world is that a sportsperson gets in shape by just playing or taking part in his/her chosen sport. If a stationary level of performance, consistent ability in executing a few limited skills, is your goal then engaging only in your sport will keep you there. However, if you want the utmost efficiency, consistent improvement, and balanced abilities sportsmen and women must participate in your round conditioning programs. The bottom line in sports conditioning and fitness training is stress. Not mental stress, but adaptive body stress. Sportsmen and women must put their bodies under a certain amount of stress to increase physical capabilities.

Physical Fitness

Physical fitness refers to the capacity of an athlete to meet the varied physical demands of their sport without reducing the athlete to a fatigued state. The components of physical fitness are: Strength, Endurance, Speed, Flexibility and Body Composition.

Complex Training

The two benefits from traditional strength work are:

1. increased muscle mass
2. increased neural activity

Strength work has been shown to improve sports performance particularly for sprinters, jumpers and throwers but it is not beneficial in developing rate of force the speed with which force is achieved in a movement. For example it takes around 400 msec to develop maximum force during a squat exercise, but the foot-ground contact time in sprinting is around 90 msec so there is not enough time to produce maximum force in sprinting. Therefore for speed strength events, like sprinting, it is the rate of force development that becomes more important than absolute strength. To develop the rate of force the Type IIb muscle fibres need to be targeted as these are ones that produce force most explosively allowing for maximum power. The sort of exercises that develop the Type IIb fibres are:

1. Plyometric exercises e.g. bounding.
2. Speed strength exercises e.g. weighted squats jumps

Many athletes include plyometric exercises in their training programs and are were aware of their benefits. However, it is slightly less well known that the combination of traditional strength with power and plyometric exercises together results in greater Type IIb recruitment and consequently greater improvements in power and rate of force development.

Definition of Fitness

Exercise scientists have identified nine elements that comprise the definition of fitness. The following lists each of the nine elements and an example of how they are used:–

1. Power — the ability to exert maximum muscular contraction instantly in an explosive burst of movements

2. Strength — the extent to which muscles can exert force by contracting against resistance

3. Agility — the ability to perform a series of explosive power movements in rapid succession in opposing directions

4. Flexibility — the ability to achieve an extended range of motion without being impeded by cxcess tissue, i.e. fat or muscle

5. Cardiovascular Endurance — The heart's ability to deliver blood to working muscles and their ability to use it

6. Coordination — the ability to integrate the above listed components so that effective movements are achieved.

7. Balance — the ability to control the body's position, either stationary or while moving

8. Local Muscle Endurance —a single muscle's ability to perform sustained work

Of all the nine elements of fitness cardiac respiratory qualities are the most important to develop as they enhance all the other components of the conditioning equation.

Quality not Quantity

To get the best from these training workouts you need to be physically fresh and motivated. Type IIb fibres are not magically recruited by just doing the workout, you have to be focused on the exercises and perform them as explosively as possible. Try to avoid hard aerobic or anaerobic sessions for at least 48 hours before a complex session. Once a complex session has started do not perform any static stretching exercises as this will relax the muscles and reduce force production potential. It is the quality of execution o f each exercise that is important, not the quantity. To ensure quality is maintained have the correct rest periods.

What is complex training?

Complex training is a workout comprising of a resistance exercise followed by a matched plyometric exercise e.g:

1. bench press followed by plyometric press up

2. squats followed by squat jumps

The logic behind these matched pair of exercises is that the resistance work gets the nervous system in to full action so that more Type IIb fibres are available for the explosive exercise, hence a better training benefit.

Plyometrics

Speed and strength are integral components of fitness found in varying degrees in virtually all athletic movements. Simply put the combination of speed and strength is power. For many years coaches and athletes have ought to improve power in order to enhance performance. Throughout this century and no doubt long before, jumping, bounding and hopping exercises have been used in various ways to enhance athletic performance. In recent years this distinct method of training for power or explosiveness has been termed plyometrics. Whatever the origins of the word the term is used to describe the method of training which seeks to enhance to explosive reaction of the individual through powerful muscular contractions as a result of rapid eccentric contractions.

Choose the method to fit the sport

The golden rule of any conditioning programme is specificity. This mans that the movement you perform in training should match, as closely as possible, the movements encountered during competition. If you are rugby player practising for the line-out or a volleyball player interested in increasing vertical jump height, then hop jumping or box jumping may be the right exercise. However if you are a javelin thrower aiming for a more explosive launch, then upper body plyometrics is far more appropriate.

Muscle Mechanism

The maximum force that a muscle can develop is attained during a rapid eccentric contraction. However, it should be realised that muscles seldom perform one type of contraction is isolation during athletic movements. When a concentric contraction occurs immediately following an eccentric contraction than the force generated can be dramatically increased. If a muscle is stretched, much of the energy required to stretch it is lost as heat, but some of this energy can be stored by the elastic components of the muscle. This stored energy is available to the muscle only during a subsequent contraction. It is important to realise that this energy boost is lost if the eccentric contraction is not followed immediately by a concentric effort. To express this greater force the muscle must contract within the shortest time possible. This whole process is frequently called the stretch shortening cycle and is the underlying mechanism of plyometric training.

Plyometric Exercises

The following are examples of lower body and upper body plyometric exercises.

Upper body

A variety of drills can be used to make the upper body more explosive:

Medicine Ball

Another means of increasing upper body strength popular with throwers is to lie on the ground face up. A partner then drops a medicine ball down towards the chest of the athlete, who catches the ball and immediately throws it back. This is another high-intensity exercise and should only be used after some basic conditioning.

Press ups and hand clap

Press-ups with a hand clap in between is a particularly vigorous way to condition the arms and chest. The pre-stretch takes place as the hands arrive back on the ground and the chest sinks, and this is followed quickly by the explosive upwards action. Once again, to get the best training effect keep the time in contact with the ground to a minimum.

Lower Body

Bounding and hurdling

If forward motion is more the name of your game, try some bounding. This is a form of plyometric training, where over sized strides are used in the running action and extra time spent in the air. Two-legged bounds reduces the impact to be endured, but to increase the intensity one legged bounding, or hopping, can be used.

Bounding upstairs is a usefulway to work on both the vertical and horizontal aspects of the running action. Multiple jumps over a series of obstacles like hurdles is a valuable drill for athletes training for sprinting or jumping events. Examples of lower body plyometric exercises with intensity level:

1. Jumps from standing –Standing long jump, Standing hop, standing jump for height

2. Multiple jumps with run in – 11 stride run +2 hops and a jump into sandpit, 2 stride run in + bounds

3. Eccentric drop and hold drills – hop and hold, bound/hop/bound/hop over 30m, drop and hold from a height > one metre

4. Standing based jumps performed on the spot – Tuck Jumps, Split Jumps

5. Depth jumping – jumps down and up off box, bounding up hill

6. Multiple jumps from standing – bounds, bunny hops, double footed jumps over how hurdle, double footed jumps up steps

Drop Jumping

This exercise involves the athlete dropping to the ground from a raised platform or box, and then immediately jumping up. The drop down gives the pre-stretch to the leg muscles and the vigorous drive upwards the secondary concentric contraction The exercise will be more effective the shorter the time the feet are in contact with the ground. The loading in this exercise is governed by the height of the drop which should be in the region of 30–80 cm. Drop jumping is a relatively high impact form of plyometric training and would normally be introduced after the athlete had become accustomed to lower impact alternatives, such as two-footed jumping on the spot.

Planning a Plyometric Session

The choice of exercises within a session and their order should be planned. A session could:

1. work through exercises that develop concentric strength

2. begin with exercises that are fast, explosive and designed for developing elastic strength

3. finish with training for eccentric strength.

An alternative session could be:

1. progress to bounding and hopping,

2. finish with medicine ball work out for abdominals and upper body.

3. begin with low hurdle jumps

4. continue with steps or box work

Example plyometric sessions for the arms and legs are detailed on the Leg Plyometric page and the Arm Plyometric page.

Conditioning for Polymetrics

Higher than normal forces are put on the musculoskeletal system during polymetric exercises so it is important for the athlete to have a good sound base of general strength and endurance. Most experts state that a thorough grounding in weight-training is essential before you start polymetrics. It has been suggested that an athlete be able to squat twice his body weight before attempting depth jumps. However, less intensive plyometric exercises can be incorporated into general circuit and weight training during the early stages of training so as to progressively condition the athlete. Simple plyometric drills such as skipping hopping and bounding should be introduced first. More demanding exercises such as flying start single-leg hops and depth jumps should be limited to thoroughly conditioned athletes. Conditioning programmes to develop leg strength are detailed on the Lower Leg Conditioning page and the Leg Conditioning page.

Warm up

A though warm up is essential prior to plyometric training. Attention should be given to jogging, stretching, striding and general mobility especially about the joints involved in the planned plyometric session. A cool down should follow each session.

How many?

It is wise not to perform too many repetitions in any one session and since it is a quality session, with the emphasis on speed and power rather than endurance, split the work into sets with ample recovery in between.

Young athletes

Some authors suggest that moderate jumps can be included in the athletic training of very young children. However, great care needs to be exerted when prescribing any training procedures for pre-adolescent children. Because of the relatively immature bone structure in pre-adolescent and adolescent children the very great forces exerted during intensive depth jumps should be avoided.

Where to do it and what to wear

For bounding exercises use surfaces such as grass or resilient surfaces. Avoid cement floors because there is no cushioning. Choose well-cushioned shoes that are stable and can absorb some of the inevitable impact. All athletes should undergo general orthopedic screening before engaging in plyometric training. Particular attention should be given to structural or postural problems that are likely to predispose the athlete to injury.

Arm Plyometrics

This page contains a selection of plyometric exercises designed to develop the elastic strength of the arms.

How to perform the drill

1. Stand facing each other with your feet shoulder width apart and your knees slightly bent

2. Pass the ball to your partner, pushing it off your chest and ending with your arms straight

3. This drill requires a partner

4. Try to anticipate the catch and return the ball as quickly as you can

5. Begin by holding the medicine ball with both hands at chest level, elbows pointing out

6. Keep the catch time to the shortest time possible

7. Your partner catches the ball, allows the ball to come to the chest before passing it back to you

Incline Push up depth jump

1. Face the floor as if you were going to do a push-up, with your feet on the box and your hands between the mats

2. Two mats, three to four inches high, placed shoulder width apart

3. Push off the mats with both hands and catch yourself in the starting position

4. A box high enough to elevate your feet above your

shoulders when in a push-up position

5. Push off from the ground with your hands and land with one hand on each mat

How to perform the drill

1. Lie supine on the ground with your arms outstretched

2. Your partner drops the medicine ball into your hands.

3. This drill requires a partner

4. Your partner stands on the box holding the medicine ball at arm's length

5. Catch the ball with elbows bent

6. Extend the arms to propel the ball back to the partner on the box

7. Keep the catch time to the shortest time possible

8. Allow the ball to come towards your chest

How to perform the drill

1. Lean back at a 45 degree angle, keeping your abdominals tight

2. Work with a partner and sit facing each other

3. Pass the ball to your partner, pushing it of your chest and ending with your arms straight

4. Try to anticipate the catch and return the ball as quickly as you can

5. Being by holding the medicine ball with both hands at chest level, elbows pointing out

6. Your partner catches the ball, allows the ball to come to the chest before passing it back to you

7. Keep the catch time to the shortest time possible

Young athletes

Some authors suggest that moderate jumps can be included in the athletic training of very young children. However, great care needs to be exerted when prescribing any training programmes for pre-adolescent children. Because of the relatively immature bone structure in pre-adolescent and adolescent children the very great forces exerted during intensive depth jumps should be avoided.

Where to do it and what to wear

For bounding exercises use surfaces such as grass or resilient surfaces. Avoid cement floors because there is no cushioning. Choose well-cushioned shoes that are stable and can absorb some of the inevitable impact. All athletes should undergo general orthopaedic screening before engaging in plyometric training. Particular attention should be given to structural or postural problems that are likely to predispose the athlete to injury.

Bounds

1. Push off with your left foot and bring the leg forward, with the knee bent and the thigh parallel to the ground

2. Hold this extended stride for a brief time, then land on your left foot

3. Make each stride long, and try to cover as much distance as possible

4. Jog into the start of the exercise

5. At the same time, reach forward with your right arm. As the left leg comes through, the right leg extends back and remains extended for the duration of the push-

off

6. The right leg then drives through to a forward bent position, the left arm reaches forward, and the left leg extends backward

7. You should land on the sole of the foot, allowing energy to be stored by the elastic components of the leg muscles, and immediately take off again.

Hurdle Hopping

How to perform the drill

1. The movement should come from your hips and knees

2. Tuck both knees to your chest

3. Keep your body vertical and straight, and do not let your knees move apart or to either side.

4. You should land on the balls of the feet, allowing energy to be stored by the elastic components of the leg muscles, and immediately take off again

How much

1. Allow a full recovery between each set

2. One to three sets using 6 to 8 hurdles

3. Hurdles should set up in a row, spaced according to ability

4. Quality of hurdle hopping is far more important than quantity

5. The height of the hurdles should be in the region of 12 and 36 inches high

Single Leg Hopping

How to perform the drill

1. Push off with the leg you are standing on the jump

forward, landing on the same leg

2. You should land on the ball of the foot, allowing energy to be stored by the elastic components of the leg muscles, and immediately take off again

3. Try to keep your body vertical and straight

4. Beginners will use a straighter leg action where as advanced athletes should try to pull the heel toward the buttocks during the jump

5. Stand on one leg

6. Use a forceful swing of the opposite leg to increase the length of the jump but aim primarily for height off each jump.

7. Keep the foot touch down time to the shortest time possible

8. Perform this drill on both legs

How much

1. One to three sets over 30 to 40 metres

2. Quality of bounding is far more important than quantity

3. Allow a full recovery between each set

Depth Jumps

How to perform the drill

1. Stand on the box with your toes close to the front edge

2. Try to anticipate the landing and spring up as quickly as you can

3. Step from the box and drop to land on then balls of both feet

Keep the feet touch down time on the ground to the

shortest time possible

How much

1. Allow a full recovery between each set

2. The height of the box should be in the region of 30 80 cm

3. One to three sets using 6 to 8 boxes

Box Jumps

How to perform the drill

1. Keep your hands on your hips or behind your head

2. Assume a deep squat position with your feet shoulder width apart at the end of the row of boxes

3. Maintaining the squat position, jump off the box onto the ground, landing softly in a squat position on the balls of the foot

4. Jump onto the box, landing softly in a squat position on the balls of the feet

5. Keep the feet touch down time on the ground to the shortest time possible

6. Jump onto the next box and so on

How much

1. Allow a full recovery between each set

2. One to three sets using 6 to 8 boxes

3. Quality of box jumping is far more important than quantity

4. The height of the box should be in the region of 30-80cm

Where to do it and what to wear

For bounding exercises use surfaces such as grass

or resilient surfaces. Avoid cement floors because there is no cushioning. Choose well-cushioned shoes that are stable and can absorb some of the inevitable impact. All athletes should undergo general orthopaedic screening before engaging in plyometric training. Particular attention should be given to structural or postural problems that are likely to predispose the athlete to injury.

Warm up

A thorough warm-up is essential prior to plyometric training. Attention should be given to jogging, stretching, striding and general mobility especially about the joints involved in the planned plyometric session. A warm-down should follow each session.

Young athletes

Some authors suggest that moderate jumps can be included in the athletic training of very young children. However, great care needs to be exerted when prescribing any training procedures for pre-adolescent children. Because of the relatively immature bone structure in pre-adolescent and adolescent children the very great forces exerted during intensive depth jumps should be avoided.

Plyometric Exercises

Emphasis on these exercises is a high knee action and height–except for speed bounding where the emphasis is speed across the ground. The upper leg should be parallel with the ground, lower leg vertical and the foot dorsi flexed.

Weight Training

Better performances can be the product of a number of factors. This product is primarily the outcome of efficient technique, the progression of speed and the maturing competitive attitude on a sound basis of general endurance, all round strength and general mobility. The development of all round strength is best achieved via circuit training and then progressing this through strength training. Weight training is the most widely used and popular method of increasing strength.

Complex Training

Specific phase of training – example 2 sets

1. Weight Exercise - 4 reps with 8 RM
2. Plyometric exercise
3. 3 min recovery
4. Weight Exercise - 4 reps with 8 RM
5. Plyometric exercise
6. 3 min recover

Repeat for next exercise

General phase of training–example 2 sets

1. Weight exercise – 6 reps with 12 RM
2. 1 min recover
3. weight exercise – 6 reps with 12 RM
4. 1 min recover
5. Plyometric exercise
6. 3 min recover
7. Repeat for next exercise

How do we get stronger?

A muscle will only strengthen when forced to operate beyond its customary intensity. Overload can be progressed by increasing the:

1. resistance e.g. adding 10 kg to the barbell
2. number of sets of the exercise
3. number of repetitions with a particular weight

Which weight training exercises?

The exercise must be specific to the type of strength required, and is therefore related to the particular demands of the event. The coach should have knowledge of the predominant types of muscular activity associated with the particular event, the movement pattern involved and the type of strength required. Exercises should be identified that will produce the desired development. Although specificity is important, it is necessary is every schedule to include exercises of a general nature – e.g.

Power Snatch

Power Clean

Back Squats

Bench Press

Sit Ups

Chest Press

Shoulder Press

Lat Pull downs

Lower Back Extensions

Calf Raise

Tricep Press

Bicep Curls

Leg Extension

Leg Curls

Leg Press

These general exercises give a balanced development, and provide a strong base upon which highly specific exercise can be built.

Muscle Fibre Hypertrophy

Resistance training will increase the muscle size. Muscle growth depends on the muscle fibre type activated and the pattern of recruitment. Muscle growth is due to one or more of the following adaptions:

1. Increased number of and size of myofibrils per muscle fibre
2. Increased enzymes and stored nutrients
3. Increased contractile proteins
4. Increased amounts of connective, tendinous and ligamentous tissues

Olympic Lifts

The Olympic Lifts are recommend exercises for inclusion in power and speed training programs. The objective of these exercises is to develop the large muscles of the body in an explosive action which requires the use of many joints and muscle groups in a coordinated movement. The Olympic Lifts comprise of the Clean and Jerk and the Snatch. The Power Snatch and Power Clean are auxiliary lifts that aid in the training of the Clean and Jerk and the Snatch.

1. Jerk
2. Power Snatch
3. Power Clean

How Much?

The amount of weight to be used should be based on a percentage of the maximum amount of weight that can be lifted one time, generally referred to as one repetition maximum. The maximum number of repetitions performed before fatigue prohibits the completion of an additional repetition is a function of the weight used, referred to as repetition maximum, and reflects the intensity of the exercise. A weight load that produces fatigue on the third repetition is termed a three repetition maximum and corresponds to approximately 95% of the weight the could be lifted for 1 RM. For maximum results athletes should train according to their genetic predisposition.

An athlete with a greater proportion of slow twitch muscles would adapt better to an endurance training and a muscular endurance program using more repetitions of a lighter weight. An athlete with a greater proportion of fast twitch muscles would benefit from sprint training and a muscular strength program using fewer repetitions of a heavier weight.

Rest Interval between sets

The aim of the recovery period between sets is to replenish the stores of ATP and Creatine Phosphate in the muscles. An inadequate recovery means more reliance on the Lactic Acid energy pathway in the next set. Several factors influence the recovery period, including:

1. Type of strength you are developing
2. Number of muscle groups used in the exercise
3. The load used in the exercise
4. Your weight
5. Your condition

A recovery of three to five minutes or longer will allow almost the complete restoration of ATP/CP.

Load - Repetition Relationship

The strength training zone requires you to use loads in the range of 60% to 100% of 1 RM. The relationship of percentage loads to number of repetitions to failure are as follows:

60% - 17 reps

65% - 14 reps

70% - 12 reps

75% - 10 reps

80% - 8 reps

85% - 6 reps

90% - 5 reps

95% - 3 reps

100% - 1 reps

How Many

The number of repetitions performed to fatigue is an important consideration in designing a strength training program. The greatest strength gains appear to result from working with 4 - 6 RM. Increasing this to 12-20RM favours the increase in muscle endurance and mass. One set of 4-6RM performed 3 days a week is a typical strength training program. The optimal number of sets of an exercise to develop muscle strength remains controversial. In a number of studies comparing multiple set programs to produce greater strength gains than a single set, the majority of studies indicate that there is not a significant difference. Handling heavy weights in the pursuit of strength will require a recovery of 3-5 minutes between sets, but only minimum recovery should be taken if strength endurance is the aim.

The majority of athletic events are fast and dynamic, and therefore this quality must be reflected in the athlete's strength work. Muscular strength is primarily developed when 8 RM or less is used in a set. How much load you use depends upon what it is you wish to develop:

1. 1 RM to 3RM - neuromuscular strength

2. 4RM to 6 RM -maximum strength by stimulating muscle hypertrophy

3. 6 RM to 12 RM -muscle size with moderate gains in strength

4. 12RM to 20RM-muscle size and endurance

Rest Interval between sessions

The energy source being used during the training session is probably the most important factor to consider. During the maximum strength phase, when you are primarily using the ATP/CP energy pathway, daily training is possible because ATP/CP restoration is completed within 24 hours. If you are training for muscular endurance then you require a 48 hour recovery as this is how long it takes to fully restore your glycogen stores. As a 'rule of thumb' 48 hours should elapse between sessions. If training strenuously, any athlete will find it extremely difficult to maintain the same level of lifting at each session, and the total poundage lifted in each session would be better to be varied each week.

Training Systems

Pyramid System

Here the load is increased and the repetitions are reduced. Pyramid lifting is only for experienced lifters who have an established good technique.

Simple sets

3 × 8 with 70% -meaning three sets of eight repetitions with a weight of 70% of maximum for one repetition. This is the system that all novice lifters should work on, because the high number of repetitions enables the lifter to learn correct technique, and thereby reduce the risk of injury.

Super Setting

This consists of performing two or three exercises continuously, without rest is between sets, until all exercises have been performed. The normal 'between sets' rest is taken before the next circuit of exercises is commenced.

What sort of weight lifting equipment?

There are variable resistance machines and free weights. Variable resistance machines are effective tools for building strength and muscle tone and are designed to work the target muscle in isolation, without the assistancc of the surrounding muscles. Free weights and machines that provide the same equal resistance to a allow you not only to target a particular muscle group but to engage other muscles that assist in the work. Once they are conditioned, these assisting muscles help you to increase the weight you use in training the target muscles in order to stimulate the most growth in muscle fibres. The assisting muscles help stabilize the body, support limbs and maintain posture during a lift. Lifting free weights improves your coordination by improving the neuromuscular pathways that connect your muscles to the central nervous system.

Training Programs

Use the above notes to assist you in the preparation of a general strength training program, to develop your general strength, and a specific strength training program to develop your specific strength to meet to the demands of your event/sport. If weight training facilities is limited to your home and a set of dumbbells then it is still possible to construct a dumbbell weight training program. To monitor progress in training you should conduct strength and muscle balance tests.

Circuit Training

Circuit training is an excellent way to simultaneously improve mobility, strength and stamina. The circuit training format utilizes a group of 6 to 10 strength exercises that are completed one exercise after another. Each exercise is performed for a specified number of repetitions or for a prescribed time period before moving on to the next exercise. The exercises within each circuit are separated by brief, timed rest intervals, and each circuit is separated by a longer rest period. The total number of circuits performed during a training session may vary from two to six depending on your training level, your period of training and your training objective.

Safety in the Weight Room

Strength training is safe when properly supervised and controlled. Every weight room should have a set of rues and regulations pertaining to safety and they should be on public display. Rules may vary from one weight room to another but some very basic rules apply to them all:

1. Follow your training schedule
2. Train only when a qualified coach is present
3. Work in pairs – one lifting the other spotting
4. Wear the correct clothing and shoes
5. No personal stereos with headphones

6. Only athletes who are working out should be in the weight room

7. No horseplay

8. No eating, drinking or smoking

9. Help and respect other athletes

Make sure you and your athletes are fully aware of the safety rules applying to the weight training room you use.

Example sessions from Owen Anderson

Warm up with 10 to 15 minutes of easy jogging, swimming or cycling, and then perform the following exercises in order. Move quickly from exercise to exercise, but don't perform the exercises themselves too quickly.

- Run 400 meters at current 5k race pacc
- Complete 36 abdominal crunches
- Do 5 chin-ups
- Do 15 press-ups
- Perform 15 squat thrusts with jumps
- Run 400 metres at 5k pace again
- Complete 30 body-weight squats
- Do 12 squat and dumbbell presses
- Perform 36 low-back extensions
- Complete 15 lunges with each leg
- Repeat steps 2–13 one more time, and then cool down with about 15 minutes of light jogging, swimming, or cycling.
- Do 15 bench dips

• Run 400 meters at 5k pace again

Once your fitness and strength have increased so much that the above circuit sessions are no longer challenging, you can then move on to a more challenging circuit workout, as follows: Warm up with two miles of easy running, and then perform the following exercises in order. Move quickly from exercise to exercise, but don't perform the exercises themselves too quickly.

• Complete 8 high bench step ups with jumps

• Perform 3 series of the 6 way lunge with arm drop

• Perform 8 prone trunk extensions with arm raises

• Run 400 meters at 5k race pace

• Do 6 plyometric press ups

Repeat steps 2 to 8 once more, and then cool down with 2 miles of easy ambling.

• Complete 8 reps of the hanging scissors plus double knee raise

• Run 400 metres at 5k race pace

Half Marathon Circuit

Warm up with two miles of easy running and follow with some stretching routines and then perform the following activities in order. Move quickly from exercise to exercise, don't perform the exercises themselves too quickly.

• Run one mile at your goal half-marathon velocity

• Do 70 ab crunches

• Carry out 70 low back extensions

• Complete 15 one leg squats with your right leg and then 15 more with your left

• Carry out 30 bench dips

• Jump 100 times in place, getting your propulsive force from your ankles, not your knees, and carrying out the last 30 jumps at an especially quick tempo

• 5 × 100 meters at close to top speed, with short recoveries

• Complete 20 squat thrusts with jumps

• Perform 20 lunges with each leg, with your non lunging foot on a step or platform which is about six inches off the ground.

• Do 20 press-ups

• Run one mile at goal half marathon velocity

• Carry out 30 cross body leg swings with each leg. To do these, lean slightly forward with your hands on a wall and your full body weight on your left leg. Then, swing your right leg to the left in front of your body, pointing your toes up as your foot reaches it final point of movement. Repeat this overall motion 30 times before performing 30 reps with your left leg.

• Repeat steps 3 to 14 one more time, and then cool down with two miles of light jogging

• Run one mile at goal half-marathon velocity

Marathon Circuit

Warm up with two miles of easy running and follow with some stretching routines and then perform exercise to exercise, but don't perform the exercises themselves too quickly.

1. Complete 15 burpees

2. Do 12 one leg squats with each leg

3. Carry out 50 abdominal crunches

4. Perform 50 low back extensions

5. Do 12 feet elevated press ups

6. Carry out 12 high bench step ups

7. Repeat steps 2 to 13 twice more

8. Run 800 metres at what feels like 10K intensity

9. Perform 12 press ups

10. Run 800 metres at a little faster than marathon speed

11. Complete 12 lunges with each leg

12. Run 800 metres at a little faster than goal marathon speed

13. Cool down with two miles of easy running

14. Do 15 bench dips

15. Run 1600 metres at a little faster than goal marathon speed

These circuits build a tremendous foundation of whole body strength and fatigue resistance, both of which are critically important for marathon running. The circuits also improve efficiency while running at marathon intensity and help to raise lactate threshold.

15

WEIGHT TRAINING FOR FITNESS

The use of weights to improve the functional efficiency of the human is probably as old as sport itself. The celebrated Milo of Croton is reputed to have started his athletic training by raising a new-born calf over his head and continuing the practice daily, he grew in strength until the animal reached maturity. He provides a good illustration of the use of progressive resistance exercise. In subsequent centuries man has continued to search for ingenious methods of resisting muscle action to enhance his function as well as derive a variety of lifting and throwing competitions.

This chapter outlines some common uses of weight training and suggests ways that injuries associated with the practice may be avoided. It is first necessary to distinguish between weightlifting and weight training. Weightlifting is a competitive sport contested in the Olympic Games whereas weight training describes the employment of weights in the training regimes of non-athletes as well as athletes. The two Olympic lifts most commonly demonstrated to illustrate the sport are the snatch and the clean and jerk. These are known as the quick lifts because of the agility and coordination required for their execution. The rules for each event determine how the lift is performed.

The clean and jerk

This is performed in two phases. The clean requires that the weight be pulled to the chest in an uninterrupted motion. This has some similarity with the snatch though heavier loads can be lifted. Preparatory to the next phase the lifter stands with the load at his chest. He flexes his knees, then jumps upwards with the weight, throwing it to an overhead position as he again parts his legs to get underneath the ascending weight. Here also the upright position must be assumed with the weight held overhead to achieve a valid lift. There are a few observations about weightlifting that also help to illuminate the field of weight training. Weightlifting is a heavy resistance weight-bearing action, necessitating great explosive power and the ability to hold great weights momentarily under control.

The lifter uses maximal efforts against extremely heavy loads in training and in competition. It is at.these intensities that stresses on the articulo-skeletal system are greatest. The lifts are rapidly executed, taking in toto less than six seconds per lift. Studies of weightlifters show that over a two-hour training session they may be actually working for only two to six minutes, though this work will be extremely strenuous. It is essential that correct techniques be applied to reduce the strain at body sites of greatest vulnerability–the knee, the back and the wrist. The knee joint is particularly vulnerable at the initiation of the lift before the quadriceps contract powerfully. The back experiences high levels of strain, the force acting on a lumbo-sacral disc being calculated to exceed 1000kg in the study of Morris and co-workers.

The load on the spine is to an extent alleviated by

the intra-abdominal pressure induced. For these reasons it is essential that the lift be carried out in a manner that minimises mechanical strain on the spine. Frequently the annulus fibrosus cartilage is strained. Efficient lifting actions should be practised, imperfections being corrected during the early stages of learning the techniques. Deterioration at the wrist may occur due to hyperextension associated with repetitive lifting and holding weights overhead. Fractures of the distal radial epiphysis have been reported in adolescent weightlifters executing the military press. Rowe reported a comminuted fracture of the distal end of the radius and fracture of the ulnar styloid process on sudden hyperextension of the wrist of losing control of the weight.

Finally, it is important not to suspend breathing during the moment of extreme exertion. With the breath held and the epiglottis closed the chest is compressed and intrathoracic pressure builds up. This precipitates the Valsalva manoeuvre, resulting in a reduced venous return to the heart and consequent rapid drop in blood pressure with possible loss of consciousness. International weightlifters have fainted during competition as a result of failure to time their breathing correctly.

The Snatch

In the snatch, the weight must be brought from the floor to a position overhead without interruption. This action involves pulling the weight as high as possible, then splitting the legs apart in the sagittal plane to nip underneath as it ascends. The arms must lock straight promptly as the weight reaches the peak of its ascent. The lifter must then stand upright with the weight held overhead.

ACCOMMODATING RESISTANCE MODES

Nautilus equipment

An alternative form of accommodating resistance is provided by Nautilus equipment. This is not isokinetic machinery since the speed of contraction may vary. The apparatus provides stretching the involved muscle group in the starting position and resistance throughout the range of movement correlated to the force exerted. A specially shaped cam compensates for the variations in force by changing the moment arm and the resistance is increased or decreased even though the machine loading remains constant. The machinery allows a rotary movement in 17 different stations for various exercises. The cams for each machine are designed according to the strength curves of the different muscle groups with varying angles. As a result the resistance is lowest at the joint's weakest position and greatest in its peak strength position.

Isokinetics

Isokinetics describes the form of exercise permitted by machinery with the facility to adapt resistance to the force exerted. Normally when weights are lifted through a range of movement the maximum load is limited to that sustainable by the muscles involved at the weakest point in the range. Consequently other points within the range undergo sub-maximal training stimuli. With isokinetic machines this problem is overcome as the speed of contraction is pre-set, a speed governor in the apparatus allowing the resistance to adapt to the force applied. In this way, the greater the effort exerted the greater is the resistance, and maximal effort can be performed throughout the complete range of movement.

Where comparisons have been made, training programmes using isokinetic machines have proved superior to isometric and typical progressive resistance programmes with high speeds producing best results. Using Mini-Gym, Lumex or Cybex isokinetic apparatus, the weight-thrower can go through the pattern of shoulder and arm motion of his competitive event, so getting a training effect suitable for his specific purpose. Accessory equipment can be attached to the machine to accommodate specificity training for a range of sports. A limitation of isokinetic exercise of that it may interfere with the natural pattern of acceleration employed in the competitive action. Additionally it provides opportunity for just concentric work.

CONVENTIONAL WEIGHT TRAINING EXERCISES

Quite apart from the Olympic lifts used at the International Weightlifting Federation's competitions, the British Amateur Weightlifters' Association recognises 31 lifts. From this battery a number have been adopted over the last two decades or so by athletes for use in general conditioning. In most cases the lifts have been modified to provide an action compatible with the athlete's specific requirements. A typical sample of such exercises, which can also be used by sedentary individuals for positive health purposes follows. These exercises are divided according to the degree of skeletal muscle involvement into light muscle group or large muscle group work.

Large muscle-group work

Squats

A loaded barbell is supported on the back of the neck. Sometimes a piece of foam rubber or a towel is used to alleviate pressure on the cervical vertebrae. The body is lowered from standing to a squat position, form which its weight plus the loaded barbell must be lifted by powerful contraction of the knee extensors. This exercise has come in for much criticism because of the risk of knee joint degeneration from strain on the patellar bursae. During deep knee bending without attendant weights the patello-tendon force has been calculated by Reilly and Martens to reach 7.6 times bodyweigth. In the full squat position with posterior aspects of thigh and calf in contact, the knee, ligaments are overstretched and long-term ligamentous damage may be caused.

In this position the lateral meniscus may also suffer from being caught between the femoral condyle and the tibial plateau. For these reasons performance of partial squats is advised, though full squats may be permitted at much less frequent intervals to provide maximum overload and maintain the joint's range of movement. Maintenance of stability may present a problem during this exercise. Initially the athlete assumes a starting position with feet apart underneath the hips to best support the bodyweight. Stability is achieved by keeping the line of gravity within the base of support.

This is effected by pushing the hips back slowly as the bodyweight is lowered. By retaining heel contact with the ground the base of support is kept relatively large and stability facilitated. One manoeuvre to assist balance is to elevate the heels by means of an inclined board or to perform the exercise with a board placed underneath the heels. A more satisfactory procedure is to use a steel rack which arrests movement of the bar in the fore and aft direction and which incorporates obvious additional safety factors. These racks are installed in all well-equipped gymnasia. Since greater weights can be lowered than lifted, a useful modification of the half-squat is to overload the individual beyond his lifting capacity and allow him to slowly lower the weight under eccentric muscular control.

Sit-UPS

The resistance is normally provided by approximately half the body mass which the abdominal muscles must move against gravity. The load on the abdominals in a sit-up action from supine lying can be increased by holding a loaded barbell on the chest. This is preferable on comfort criteria alone to holding a disc behind the neck. An assistant is needed to hold the ankles of the athlete to facilitate the action. Another variation is to sit-up with a twist, arms behind the head, to touch each knee alternately with contra-lateral elbows.

Squat Jumps

Here the athlete jumps high into the air from a squat or partial squat position with a loaded barbell supported on his shoulders. Good coordination is essential to prevent overbalancing on landing. Frequently a towel is used underneath the bar to cushion its jarring effcct. When ascending it is necessary to pull down hard on the bar to avoid its bouncing against the back of the neck. It is particularly beneficial to athletes who during performance move the body explosively against gravity.

Power Cleans

This exercise involves approximately the same energy demands as a full squat. The weight is lifted from the floor to above head height in one complete movement. Special attention to technique is needed in the initial lifting movement. There has been considerable discussion for many years of the relative demerits of the back-lift with knees straight (the derrick lift) and with the trunk erect and knees flexed (the knee action) in various industrial contexts. Whitney (1962), for example, compared the strength of the lifting action in both types of lift. The knee lift is preferable, with the back straight to prevent the turning of the spine into a cantilever with consequent spinal strain. Correct placement of the feet is essential prior to attempting the lift.

The athlete should become accustomed to performing the action with the head erect and looking directly ahead and so avoid the natural temptation to look down at the weight as he attempts to overcome its inertia. As the forces on the spine are a function of the distance the weight is away from it, is recommended to keep the weight close to the body as it is being lifted.

<u>Bench Step-UPS</u>

Bodyweight plus a weighted barbell provide the resistance as the athlete steps repeatedly on to a bench with load supported on the shoulders. Ideally the bench height should be matched to the stature of the individual, otherwise quadriceps tear is a risk where the smaller athletes operate with a high bench. With too heavy weights the rhythm of stepping may be disrupted with consequent danger of overbalancing and injury.

<u>High Pulls</u>

This involves basically the same gross muscular action and equivalent energy expenditure as power cleans. The barbell is taken from the floor to a height roughly in line with the clavicles. The athlete may increase the work done by coming up on to his toes to complete the lift, good coordination being demanded for this. The elbows are raised above the bar at its high-point, which does not go overhead. Again it is important to keep the back straight during the left as jerking into back extension, particularly during the early phase of the action, can be damaging.

Arm and shoulder work

<u>Overhead Press</u>

Overhead press can be performed standing upright or sitting on a bench. The starting position can be from the chest but usually the weight is pressed vertically from behind the neck until the arms are at full stretch overhead, an inflated chest acting as a platform from which the action takes place. In the standing posture heavy weights may produce compensating movements in the legs or trunk to allow the action to be completed. In younger individuals acquiring the technique, an assistant can apply light pressure at the scapulae to prevent swaying. Alternatively, it may help if the action is performed with immediate visual feedback from a mirror. If dumb-bells are used the line of action of the specific competitive performance can be employed. Shot putters, for example, may use one or both arms alternately or simultaneously at an angle of release of release in the sagittal plane of approximately 45°.

Overarm-Pulls

This exercise may be performed with the athlete lying supine on a bench and feet supported on the ground. The arms may be held straight or flexed. A mild flexion is recommended to reduce strain on the shoulder joint. The weights lifted should not be unduly heavy, otherwise they will be difficult to control at the outer ranges of movement. The barbell may be taken from a position on the ground in a circular motion forward to a position over the chest or continued further to rest on the thighs. Endurance athletes can usefully employ this exercise because the serratus anterior is stretched as the weight is lowered to recommence the movement. Correct timing or breathing is important, inhalation occurring as the weight descends towards the ground and exhalation as the load is taken back up.

Bench Press

The athlete lies supine on the bench with feet apart and supported on the ground on either side. Two spotters are used for precautionary reasons. The bar is taken from supporting stands by the spotters and handed to the athlete on his upper chest. Taking the bar in too high near the throat is to be avoided on safety considerations. Normally a wide handle greater weights, though this defeats the purpose anterior deltoids and triceps. However, care must be taken that the grip is sufficiently wide not to jeopardise spotters as 40kg is sufficient to lacerate the facial bones from a fall of half a metre. The weight is pushed vertically from the chest. Prior to the movement it is necessary to have the chest full of air to provide a rigid exhales base from which the weight is moved. The performer exhales after the weight ascends.

The bar should be lowered slowly so as to permit complete control of the weight throughout. Altering the hand spacing affects the pattern of muscular involvement. Dumb-bells may be used to replace the barbell and, though this invariably means a lower resistance, it allows movement through a greater range. An alternative procedure is to have the assistants lift the barbell, the athlete's task being to control its lowering by eccentric muscle contractions. This overcomes the limitation of performing only un-directional work. Heavier loads can be handled than in concentric work. The benefits of the training programme are enhanced when both concentric and eccentric action are employed. Bench pressing is ubiquitous in the weight-training programmes of sportsmen. It has been widely accepted by runners, jumpers and games players.

Rowing

Rowing may be performed from an upright or a bent forward posture. The action should be restricted to the arms and shoulders, with careful attention given to the exclusion of the back and trunk. In both forms, the downward movement of the bar should be controlled. An observer can ensure the posture does not get progressively higher with each succeeding effort in bent forward rowing. This can indicate the performer is tiring and it is when fatigued that he is most likely to handle weights incorrectly. Again, the use of a mirror in learning the technique is recommended. A partner may be used to exert light pressure on the upper back to prevent accentuation of the lordotic curve. If performed in a quick jerky manner with the knees locked, damage to the intervertebral discs can occur with pressure on the disc forcing its fluid-like centre, the nucleus pulposus, to project posteriorly causing medical complications.

This can be avoided either by resting the forehead on a padded table while the lift is performed or bending the knees to about 15° flexion. This releases tension from the muscles of the posterior thigh and back and allows the lumbar spine to retain a normal curvature. The muscles isolated in this exercise are the latissimus dorsi, teres major and rhomboids. In upright rowing a narrow grip is used with the elbows pointing upwards. In bent-forward rowing the elbows assume a more lateral orientation.

USES OF WEIGHT TRAINING

Weight training can be exploited to achieve different results. Since the classic report of De Lorme it has been known that few repetitions of high intensity work produce a strength training stimulus while many repetitions at low or moderate intensity improve local endurance. Skeletal muscle is an extremely adaptable tissue and exercise of an endurance nature, although it produces biochemical changes leading to greater oxidative capacity, leaves the size of the musculature relatively unchanged. Maximal intensity of relatively short its connective tissue and tendonous attachment. The important ultra-structural change in muscle hypertrophy is increase in the myofibril content of the cell. It appears that an important factor determining the extent of hypertrophy is the speed of contraction as well as the work intensity. There is, as yet, no exact demarcation in physiological terms between a strength training stimulus and a power training stimulus.

In studies of women throwers, appreciable gains in strength using maximal resistance are found without evidence of the muscle hypertrophy that might be unwanted in females for social reasons. There is ample evidence that weight training can improve speed of limb movement and muscular coordination in addition to strength and enhances conventional conditioning programmes. Masley et al showed that performance in fencing could be improved by engaging in specific weight training exercises. Undoubtedly weight training aptly used can have manifold benefits beyond the seasoning of muscular strength. Caution is needed in the early stages of a weight training programme. At first the athlete starts off with modest loads during familiarisation with the exercises.

Then the principle of progressive resistance is applied to scheduling the programme. The load is gradually increased as the individual adapts to meet the demands the schedule imposes. To improve further a higher load is needed. This procedure is continuously applied as strength develops. Normally the athlete will perform, say, six repetitions at high intensity, rest completely and repeat a few times before progressing to another exercise. An alternative is the pyramid system where after the first six repetitions or first set, the load is actually increased. This necessarily reduces the number of repetitions the athlete can perform. The load is progressively increased until it is too heavy to be overcome. Equipment for leg pressing provides an ideal set-up for most athletes working on a pyramid system to improve leg strength —even when the load cannot be moved an isometric contraction can be held for a fixed period to terminate the sets. Another use of weight training is its incorporation in circuit-training for the purpose of conditioning the circulatory system. Circuit-training designed by Morgan and Adamson is so called because a series of separate exercises is organised for performance in a circle.

Individuals rotate around the circle as they progress through the training session. The circuit should allow variation of muscle-groups involved between work stations to avoid cessation of work due to local muscular fatigue. In theory this method is ideal for team training provided the number in the group does not exceed the number of work stations laid out. In practice group organisation invariably presents some problems as do inter-individual differences. Where weight training is included in the circuit, a fixed load may not be suitable for all or many of the group while altering the loads slows up the performance and allows untimely recovery. Ideally a homogeneous group, a thoroughly well organised routine and repetition of the circuit or supplementary training are necessary to achieve objectives. Multi-station exercise machines overcome the organisational problems of circuit-training and the injury risks of weight training using traditional resistance modes.

Muscle groups change from station to station and use of the machine involves abdominals, leg, shoulder, arm, and back muscle work. Physiological studies have shown the training stimulus to the circulatory system is significantly greater than conventional circuit-training routines. However, as delay in altering loads at any one station is minimal the circuit of 12 stations can be repeated to perform two or more sets in a training session. Safety factors are inherent in the design of each station which accommodates a wide range of physiques and capacities. Over a lengthy validation period no accidents or injuries were found with extensive use of the machine. Additionally individual stations provide the facility for training of specific muscle groups.

This type of equipment is in use in many professional sports clubs and sport centre complexes. The use of heavy weights in resistance training emphasises the need for teaching lifting techniques correctly. Most injuries occur when heavy weights are lifted and most back injuries occur when spinal flexion is permitted. This is manifested in the relatively much larger proportion of injuries in male than in female athletes using weight training, releases tending to operate at intensities permitting greater safety margins. Special care should be given to young athletes to prevent undue over-exertion in lifting weights.

This should be an important consideration before the epiphyses of the long bones close as further growth might be affected. Safety considerations should override all others where large groups are involved. This may require more careful programming of the gymnasium timetable. Spotters and weight-racks should be used where appropriate. Use of commercially available chalk blocks can ensure a continuing good grip on the bar once the palms commence to sweat. In addition a suitable surface is needed, most lifting exercises being conducted from rubber mats. Appropriate footwear is required to provide sufficient frictional contact with the floor, in most cases the orthodox multi-purpose gymnasium shoe is inadequate. Collars must be used to firmly fix the discs to the bar as many injuries arise from insecurely attached equipment falling on the feet.

On the 'cosmetic' side of fitness, a reasonably symmetrical and muscled body may be desired, and this can only be gained by muscle-building work. A feeling of strength is an essential part of the business of feeling fit. When the muscles are regularly worked to the limits, there is often a resulting undefinable feeling of compactness, springiness, and all-round well-being. It feet good to be strong. Many people prefer to exercise in a gymnasium rather than jog or join an exercise class. This chapter explains how both strength and stamina can be achieved using gym equipment and weights. The various aspects of strength are achieved in different ways. Maximum strength is increased by working the muscles at about 80 to 90 per cent of maximum. Strength-endurance is developed by repetitive work against resistance outside the force-duration profile or above twenty-five repetitions. It can be achieved by raising maximum strength or, most commonly, by increasing the repetitions at the desired weight. Power is increased by raising maximum strength and moving weights of above 60 per cent of maximum, as fast as possible.

This power aspect of strength, however, does not affect the average person is quest of fitness, but athletes who have to define their sport very narrowly may need to work on it. Strength is built up by gradually increasing the resistance against which the muscles have to work. This is generally done in two ways, piece of resistance equipment. The weight of the body can be used in many different ways depending upon whether maximum strength or strength-endurance is being developed. If all the body weight can be concentrated on one small muscle group it may be capable of only a few movements, for example, one arm press-ups or one legged knee bends.

This would develop maximum strength in that muscle group. On the other hand, in press-ups the body weight is only partially on the arms and more than twenty-five repetitions may be possible, in which case strength-endurance is tested and worked upon. The ability to use body weight alone to build up strength also depends upon age and sex. Whereas a young adult male would find body weight alone insufficient for maximum-strength training, an older or much younger person or female might well find body weight enough. A young adult male might also find that body weight alone was insufficient for strength-endurance work as he could build up to several hundred press-ups, for example, but would always be working against the same resistance.

If he wanted to build up against a higher resistance he would have to use an external weight. This chapter may therefore be of most interest to men, since the strength training methods described involve the use of weights. Although increasing numbers of women are becoming bodybuilders, the majority will probably get as much strength as they need from calisthenics or yoga. For those who do need to build up real strength, and not just body-tone, weight training is very suitable. Many women fear that exercise will create large muscles. Although any exercise stimulates growth in muscle fibre, women do not respond in exactly the same way as men.

The dominant hormone of the male sex hormones, testosterone, is responsible for gains in muscle size in men. Growth in muscle size is associated with lifting heavy weights, as when men lift heavy loads there is an increase in testosterone secreted. However, significant increases have not been found in women lifting heavy loads. Whatever muscle growth is stimulated it is usually masked by the thicker layers of fat beneath the skin that women have, so the contours stay the same. Slight gains in weight due to muscle fibre increase are more than offset by fat loss, and the tape measure will actually show a decrease in size, as fat is bulkier than muscle. As with all forms of fitness training, those starting weight training or joining a gym are advised to undergo a thorough physical examination to determine cardiac, abdominal or any other weaknesses.

Equipment

A variety of equipment is now available for strength training in its various forms. The weights may be attached to pulleys, or fixed in a rigid frame and moved by leverage. Weights may not be used at all, as with steel springs or rubber cables and pneumatic valve equipment. There are advantages and disadvantages with all this equipment. Fixed frame apparatus is extremely convenient. The weight that is moved can be increased just by moving a pin. In contrast to this, free weights such as barbells and dumb-bells can be very fiddly when increasing or decreasing the weight and manoeuvring the equipment into position for the exercise.

With the free weights however, the path of the movement is not fixed, as with the fixed frame equipment, and more muscles are called into play. Equipment where work is against a pneumatic valve, or similar resistance-varying devices, is said to be the best for producing strength. The muscles have to work fully throughout the whole movement as compared to working with free weights, where a lot of effort is at the beginning of the movement, when the weight is jerked into motion. This type of equipment and movement is usually known as isokinetic. When using isokinetic equipment, the best strength gains are made by doing only one set of about fifteen repetitions, taking about four seconds to make the full movement.

The results of this are about the same as doing three sets of five repetitions with weights. Steel springs or rubber cables when used in such items as 'chest expanders' are very useful. There are a large number of upper body exercises that are easily done with the chest expander which are difficult to do with the free weights. However, the chest expander is not very good for leg, stomach, or lower back work. In addition to the above, a gymnasium may contain a variety of machines for working different parts of the body, either moving the weight by pulley, leverage or isokinetically.

Using weights

Weight training is the main form of developing strength using an external load. It is mostly done using a barbell or dumb-bells, so the weight can be increased or decreased by adding or removing the iron discs at each end. The advantage or this, and other types of weight-training equipment, is that the increase in weight can be accurately measured, and so a gradually increasing resistance can be applied to the muscles. The principle of weight training is progressive overload. That is, the muscles are progressively given more and more work to do. This is achieved by working to a formula of sets times repetitions maximum. For many years the standard formula has been three sets of ten repetitions.

A weight is moved ten times in a particular exercise. Then a brief rest is taken and the exercise is repeated. A final rest is taken, and the exercise is repeated for the last ten times. There are two points that must be understood with the sets × RM formula with regard to increasing strength. Firstly it is a target. When you can do three sets of ten repetitions, you have reached your target, and it is then time to increase the weight. Usually about a 5 per cent increase is made. For a while after you have increased the weight, you will not be able to achieve the number of movements. In the first set you may achieve ten movements, in the second set you may only be able to do eight, and in the final set you may only be able to do six movements. Over the following weeks you must keep working to achieve three sets of ten repetitions.

When you do, you have made an increase in load by another 5 per cent or so. The second point about the formula is that the weight used is the maximum. If you pick up a bar and move it ten times in three sets, but are in fact capable of moving it for three sets of fifteen repetitions, then you would not have been working at ten repetitions maximum. This refers to the maximum amount of weight you can move for the given number of repetitions. An exercise would progress with the first set comfortably performed, but with a slight feeling of 'burn' in the muscles. The second set would be done with probably a bit of struggle in the last two repetitions. The third set would be done with considerable struggle in the last four repetitions and a lot of 'burn' in the muscles. It is the number of repetitions you set yourself that determines the weight used.

A period of experimentation is necessary at the start of any weight training programme to find what weight you can move. Within the sets × reps formula considerable variations are found. Sets or repetitions may be higher or lower and the weight on the barbell may be decreased or increased during the sets. Despite all the variations, recent research seems to show that the greatest gains in strength are made with a formula of about three sets of about six repetitions with the same load on the barbell, and sufficient rest between sets. When an increase in maximum strength is not the training objective, the sets × repetitions formula will differ. You may want to use the weights for a general workout – in other words to get the muscles toned-up, and have a sweat and a puff. Light to medium weights with high repetitions and sets, with not too much rest between the sets, will start to turn the session into an aerobic workout.

This type of workout can be quite strenuous, as resistance may be quite high, compared with just moving the body weight as in running, and also may be prolonged. Pulse rates are pushed very high and trainees may develop extremely strong hearts despite the fact that there is a lot of anaerobic work going on. This level of training would have to be achieved gradually. If, on the other hand, you already do stamina work such as running, you may only need the weights to balance up your body strength. In this case the training could be done to a formula of three sets of ten repetitions with plenty of rest in between the sets. If the training objective is to develop strength-endurance, then sets, reps, weights, and periods of rest will reflect the amount and type of endurance desired.

There is no set point at which you acquire strength-endurance. Three or four sets of 15 to 25 RM with little rest in between may be all that is required. Alternatively, the trainee may just need to move a given weight many times continuously. He would then do a single set, gradually pushing the repetitions up to the desired number. One of the advantages of training in sets is that between the sets the muscles have time to recover and replenish their energy stores. So, in a sense, the use of sets trains recovery as well. A quicker recovery would be gained by training with quite short intervals of rest between the sets. Finally, your objective may be to build up your body, and to put on more muscle. Training advice to body-builders varies considerably. Some body-builders use very heavy weight at low repetitions, while others do many sets and higher repetitions. A lot depends on the individual body, as some will respond quickly to almost anything, and others will not respond without a lot of effort.

However, one thing is very clear – all the methods advocated by the champion body-builders require an enormous amount of work. If you do a lot of exercises, and 'pump a lot of iron' in whatever formula, your muscles will respond. The particular exercises for 'sculpting' the body for body-building competition are not included in this section, although any of the exercises will build you up considerably if enough work is done.

Technique

Always warm up before you go into your weight training routine proper. If you train in a gym, use an exercise bike for about five minutes. Another useful warming-up exercise with a weight is the dumb-bell swing. Take a light dumb-bell in one hand, drop into shallow squat and swing it between your legs. Straighten the legs, swinging the dumb-bell high over your head, then swing it down between the legs again, and so on. Do fifteen swings with one hand; then fifteen with the other. Go into a deeper squat as the exercise continues, and get a good stretch when it swings high. When pushing a heavy weight there is always the danger of tearing a muscle if you are stiff or not properly warmed up. One way to avoid this is to do a few yoga-type stretching exercises at the start and finish of a session. Also do a few light repetitions of any particular exercise before you load the bar properly. Before using a bar or dumb-bell, check that there is the same amount of weight on each end of the bar, and that the collars that hold on the weights are firmly tightened. Hold the bar with your hands evenly spaced so that the weight is evenly balanced when you lift it.

If using a bar regularly, mark off the exact middle and half-way to each side with a piece of tape. When lifting a weight, lift with a flat back— never lift with a humped back. Also check that your feet and body are symmetrically placed. If using very heavy weights, get somebody to stand by to catch or support the bar, should you start to fall or fail in the exercise. When doing any exercise, concentrate on doing it in the correct form. Do not use weights that are too heavy and cheat on the movement. Try to work the muscles through their full range every time, and keep a record of what you do.

Limb and trunk exercises

Arm pulling exercises

As with the extension exercise, the arm can be moved in to the body at many different angles. In these exercises, the muscles at the front of the upper arm are strongly affected, as well as the muscles of the upper back and shoulders.

1. Bent-over rowing

This is opposite exercise to the bench press. The trainees bends forward from the waist, preferably resting his head on something about waist height. The barbell hangs down at arms' length and is then pulled up to touch the chest. The hands should grip the bar about shoulder-width apart. When doing the exercise take care not to cheat by jerking the head and upper body up, as this then involves the lower back. Resting the head on something is a good way to avoid such cheating. The exercise can also be done with dumb-bells, with the hands turned in various positions. Some exercise machines have low-level pulleys, where the trainee sits on the floor and pulls towards his chest. This has virtually the same effect as the bent-over rowing.

2. Pull-ups

The trainees hangs from a bar, then pulls himself up to it. This can be done in a number of ways. Firstly, he can pull himself up so that his chin or chest touches the bar, or, secondly, touches the back of his neck to the bar. The grip can be either with both hands facing away from or towards the trainee, or alternated, with one forward and one backward. Depending upon which handgrip is taken, the grip can be wide, shoulder width, or narrow. This is a strenuous exercise and most people will find body weight morc than enough. The very strong can overload by tying discs to the waist.

3. Upright rowing

The trainees stands upright holding the bar hanging at arms' length in front of the body, with a grip narrower than shoulder width. The bar is pulled up along the front of the body to stop under the chin, and down again. When the bar is brought up under the chin, the elbows should be higher than the bar, sticking up in the air. This exercise can also be done on low pulleys. A similar exercise is with two dumb-bells hanging at the side, and then lifted up under the armpits.

4. Lat pull-down

This exercise has a similar effect on the muscles. It may be done on a separate overhead pulley or on a fixed-frame machine, and the bar is pulled down to the shoulders exercising the lattisimus dorsi muscle from which the exercise gets its name.

Arm pushing exercises

The hands can move out from the shoulders in a pushing action at many angles. When the arms extend in this way, the muscles at the back of the arms are brought strongly into play and, depending upon the angle, the various muscles of the chest and shoulder girdle are involved.

1. Press behind neck

In this exercise the starting position is with the bar held high, and it is then lowered behind the head to touch the nape of the neck, then pushed overhead again. The grip must be fairly wide, and the wrists and elbows should stay below the bar, as in the previous exercise. Both exercises can be done seated which throws some stress on the stomach as well. Dumb-bells can also be used for the overhead pressing movements, in which case they can be pushed up together or alternately, with the hands either held palm of rewards or facing each other.

2. Standing press

The exercise starts with the weight supported at chest height, wrists and elbows under the bar. From this position the weight is pressed overhead to a full arm extension, then lowered to the chest again. As the weight is pushed up, the trainee looks straight ahead. When pushing a heavy weight, care should be taken that the stomach is not pushed forward with a lot of stress thrown on the lower spine. For such occasions, a wide leather training belt fixed tightly round the waist acts as a good support. There are a number of variations on this exercise. A similar one is the press behind the neck.

3. Sideways extension

The best piece of equipment for this exercise is the

chest expander. Rubber cables are preferable to steel springs, since they do not catch the hairs on the chest or interlock. The expander is held across the chest or back, and the arms pushed directly out to the side. This is excellent for shoulder griddle development.

4. Bench press

In this exercise the trainee lies flat on a bench. The weight is pushed up from the chest till the arms are straight, then lowered, taking care not to bounce it off the ribs. When doing the exercise take care not to change the angle of the body, as there is a tendency when pushing a heavy weight for the hips to rise off the bench. Keep your back pressed flat to the bench, or do the exercise with both legs lifted and folded so that the thighs are vertical. The grip on the bar can be shoulder width or much wider. The change of grip affects the muscles in a slightly different way. The muscles affected are chest, front deltoids and the triceps.

5. Dips

This is an exercise that extends the arms downwards. The trainee supports himself between two parallel bars, arms straight, then lowers himself as far as the arms allow, then pushes himself up. Since this exercise uses body weight alone, and high repetitions are eventually possible, it later becomes necessary to tie some discs round the waist to overload.

6. Dumb-bell bench press

The previous exercise can also be done with dumb-bells, with the hands in the same position as with the barbell, or turned forward.

Straight arm exercises

When the arm is not bent and is lifted out and up, all the weight is thrown on to the shoulder muscles, particularly the deltoids. The muscles of the arm merely lock tight. Dumb-bells or chest expanders are ideal for this sort of exercise.

1. Expander lateral pull-down

This is the reverse movement to the previous exercise. The expander is held above the head, and the arms pull down straight and out wide to the sides.

2. Dumb-bell lateral raise

The dumb-bells are held hanging down by the sides and are then lifted up sideways, either to go just higher than the shoulders or right the way up to touch at the top. In the second case, the palms must be turned in to face each other when about shoulder height to make the full movement. A similar move can be made with the chest expander held in behind or in front of the body.

3. Straight arm pull-over

This is the reverse movement of the previous exercise. The trainee lies on a flat bench, or on an inclined board with the feet higher than the head, and the barbell is lifted with straight arms from behind the head right round to touch the stomach.

4. Expander side-pulls

The expander is held out at arms' length straight in front of the body, and then the hands pull out and round to the side on the same plane. A similar exercise can be done with dumb-bells, bending forward from the waist, then lifting them out and up.

5. Dumb-bell front raise

The dumb-bells are held hanging down at the side, and are then lifted up to the front, arms straight, then above the head. Care must be taken that the weight is not swung up with a rocking motion of the body. Do the exercise fairly slowly and keep it well under control.

6. Bent arm pull-over

In this variation, the arms are bent, so that much more weight can be handled. The body position is much the same, but the hands may grip the barbell much closer together. In this exercise the arms stay bent throughout the movement, and the weight is moved from behind the head, round close to the head, to touch the chest. This exercise combines well with a breathing exercise. When the weight is lowered behind the head the ribcage is lifted, and this should combine with a deep in-breath. As the weight is swung over the head, breathe out.

7. Dumb-bell bench side raise

This is the reverse of the previous movement. The trainee lies on a bench with dumb-bells held above the body at arms' length. The dumb-bells are lowered down and out to the side, then up again.

8. Dumb-bell rear lift

The trainee bends forward from the waist with the dumb-bells hanging down at arms' length. The arms are then lifted back and up past the side of the body. This has a limited range of movement, and strongly affects the deltoid muscles at the rear.

9. Bent arms side raise

A slightly more popular variation of the previous exercise is the bent arm side raise, when heavier dumbbells may be handled. The arms stay bent, and the weight is lowered to the side and up again. This variation can also be done on an inclined bench with the feet higher than the head, or vice versa.

Arm twisting exercises

If you think of the action of using a screwdriver, you

may recall how quickly the arm tires in the motion. No equipment exists for this type of exercise. Wringing out a wet cloth is a very similar movement, and can in fact be used for strength training if so desired. Do not forget to practise wringing out the cloth in both directions.

Trunk movements

If you sit in a chair and experiment with movement of the trunk from side to side, or front to back, you will see that it does not have a great range of movement. Of course it is possible to fold the body forward, or sway right back, but in these cases the trunk itself is not moving much, only folding from the hips, which means that the muscles around the hips and upper thighs are the ones affected. Weight-training exercises for the trunk usually involve folding movements from the hip area.

1. Side sit-up

The muscles at the side of the trunk can be worked in a similar way in the side sit-up, which is a strenuous exercise. The trainee lies along a bench, but on his side, with the upper half of the body from the hips hanging off the end. So as not to over-balance, somebody must sit across the legs to hold them firmly in place. The exercise in done by clasping the hands behind the head and lowering the upper body towards the floor and up again.

2. Sideways bend

Stand with the feet nearly shoulder-width apart, holding a dumb-bell in one hand. The other hand can either hang at the side, or the hand can be placed at the back of the head. When doing this exercise, imagine that you are sandwiched between two sheets of fragile glass, so that no forward or backward movement is possible. The exercise is done by swaying to the side and letting the dumb-bell drop down the outside of the thigh, then swaying back the other way, and pulling the weight back up the thigh as high as it will go without bending the arm. The work is done when the weight is lifted, and it is the muscles of the trunk on the opposite side to the dumb-bell which are doing the work.

Another way to work the muscles at the side of the trunk is to stand, feet about shoulder-width apart, with a barbell across the shoulders. Then just sway from side to side.

Curls

All of the previous exercises work the arms and shoulder girdle considerably. However, by fixing the movement of the elbow, certain exercises can throw a lot more weight on to certain upper arm muscles, and so give them a more intense workout.

1. Triceps curl

This exercise works the muscles at the back of the arm in the same manner as the previous exercise. There are not quite as many variations as with the biceps curl. A simple way to do the triceps curl is with a dumb-bell. Hold a single dumb-bell above the head, then keeping the elbow high and immobile, drop the dumb-bell down behind the head, then up again. A chest expander can also be used in various positions to work the triceps in a similar manner.

2. Biceps curl

This is an exercise that can be done in many different ways. The simplest method is to use a barbell, when standing upright, with the bar hanging down at arms' length, palms facing forward, across the upper thigh. The bar is then 'curled' up with the elbows in a fixed position at the side of the body. By fixing the elbows, the muscles of the front upper arm take all the strain. This exercise can be done with dumb-bells with the hands turned in different positions – either knuckles forward, to the side, or to the rear. Each slight change of position affects different muscles in the arms. There is a tendency to 'cheat' in this exercise, as the body rocks back and forwards assisting the upward movement of the weight.

When this is done deliberately, a lot more weight can be handled, and it is called a cheat curl. The upper arm can be immobilised in various ways to avoid any cheating. For example, the exercise can hanging off the end, grasping the bar with the arms touching the supports of the bench. The weight is curled up as before, and the bench supports stop any movement of the elbows and upper arms. Body-building gyms have specialist benches for this sort of work. When the exercise is done with a barbell held with knuckles forward, a lot more strain is thrown on to the forearms. This is sometimes known as the French curl.

Safety hint

The following three exercises, back arch, good morning exercise and dead lift, are all very strenuous, and care should be taken that each exercise is first tried with very light weights, and that it is correctly done. Foot positioning and hand spacing on the bar must be symmetrical, and the movements must be done smoothly, in good form, and under control. Take care not to arch the back, but to keep it flat. Those with back problems should avoid these exercises altogether.

1. Good morning exercise

Stand with the feet about shoulder width apart and hold a barbell across the shoulders. Keeping the legs straight and the back flat, bend forward from the waist till the trunk is nearly parallel with the floor, and the lift up.

2. Back arch

The muscles of the lower back are very strong, and so some of these lower back exercises can take a lot of weight. In this exercise the trainee lies stomach down on a bench, with the upper body down to the hips hanging of the end. The legs must be secured so as not to overbalance, usually by someone sitting on them. The hands are clasped behind the head, or kept at the side if that is too difficult, and the upper body is lowered to the floor and than raised as high as possible. When the upper body is lifted, the trainee must try to look at the ceiling, thus using muscles of the lower and upper back. This exercise is also known as hyperextensions or dorsal raises.

3. Dead lift

The barbell is placed on the floor. The trainee bends forward from the waist, keeping his legs straight, and lifts the bar up as high as it will go, without bending his arms or legs, so the bar will go no higher than the tops of the things. The weight is then lowered, not to the floor, but to a comfortable hanging position just above the floor, then raised again.

Composite power movements

There are few exercises in which the weight, barbell or dumb-bell, is lifted up to the chest or above the head in one heave. These exercises involve a number of muscle groups, which makes them quite strenuous. Since the whole body is used, a lot of weight can be lifted. However, heavy weight cannot be lifted slowly, and these movements are done explosively, combining strength with speed, and so demanding power. These are the sort of movements used in Olympic weight lifting.

1. Snatch above head

In this exercise the weight is lifted in one smooth movement right above the head to a full outstretched arm position. The body can be dropped lower under the bar either by going into a deep squatting position or into a wide front to back lunge position. However the legs are placed, the weight must be lifted to a full outstretched arm position above the head in one continuous fast movement. Dumb-bells may also be used for this exercise.

2. Barbell clean to chest

The trainee squats slightly, grasping the bar symmetrically. A deep breath is taken, then the bar is swiftly lifted up to the chest in a standing position, locking briefly in position with the elbows and forearms under the bar, then dropped to floor, not to crash down, but to touch lightly before being lifted again. Care must be taken that the legs are bent to start with, that the back is kept flat and not humped, and that the legs, back and arms work together in one big explosion to blast the weight high. A similar exercise can be done with one or two dumb-bells.

Leg exercises

The legs are not as dextrous as the arms, so have correspondingly fewer exercises. However, they are much stronger than the arms, and can take a lot more weight. Some people find this daunting, and avoid leg work somewhat. However, the squat is often called the 'king of the weight-training exercises' and should never be missed out.

1. Calf raise

The trainee stands with a weight across the shoulders and then rises on to the tips of the toes. To increase the range of movement, it is usually done with the toes on a block. The heels are then dropped as low as possible, then raised. Throughout the exercise the body and legs stay straight, so only the feet move to raise and lower the body and weight. Standard weight-training machinery exists for this exercise.

2. Squat

In this exercise the barbell is held across the shoulders, and the trainee squats, that is, he drops his buttocks and body close to the floor, then straightens up again. Sometimes it is necessary to put a block under the heels to make the movement comfortable. When doing the exercise, take care to push the chest out and pull the head back. Since it is believed that a full squat, that is, squatting as low as possible, losses the ligaments of the knee, it is not done very often. Usually the exercise is done to a point where the thighs are parallel with the floor. Putting a lowish bench behind and squatting down far enough to touch it lightly helps to prevent going down all the way. First, there is the front squat, where the bar is held resting across the upper chest, elbows locked under the bar.

Then there is the Hack squat where the bar is held down behind the back, hanging at arms length across the buttocks. Blocks under the heels will be necessary for these exercises. The squat can also be of varying depths; the shallower the squat, the more weight can be handled.

Various machinery exists for the leg squatting movement. In the leg press machine the trainee lies on the back, feet up in the air, pushing up a weighted bar which slides up and down on two poles. When done this way, quite a lot of weight can be pushed up without the discomfort of supporting a bar across the shoulders as in the ordinary squat.

3. Leg curl

Here the curling action is the reverse of the previous one, so that it is the muscles at the back of the thigh which are worked. The trainee lies flat down on his stomach, and hooks his heels under the pad of the leg-curl machine. The pad is then curled back with the trainee pulling his feet round to his buttocks.

4. Leg extension

This is the leg equivalent of the arm curls, as again, one portion of the limb is fixed, and the other moves against the extra resistance. Standard machinery exists for this movement, although it can be done without. The trainee sits on the leg extension machine and, holding the upper body and thigh still, pushes the pad against his ankles to maximum extension of the leg. This is an excellent exercise for weak knees, and is much used by footballers in training, or in recovering from knee injuries.

Miscellaneous exercises

There are a number of exercises for the neck, hands, and feet, although these are mostly done without weights. A few strength exercises, done with weights, do exist, and these are described here:

Wrist exercises

The wrist itself does not have muscles to exercise, as it is a joint. Usually this heading refers to exercises that involve wrist movements, but which in fact work the muscles of the forearms.

1. Wrist curl

Another exercise for the forearms is the wrist curl. In this exercise the trainee rests his forearms on a flat surface such as a bench, with his hands, palm upwards, hanging over the side holding a barbell. The exercise is done by lifting the weight as high as it will go, knuckles curling in towards the forearms, then lowering it, unclenching the hands so that the bar rolls down to be held by the last joint of the fingers.

2. Wrist-roller

The wrist-roller is a simple and common piece of equipment. A short length of rope is fixed to the middle of a short round pole. A weight is attached to the other end of the rope and the weight is then wound up by rotating the pole. The arms stay fairly straight through the exercise with just the hands turning the pole, first one way, then the other.

Neck exercises

1. Head harness

Another way to work the neck is with a head harness. This is a webbing device which fits over the head and has straps hanging down to which weight can be attached. The weight is then lifted by raising or moving the head.

2. Wrestler's bridge

The Wrestler's bridge is a very common way to work

the neck, and can also be done using extra weight. The trainee lies down on his back on the floor, and draws his feet close in to his buttocks.

Something soft must also be placed under the head. The exercise is done by bridging up — that is, by lifting the body right off the floor so that is supported on the head and feet, and then lowering it again. When the neck is strong enough, the bridge can be done supporting a barbell above the body at arms length.

The neck responds very quickly to exercise and can thicken considerably. This is worth bearing in mind when it comes to buying shirts — the collar may soon be too small.

16

TIPS FOR HEALTHIER LIVING

WALKING AIDS

Walking sticks can be very helpful to those with a one-sided weakness or with a painful knee or hip joint on one side. The correct length allows an upright stance with the tip of the stick on the ground and the arm bent a little at the elbow. Walking sticks can be used in two ways. Usually the stick is held on the strong side, so that it is forward when the food on the weak side is also forward. But if one leg is particularly weak it may be better to hold the stick close to the leg on that side so that it acts as a kind of splint. People suffering from a degree of vertigo or instability may benefit from a walking stick with a broader base consisting of three or four small feet. For those with an even greater tendency to fall, the light alloy frame 'walker' can be a useful aid to mobility.

Progress must necessarily be slow and tedious, but a walker will often allow an person with severe weakness or disability to get around and perhaps gain strength for greater mobility. The older design of arm-pit crutch, which could injure the nerves under the head of the upper arm bone, has now been replaced by light forearm-support or elbow crutches. These can offer surprisingly good mobility to the active and can be used in several ways. For the most disabled, 'four point' walking is used in which only one foot or one crutch tip is moved forward at a time. In 'three point' walking, both crutches are moved forward together, then, while the weight is supported, one foot is moved and then the other.

For the more agile, the crutches can be used to support the whole weight of the body while both legs are swung forward together. Walking callipers are splints used to add strength to a leg weakened by muscle disorder or injury, so that standing and walking become possible. The calliper is a steel rod, usually passed through the heel of the shoe and bent upwards on each side to be held in place by a padded ring or strap, below or above the knee.

TRY TO BE CONTENTED

The standard of health of people in the Western world has improved progressively from the earliest times. In the last fifty years or so there has been a dramatic improvement in life expectancy and a reduction in mortality in most of the major disease groups. In the last fifteen years there has been a considerable improvement in health due to changes in lifestyle—better diets, decline in cigarette smoking and an increase in exercising. In spite of all this, there is ample evidence that people are less satisfied with the state of their health, as they perceive it, than they used to be.

There is less acceptance of disease and disability, more complaint about minor disorders, more attendance on doctors, increased consumption of drugs, and less satisfaction with the quality of medical care provided by doctors. So much publicity has been given to the very real advances in medical science that many people now assume that nothing is impossible, and often resent being told that certain problems cannot be resolved. Litigation against doctors is soaring to the point at which doctors are avoiding the more vulnerable specialities and are having to pay crippling insurance premiums against damages. Cosmetic surgery is becoming a major industry. Bodily disfigurement, real or imagined, is often regarded as a disease requiring treatment.

The same applies to anomalies of behaviour, which are now being reclassified as diseases—drug addiction, alcoholic excess, wife beating, child abuse, paedophilia. By some, these are no longer regarded as being within the province of the law, ethics, morality or religion, but rather as medical disorders correctable by treatment. There is a demand for medical intervention to enhance or modify normal characteristics. People demands stimulants, to suppress normal fatiguc, usc anabolic steroids to aid in body-building and improve athletic performance, want sex-change operations for the alteration of normal sexual characteristics.

This lack of correspondence between health improvement to enhance or modify normal characteristics. People demand stimulants, to suppress normal fatigue, use anabolic steroids to aid in body-building and improve athletic performance, want sex-change operations for the alteration of normal sexual characteristics. This lack of correspondence between health improvement and subjective satisfaction suggests that we in the materially advanced societies may have allowed our values to become defective. It may be that we are losing sight of the real elements that make for satisfaction human relationship, love, the cultivation of the mind, hard work, creativity and humanity.

TRY TO BE HAPPY

It is widely held that happy people are healthier and that a positive attitude, optimism, good humour and friendliness towards one's fellow men and women promotes good health. More than 100 separate studies have established, statistically, that there is a positive correlation between a satisfactory and happy state of mind and good physical health. The claim, or assumption, that the state of mind causes the good health has, nevertheless, been sharply criticized by some who insist that there is no evidence that disease is a direct reflection of the mental state of the individual. No one denies that good health promotes happiness and that bad health often damages it, but it is the claim that happiness promotes health that is in question. Unfortunately, this is a more difficult thing to prove.

Happiness, is an elusive concept and many people define it in terms of physical well-being or general satisfaction with life. People who are able to cope well with life are both happier and healthier and are often too busy looking outwards to give much time or attention to minor ailments. Pessimism and hypochondriasis go hand in hand. None of these considerations support the proposition, but all emphasize the intimacy of the inter-relationship of mind and body and the impossibility, in the final analysis, of separating the effects of one from those of the other.

TAKE EXERCISE EVERY DAY

Fitness is a simple concept involving some very complex physiology. Essentially, the term means what it is says—the ability to do something. A commonly used, however, the 'something' is a physical task, such as running a certain distance in a certain time. No one has laid down 'official' standards fro fitness and these obviously vary considerably depending on the occupation or the sporting interests. For people other than athletes, a standard somewhat higher than the lifestyle would normally demand is desirable, but to go on raising this standard, in an obsessive kind of way, is, for the ordinary person, rather pointless. The body is highly adaptable and will usually, within a matter of a few weeks, adjust its ability to perform, with reasonable ease, most physical tasks demanded of it.

But this will happen only if the demand is constant and sustained. The most obvious changes which occur are in the bulk and strength of the voluntary muscles, the force and pumping efficiency of the heart muscle, and the effectiveness of the respiratory muscles. But more subtle changes also occur and these involve:

1. The ability of the muscles to utilize the fuels glucose and fatty acids in the presence of lowered insulin level in the blood the increase in the size and number of the energy-producing elements in the muscle cells;

2. The speed with which the body recovers from fatigue;

3. The ability of the liver to maintain the supply of glucose to the blood, and hence to the muscles, during strenuous exercise.

4. The ability to perform more work without using up oxygen faster than the lungs and circulation can supply it;

5. The degree of attainable tension in the muscles;

All these and other factors may be involved in the changes brought about by the radical change in the pattern of activity we call 'training'. Fortunately, these subtleties need concern only the exercise physiologist.

For the man and woman in the street, or the park, it is sufficient to enjoy the growing sense of physical and mental well-being and the ease with which daily physical tasks are performed.

Jogging

By regularly engaging in jogging to be point of breathlessness, an adult of any age can increase his or her capacity for exertion, can lose weight, can lower the blood pressure, diminish the progress of arterial disease and look and feel better. The body is remarkably responsive to demands made upon it and, even in old age, will increase in efficiency and physical capability if sustained effort, in excess of the normal, is made. But jogging is not entirely without hazard, and people beyond the first bloom of youth, and especially those who smoke or are overweight, should beware. They should remember that even a modest initial indulgence may involve demands on the power of their limb muscles, on the efficiency of their hearts and on the blood oxygenating capacity of their lungs, in excess of what these systems can provide. So a very gradual build-up is important.

Most publications on the subject recommend a full medical check-up before starting, and there may be something to be said for this, but one should not expect doctors to give a certificate of safety. Orthopaedic injuries—sprains, torn ligaments, stress fractures of bones—are also a hazard, but the risk of these can also be minimized by a very gradual build-up and common-sense limitation of the duration of the running period, to begin with. Physical stress applied too early or too forcefully causes fatigue and injury. Most experienced runners also do warm-up exercises that include stretching the major muscle groups. A good, well-fitting, and supportive pair of running shoes is important, as the stresses on the feet and spine from pounding hard pavements can be considerable.

More about exercise

The evolutionary environments of early humans provided little in the way of passive transportation—apart, perhaps from floating logs or primitive boats. The use of horses came well after the present bodily from had evolved. So humans must be considered creatures naturally dependent on their own muscular ability for movement, even survival. Exercise is natural and normal to humans and they neglect it at their peril. Much of the bodily disorder suffered by contemporary people can be attributed to the use of 'artificial' energy sources to replace the use of their own muscles. But it is basic mistake to think that exercise is concerned only, or even primarily, with the muscles. No muscle can contract without an adequate blood supply to bring it oxygen and fuel in the form of glucose. Nor can it continue to contract without a good blood supply to carry away the waste products of fuel consumption the exhaust. A good blood supply requires an efficiently beating heart and a good oxygen supply requires an efficiently operating air intake system—the lungs and the muscles of respiration.

These three systems—the muscles, the heart and blood vessels and the respiratory system—are so intimately interrelated, both functionally and in terms of their physiological control mechanisms, that it is impossible to change one without changing the others. The body, as a whole, is a uniquely responsive entity and will, within the limits of our heredity, modify itself in order to deliver what we ask of it. Athletes reach their level of performance by very hard work, demanding and obtaining a response from their bodies. The top athletes are not those with the best bodies, but those with the best motivation, character, determination. The body will also, very quickly drop its capacity to a level appropriate to low demands. After six weeks in bed, it takes a minimum of six weeks, usually longer, of normal physical activity to return to the former level of fitness. The changes which occur on demand are not simply changes in muscle bulk and power—they are changes in the heart, in the respiratory muscles, in the blood vessels, even in the brain.

They are universal and their effect is widespread. Sustained exercise improves stamina and endurance by leading to the enlargement and growth of small blood vessels in the muscles–even in the heart– and by increasing the size and number of the energy producing elements in the cells. The efficiency of oxygen and glucose fuel usage increases and the work of which the muscles, including the heart muscle, are capable, increases. The rate at which the heart has to beat to maintain an adequate circulation drops and the pulse is slower both during exercise and rest, because the stroke volume is increased. As a result, the heart has to do less work for the same level of efficiency.

These benefits are not be achieved by taking a gentle stroll once a month. Ideally, we should exercise to the point of breathlessness for a minimum of twenty minutes, at least three times a week, and the exercises should involve as many muscles as possible. If we ignore these self-evident facts and live lives of self-indulgent luxury, using our muscles only to heave our overweight bodies from bed to dining table and from table to car, it is not just our muscles that suffer. If our food intake is grossly in excess of our fuel requirements and our fuel usage rate is low, the excess is laid down in the fat storage depots of the body and some of it is laid down in the walls of our under-used and cigarette-abused arteries. Atherosclerosis, the number one killer of the Western word, is probably the gravest consequence of this biologically disastrous way of life.

It clogs or occludes the arteries, reduces the blood flow, causes coronary artery disease, and peripheral artery disease, interfering with the most fundamental of life processes and leading to an ever-worsening capacity for work of all kinds. It kills more people, often in early middle life, than any other single disease process. Exercise is not just for the young. A well exercised sixty year old should have a physical performance of about 60 per cent of that of a reasonably fit man of thirty. Exercise is highly beneficial, and body-altering, at every age, with out exception. Well-controlled studies have shown that people in their eighties and nineties become fitter and improve their performance when they take deliberate exercise, and it is clear that much of the incapacity though typical of old age is simply culturally induced but mistaken stereotype. Doctors now appreciate that, apart from its general benefits, exercise under medical supervision can reduce the severity of angina pectoris, intermittent claudication, some forms of lung disease and depression.

Longevity

Physically active people live longer than sedentary people. Walking, stair-climbing and sports play relate inversely to mortality, chiefly from heart and lung diseases. Death rates decline steadily as the amount of energy expended on these activities increases, from less than 500 calories per week to 35 calories per week. People expending 2000 calories or more per week have death rates one-quarter to one-third lower than those among the less active, of comparable age. Walking half a mile equates to about fifty calories; climbing seventy steps to about thirty calories; light sporting activity equates to about five calories per minute and vigorous sport to about ten calories per minute. Seventy-three per cent of physically active men of sixty survive to eighty; only 63 per cent of man of sixty survive to eighty if they are not physically active. Even after the age of eighty, over two years of extra life can, on average, be expected from earlier increased physical activity.

Aerobic exercise

In intense, strenuous exercise, such as a 100-metre sprint, oxygen is used up faster than it can be supplied to the muscles. The comparatively small amount stored is rapidly consumed, and the exercise can be maintained for only a short period. Breathing is unnecessary during the ten seconds or so of the race. In aerobic exercising, such as walking, jogging, swimming, cycling, etc., the rate of oxygen consumption is such that the supply from the lungs, via the bloodstream, is adequate to meet the need. The exercise may therefore be maintained for long periods.

DRINK ONLY IN MODERATION

Alcohol has consoled and relaxed mankind since the down of history, and moderate usage is generally deemed to be valuable and to offer no hazard to health. But it is a blessing which, by the nature of its effects, is very easily abused. Its desired effects come from its depressant action on the higher functions of the brain which are bound-up with social inhibition, anxiety, tensions and the sense of responsibility. By reducing the strength of these functions, alcohol allows the drinker to operate on a simpler, more biological, and less critical level, engaging in enjoyable activity of all kinds without the restraining effect of the normal full awareness of the consequences of his or her actions. Under the influence of alcohol, many people will, for instance, engage in sexual activity which would be unthinkable if they were sober.

Alcohol also abolishes critical awareness of its own effects and the intoxicated have little consciousness of the invariable decrease in quality of judgement and the exercise of skills. Alcohol has other effects. The blood vessels are widened so that the skin becomes flushed and feels warm, the appetite is stimulated so that more is eaten than is required, and the output of urine is greater than the fluid intake so that the body becomes partially dehydrated and thirst is induced which unsatisfies further alcohol intake. This effect is especially common in beer drinkers and is one of the reasons for the often excessive quantity drunk.

The unit system

The average heavy drinker will have a daily intake of at least 80 grams of ethyl alcohol, or ten 'units'. The 'unit' system of assessing drink intake is useful. One unit of drink is a half-pint of average strength beer, or a single of 70 degree proof spirit, or one glass of wine. One unit contains 8 grams of ethanol. So someone drinking 80 grams of ethanol a day is taking about five pints of beer, or five double whiskies bout the effects of such intake.

Delirium tremens

This is a withdrawal condition occurring up to seventy two hours after the last drink. There is clouding of consciousness, then horrifying hallucinations associated with extreme terror, violently threatening behaviour, disordered action of the heart and occasional attempts to commit suicide. The attack, unless effectively treated by injections of powerful sedatives, may go on for as long as five days and the mortality—usually from heart failure—is appreciable. Excessive drinking can also cause mental illness indirectly by the effect on the kind of all the shattering social, sexual and economic consequences of alcohol dependency.

Alcohol dependence

It is sometimes thought that, as with drugs like heroin dependence on alcohol will inevitably occur if enough is taken. This, however, does not seem to be so. It is only a comparatively small proportion of drinkers who become chronic alcoholics and, in these, the dependence seems to be so. It is only a comparatively small proportion of drinkers who become chronic alcoholics and, in these, the dependence seems to be psychological rather then pharmacological. Many alcoholics have a personality inadequate in certain respects, or have major difficulty in relating effectively to others.

But the easy availability of alcohol and the encouraging social attitudes to drinking are also probably important factors. The incidence of alcohol dependence is high in people engaged in the liquor trade and in those occupations and social groups in which regular heavy drinking is an established feature. Genetic factors may also play a part but it is very difficulty to separate such effects from those of personality and the effects of early environmental influences on personality. Because the treatment of established alcohol dependence is difficult it is important to detect the problem early and try to avoid it. Alcohol dependence is probably always related to personality problem and it is likely that in most cases the personality problem causes the excessive drinking because of short-term gains from alcohol. Alcohol is a great consoler, and many turn to it out of a feeling of professional or business failure, frustration, repressed aggression, marital and sexual dissatisfaction, or severe social inhibition. All these, and other distressing elements, may be indicators of a liability to become permanently dependent on alcohol. People aware of any such factors and worried about drinking should see clearly that they may be gravely at risk of passing into a far worse state-that of chronic dependence.

Alcohol excess — the warning signs

'Moderation in everything' is an excellent maxim for all seeking health and contentment. It is especially appropriate in relation to alcohol. The following points are a clear indication that alcohol is being used immoderately. Here are the warning signs:

1. The mornings are bad. The hands shake, there is sickness, retching, gagging and depression. Ordinary sounds seem intolerably loud, there is ringing in the ears and the skin itches.

2. Undesirable social or legal effects do not deter.

3. Drinking has become a central part of life, rivalling, in its importance, other major activities.

4. About ten hours after the last drink, another one is badly needed.

5. Drinking is becoming established as a daily habit with a regular indulgence at lunchtime.

6. These symptoms can be cured by a good stiff drink.

7. The drinker believes he or she has a wonderful head for drink and can carry on 'normally' after an intake that would put the next person under the table.

It takes, on average, ten to fifteen years to reach a stage of major addiction, but the range may be as wide as from two to twenty-five years. Alcohol consumption is rising steadily in Britain and, with it, there is a progressive rise in:

1. Alcohol-related anaemia and nutritional disease;

2. The serious disease of the pancreas, chronic calcifying pancreatitis;

3. The liver disease cirrhosis;

One unit contains 8 grams of ethanol. So someone drinking 80 grams of ethanol a day is taking about five pants of beer, or five double whiskies or a bottle or wine. The box contains some useful information about the effects of such intake.

Alcoholic dementia

This comes on very gradually in heavy drinkers, usually quite late in life. The patient, often female, usually around sixty, shows a definite change in personality and severe loss of memory. He or she may seem unconcerned or may be depressed but, on being tested, will be found to have suffered severe deterioration in mental powers, with poor judgement and inability to relate socially in the normal way. She is likely to deny excessive drinking and many show some cunning in keeping up her intake inconspicuously. A CT or MRI scan will show obvious atrophy of the outer layer of the brain. This is the part concerned with the higher functions of the nervous system, including intelligence. Other effects of alcohol on the brain include the condition of Wernicke's encephalopathy which is due to a severe deficiency of the vitamin B1.

Its symptoms include paralysis of the movement of the eyes, severe loss of balance and gross mental confusion. It occurs only after very heavy, prolonged drinking. Treatment, by thiamine injections, is always urgently needed. If a person with Wernicke's is always urgently needed. If a person with Wernicke's encephalopathy does not get medical attention, the condition eventually progresses to a state, known as Korsakoff's syndrome, in which there is profound loss of memory, both for recent and remote events, so that the patient can hardly remember anything at all. There is a pitiful reaction to this in which the patient invents fictitious accounts to make up for the defect in memory but soon forgets what he or she has just said. Once Korsakoff's syndrome is established, treatment is almost hopeless. Only 14 per cent show any improvement, even on the best management, over a period of five years.

Alcohol and the heart

Alcohol does not directly affect the heart unless a great deal is drunk over a period of at least ten years. When it does, it is the heart muscle which is affected. This is called cardiomyopathy. So most of the people who develop alcoholic heart disease are chronic alcoholics. Many are employed in the liquor trade and there are fairly clear indications that the condition is caused, not only be direct alcohol damage to the heart muscle, but also by nutritional and vitamin deficiency in people who get enough calories from the alcohol not to require to eat. The first sign of trouble is gradually increasing breathlessness on effort and obvious awareness of the beating of the heart.

There is none of the acute chest pain of a heart attack or angina pectoris. If medical advice is not sought, the condition goes on to swelling of the ankles and fluid in the chest from failure of the heart to keep a sufficiently good circulation going. The heart beat becomes irregular and the pulse abnormally fast. Death may occur from severe heart failure. The extraordinary thing about alcoholic heart muscle disease is that if affected person can be persuaded to give up alcohol completely, even in an advanced stage of the disease, recovery is 100 per cent.

Ironically, persuasion often fails and the victim goes back to drinking as soon as he or she is out of hospital. So, as with alcoholic liver disease, this is yet another way in which one can literally drink oneself to death. Carefully conducted studies have also shown that moderate to heavy drinking-over six units a day–raises the blood pressure both in normal subjects and in those already known to have high blood pressure. These studies showed that a curtailed alcohol intake, specifically the change to low-alcohol beer, and improved blood pressure control can reduce the need for treatment. The reason for this effect has not been established, but it is well known that many patients attending hypertension clinics are heavy drinkers and that in these, in particular, blood pressure control is poor. It is recognized that heavy drinkers may be less reliable in taking medication, but this is not thought to be the cause of the findings.

Alcohol and the brain

This section is of special relevance to women – who are drinking twice as much alcohol as they did ten years ago. The greater sensitivity of women to alcohol applies as much to its effect on the brain as on other organs. CT scanning has been used to compare alcohol-induced brain changes in women and men. These changes include widespread shrinkage of brain tissue with enlargement of the normal spaces with the brain and widening of the grooves, and they occur after a much shorter drinking history and lower average consumption in female alcoholics than in males of the same age. Brain damage does not occur solely from the direct effect of alcohol on nerve tissue. Other factors include nutritional and vitamin deficiency, liver disease, hormonal factors and head injury from falls and blows. The deteriorated female alcoholic is often suffering from a true alcohol dementia. Men, too, suffer all these effects, but all of them occur earlier in women.

CARE OF THE ELDERLY

Ideally, elderly people should live at home enjoying the support and loving care of a devoted family. But many are necessarily solitary or choose to live alone, and it is these who are most at risk from ill-health. It is commonly assumed that a gradual loss of capacity, both mental and physical, is an inevitable feature of old age, but this is not so. Frequently decline in health is the result of unsuspected physical disorder from the gradual accumulation of damage from previous illness, degenerative disease and injury. Many diseases, are, by their nature, commoner in old age.

These conditions, which may seriously prejudice the quality of life, include atherosclerosis, cancer, cataract, depression, diabetes, fracture of the femur, malnutrition especially vitamin deficiency, under action of the thyroid gland, osteoarthritis, osteoporosis, pernicious anaemia and shingles.. Several of these conditions may co-exist. Some of them are obvious, but, unfortunately, many remain concealed and, as a result, many elderly people do not receive an appropriate level of medical care. Chronic ill-health in the elderly tends to be concealed for several reasons. Many old people expect to be frail or unwell and feel that they should not complain. Many are remarkably stoical, and the elderly often have a lowered sensitivity to pain or even a lowered level of general awareness. Most are disinclined to be a burden to others.

Sometimes failure to complain is due to genuine mental impairment, but an appearance of unconcern may be the result of physical disorder and lack of stimulation. Sensory deprivation is especially important and many old people, who could be restored to self-sufficiency by a cataract operation or the provision of a hearing aid, remain sunk in lethargy and seeming difference and require constant attention. So it is clearly important that the elderly should have full and regular medical attention. Millions of old people suffer unnecessary invalidism, distress and disability because of remediable conditions. Gradually developing anaemia, bedsores, and malnutrition may go long unnoticed and conditions such as dehydration and hypothermia may affect even those in affluent circumstances.

These are only a few of the conditions which, given reasonable standards of medical and nursing care, need never occur. Self-neglect, often with serious consequences, may be the result of dementia but it may also be due to mild confusion, forgetfulness, depression and the increasing physical difficulties imposed by organic disease. Such people should never be left unvisited for long periods. Those in greatest need of help include people recently discharged from hospital, those handicapped by poor vision and deafness, the recently bereaved and the lonely. The nature of the accommodation is important.

Adequate heating and a high level of artificial illumination make for comfort and safety and encourage reading, sewing and other useful activities. Accidental injury from falls remains a common danger to the elderly and for this and other obvious reasons, such people living alone should always be provided with an effective alarm system so that help can be summoned reliably and quickly. Voluntary agencies and Public Health authorities do much to help and full use should be made of available facilities. The home Help Service can provide more than merely domestic assistance. Home helps keep a watchful eye on their elderly charges, noting signs of difficulty and calling in professional assistance when necessary. Volunteers providing meals on wheels can also offer a valuable monitoring service. The concept of sheltered housing, in which elderly people enjoy the benefits of custom-designed accommodation while remaining under unobtrusive surveillance, is an excellent one and such housing is often preferred to a nursing or residential home. Adequate social intercourse, mental stimulation and the encouragement of activity are essential for the elderly.

These may be obtained by regular attendance at day health care centres, at which bathing, chiropody and launderette services are provided at workshops for the elderly, senior citizens clubs, and, when appropriate, stroke clubs and day hospitals. The latter are valuable institutions, offering full medical investigation and assessment, rehabilitative treatment and the means of health maintenance, on a daily attendance basis. Relatives are encouraged to participate in discussion of future management at home and to learn how maximal activity and independence may be achieved.

Because of failing vision, unsteadiness, slower reflexes, vertigo, stiffness and muscle weakness, hazards easily avoided by younger people become significant for the elderly and falls are common. These are more dangerous than is often realised and are often fatal in their long term consequence. Osteoporosis makes old people, especially women, particularly susceptible to fractures, even from quite minor injuries and the resulting immobilization and decline in the level of activity can have grave effects. Chest and urinary infections commonly supervene and these may tip the balance against survival.

Delicate skin can tear and bruise easily and muscle

injuries are slow to heal. Long periods of pain, discomfort and disability may follow an apparently trivial fall. Because of these risks, every effort should be made to avoid hazards in the environment of the elderly such as loose mats on polished floors, damaged floor coverings, carelessly disposed electric cables, poorly lit stairs or corridors and icy paths. Elderly people living alone are especially at risk, and some form of alarm system which will enable the victim to summon help, even if immobilized, in mandatory.

THE EFFECTS OF COLD

Even in the most severe winters, the numbers of cases of hypothermia in Britain is small. In only about twenty-five cases per year is hypothermia given on death certificates as the underlying cause of death. But the effects of cold on old people are very much more widespread and serious than this figure would suggest. We now know that cold is a major contributing factor to heart and lung disease in old people and in causing their death from these conditions. Every year, there is an immediate rise in the death rate among old people when mean temperatures drop below freezing, and this rise continues for over a month after the extreme cold has passed. About 40,000 more people die each average winter, in England and Wales, than during a comparable period in summer. Body heat production is defective in old people, almost all of whom have had a marked decline in the rate of using up body fuel.

Even more important, shivering is less effective in producing heat, because of poor muscles. Shivering is the most important way of raising the body temperature when this is tending to fall. Heat is normally lost by widening of skin blood vessels and conserved by constriction of these, so that less blood flows through the skin. Because of ageing changes in the vessel walls, elderly people's skin vessels are often unable to constrict, and so they are denied this means of conserving heat. The control of heat regulation in the brain is also less efficient in the elderly. These factors lead to a rise in the thickness of the blood and a rise in blood pressure. Low temperatures interfere with the efficiency of the linings of the bronchial tubes in resisting infection and can induce asthma.

The net effect is substantial increase in the death rate from serious heart and lung disorders. Old people must be kept warm, both by effective domestic heating and by insulating their bodies in order to minimize heat loss. Multiple layers of garments are more effective than heavy material and it should be remembered that considerable heat can be lost from the top of the head. There is much to be said for woolly hats, indoors, in winter.

DRIVE CAREFULLY

Road traffic accidents are a major cause of death and disablement, especially in young people. The term 'accident' is usually a misnomer, for the great majority of car crashes are not accidental but are the result of lack of imagination, foresight and knowledge. They are caused by carelessness, stupidity, aggression and ignorance. High speed is the great killer, and today's ridiculously over-powered motor vehicles allow large number of irresponsible people to use speed as a source of amusement, an expression of frustration or aggression, or balm for a feeling of inadequacy. In the case of those who have already had a crash, there is sometimes an element of accident-proneness believed by some psychologists to indicate deliberate, if half-conscious, intention to do themselves an injury.

Accident-prone people often have an aggressive and rebellious attitude to authority and rules, which arose, initially, through rebellion against their parents.

But they are also said to have a sense of guilt over their rebelliousness, which demands suffering for wrongdoing. Studies have shown that people who have had four accidents are about fourteen times as numerous as they should be by pure chance. Moreover, they tend to repeat the same type of accident. To many, high-speed driving seems a bold, macho activity worthy of the admiration of others. It is engaged in by thousands ignorant of the most elementary idea of the forces involved–of the horrifying kinetic energy possessed by a ton of matter accelerated to seventy miles per hour. The energy built up in this way is proportional to the mass of the vehicle multiplied by the square of the velocity. Every surgeon knows, from bloody experience, what this means in practice.

The ration of deaths to injuries increases more than six times when imposed speed limits increase from thirty to sixty miles per hour. Studies in the USA have shown that death rates, from car crashes, in areas of low population density, where high speeds are possible, are more than 100 higher than in areas of high population density, where speeds are better controlled. Another factor determining the probable outcome of car crashes in the wearing of seat belts. Seat belts are highly effective in minimizing injury. Alcohol usage before driving is another obvious factor.

Take note of warning signs

There are several well-recognized signs which should be known to all as they may give early warning of cancer or other serious disease. They should always be reported.

UNDERSTAND HOW INFECTIONS OCCUR

Infection is the entry into the body, and the subsequent reproduction and establishment within the body, of colonies of any organism capable of causing disease. Many organisms gain access to the body, but only a small proportion are able to overcome the basic defence mechanisms and cause infection. Most swallowed organisms are destroyed by the acid in the stomach, but some, such as the Salmonella group, are able to resist even this and establish themselves in the bowel. The intact skin provides a good barrier to infection, but cuts and abrasion allow access to areas where the second line of defence–the immune system–must operate.

Organisms may exist in certain parts of the body without causing any harm but may become extremely harmful if they gain access to other parts. Perforation of the bowel allows organisms access to the sterile region around the outside of the organs and the serious condition of peritonitis is inevitable. When organisms gain access to normally sterile areas, the outcome depends on the balance between the number and virulence of the organisms, on the one hand, and the effectiveness of the defences, on the other. Good hygienic principles–regular washing, sanitary habits, fastidiousness about food, avoidance of obvious sources fastidiousness about food, avoidance of obvious sources of infection, and a realistic cynicism about the standards of personal hygiene in others–help to reduce the strength of the attack. So every effort should be made to minimize the dose of infective organisms acquired. Here are a few tips:

1. If you do get your fingers contaminated in this way, keep them away from your face until you get a chance to wash your hands thoroughly.

2. Look out for food-handlers with dirty hands and especially those with boils or pimples on their skin. Refuse to accept food from such people.

3. In particular, do not rub your eyes or nose. Cold viruses readily gain access via the conjunctivae of the eyes or the mucous lining of the nose.

4. Invite inconsiderate colleagues to cough and sneeze into handkerchiefs.

5. Avoid eating-places where there are no obvious and adequate washing facilities.

6. Common cold viruses are spread mainly by finger contact rather than by droplet spread. Avoid shaking hands with someone with a cold and, if possible, avoid touching things they have recently touched.

7. Do not engage in causal sex. A willing partner will have been willing with others and may well have, or be incubating, a sexually transmitted disease.

8. Try not to inhale other people's coughed or sneezed air. Many organism are spread in this way.

9. Assume that handles on public transport are contaminated with virulent organisms. Wear gloves when travelling, or wash before touching your face.

Remember, also, that the pursuit of good health helps to maintain good defences.

DON'T SMOKE CIGARETTES

'Smoking cigarettes is the chief, single avoidable cause of death in our society and the most important public health issue of our time.' This statement by the United States Surgeon General expresses the views of informed medical opinion, worldwide. Here is why:

Smoking and chronic bronchitis

Aside from damaging the ciliated cells lining the bronchial tubes and eventually destroying the ciliary action altogether, chemical irritants such as cigarette smoke or other environmental or industrial pollutants also stimulate excess mucus secretion from the glands in the air passages. But because the cilia are not working properly, this mucus accumulates in the tubes. In order to clear this material from the tubes, the individual has to cough. Irritants, such as tobacco smoke, also interfere with the white blood cell mechanism which combats infection in the lungs, and the result of all this is that the stagnant material in the tubes becomes infected.

This is the condition of chronic bronchitis. People with chronic bronchitis cough up sputum, on most days, for at least three months of each year—usually the winter months. Most heavy smokers have chronic bronchitis, but refer to it simply as 'a smoker's cough'. Often the efficiency of the coughing is impeded by a tendency for the circular muscles in the wall of the bronchial tube to contract, so causing the tubes to narrow. This is called bronchospasm and it causes wheezing–another sign of chronic bronchitis. Asthma is a severe from of bronchospasm. In the early stage, chronic bronchitis is a comparatively mild disease.

But, with time and continued abuse, it is likely to progress to the very unpleasant condition called chronic obstructive airway disease, in which large numbers of the tiny lung air sacs break down to from a smaller number of larger air spaces. The trouble with this is that the total surface area now available for oxygen transfer to the blood is greatly reduced so the affected person becomes short of oxygen. In addition, the smaller bronchial tubes become inflamed, narrowed and partially blocked by mucus which cannot get out. The end result may be a constant, exhausting and irremediable state of breathlessness in which the unhappy victim, to maintain his or her laboured breathing, is forced to use the shoulder muscles to try to increase chest movement. The skin may show an ominous blueness and, in the end, the sufferer may need to wear an oxygen mask while waiting for the inevitable eventual heart failure to supervene.

Smoking and carbon monoxide

The function of the red cells of the blood is to take up oxygen in the lungs and to carry it to all parts of the body where it is needed to oxidize fuel and release energy. The link between oxygen and the haemoglobin in the red cells is a loose one, so that oxygen can easily be released when the blood reaches an area that needs it. Cigarette smoke contains a gas called carbon monoxide and this combines readily with haemoglobin. But when it does so, the chemical bond is so strong that the carbon monoxide cannot be released and remains in the blood cells for weeks. So part of the haemoglobin of the blood is unavailable for oxygen transfer.

Incidentally, the cause of death in car exhaust poisoning is this same carbon monoxide which has caused a massive conversion of haemoglobin to carboxy-haemoglobin-50 per cent is fatal. Heavy smokers have carboxy-haemoglobin levels of 5 to 8 per cent in their red cells. To compensate for the reduced availability of oxygen to the tissues, a 20 per cent increase in blood flow is necessary. Vessels narrowed by atherosclerosis may not be able to widen enough to allow this–with predictable results like thrombosis or heart attack. Carboxy-haemoglobin can tip the balance between normal tissue and gangrene, sometimes even between life and sudden death. Here is a quotation from one major textbook of medicine, in the section concerned with atherosclerosis: 'Sudden death is the most frequent clinical event associated with cigarette smoking.'

The cost of smoking

The National Health Service in Britain spends hundreds of millions of pounds every year on treating, or trying to treat, tobacco–related diseases. That money is contributed by tax-paying smokers and non-smokers alike and is wasted. Society would be greatly advantaged if these large sums could be applied to purposes of health improvement for all–welfare, medical research, public health measures, preventive medicine, aids to the disabled and so on. Unfortunately, tax revenue from smoking amounts to many times the cost of the whole National Health Service, so the Government is in dilemma.

This is the reason why Government statements on such issues as tobacco advertising always sound strange. Smoking imposes in incalculable cost on society from lost productive capacity, working time and trained expertise–which are the main source of society's wealth and prosperity. Again, all suffer. Finally, there is the terrible cost to the affected individual and the cost to families in lost income, in the health-sapping effect of having a chronic invalid in the house and in the eventual bereavement.

Smoking and lung cancer

The lining cells of the air tubes in healthy lungs are tall and the surfaces nearest the inside of the tube are covered with fine hairs which move together in a manner similar to the effect of wind blowing across a field of ripe corn. The hair movement acts to carry dust and other foreign material upwards and away from the deeper parts of the lungs. This is one of the body's protective processes and, without it, a good deal of unwanted material in the air we breathe in would find its way into the delicate air sacs. In people who smoke cigarettes, these important cells soon suffer three obvious changes. First, the cilia disappear, then the number of cells increases and, finally, the cells become flattened, so that the columnar lining is replaced by an abnormal atrophied, scaly layer. After a number of years, there is a tendency for these bald, flattened cells to begin to show signs of excessive multiplication.

The next stage, again usually some years later, may be cancer of the lung. The more cigarettes smoked, the more marked the early cell changes become. The loss of cilia and flattening of the columnar cells occur much more frequently in cigarette smokers than in those who smoke pipes or cigars. People who have given up smoking have fever affected cells than smokers, and the number of affected cells becomes progressively less as the number of years of non-smoking increases. But the number of damaged cells never reaches the low level found in people who have never smoked cigarettes.

Ironically, smokers who inhale the smoke deeply into their lungs so that it moves quickly past the ciliated cells in the main lung tubes are slightly less liable to get cancer than those who inhale less deeply. But the deep inhalers, who carry the smoke right to the air sacs, from whence many of the 3000 or so constituents can get into the bloodstream, suffer a higher incidence of the other important effects of smoking, especially heart attack. Obviously, every heavy smoker does not get lung cancer. Some simply have a natural, inborn resistance to the typical changes in the cells. Others have very powerful defence mechanisms which can minimize the effects of the tiny smoke particles on the lung tissues. But there is no way of knowing whether any particular individual will have such built-in resistance.

Smoking and the heart

The evidence linking smoking with heart disease is slightly less direct than in the case of lung cancer, because we still do not fully understand what causes heart disease. Most of the evidence comes from a series of long-term statistical studies of large population groups in which the members are examined at regular intervals. Some of these groups member over 5000 people and the studies take into account factors such as age, sex, smoking history, blood pressure, weight, amount of physical activity, blood cholesterol levels, stress, family history, the hardness of the local water, and so on. By finding out what eventually happens to these people and correlating this with the factors mentioned, it is possible to discover which factors are regularly associated with diseases.

All the studies show the same result. Cigarette smoking has invariably been found to be a major risk factor in the causation of heart attack, stroke and disease of blood vessels generally. It correlates with a raised incidence of sudden death from coronary artery blockage, and with angina pectoris and severe limitation of activity from disease of the blood vessels supplying the legs. The heavier the smoking the higher the risk. Post-mortem examination of the blood vessels of smokers shows, to a higher-than-average degree, changes in the inner layer which, instead of being perfectly smooth and even, shows irregularity and lumpiness.

The lumpy areas are caused by deposition, just under the inner lining, of fatty tissue and cholesterol mixed up with degenerate muscle cells and elastic connective tissue. This condition is called atherosclerosis, and the atherosclerotic plaques usually affect the larger and the medium-sized arteries. The plaques become larger with time and the inner surface of the vessel, at the site of these plaques, is so altered that blood in contact with it can actually begin to clot. This results in a stoppage of the supply of blood to the tissue which the vessel is feeding. The heart is a very active, hard-working, muscle and requires a substantial blood supply to keep up its considerable need for glucose fuel and oxygen.

This blood supply is provided by the coronary arteries and these are usually affected, to a greater or lesser degree, by atherosclerosis. When one of these arteries becomes blocked by atherosclerosis or by blood clotting on top of an atherosclerotic plaque, the result is sudden death or, if a small branch is involved, a dangerous and disabling illness. The significance of nicotine is not clear. Many authorities consider that none of the risks of cigarette smoking is connected with the nicotine, but others are more wary and point out that the nicotine-induced increase in the heart rate and rise in the blood pressure, and the possible constriction of the coronary arteries, are probably contributory. But there is certainly no medical argument over the proposition that patients with coronary artery disease, who continue to smoke, are dicing with death.